AF785146

~ Country Club Heritage ~

~ Country Club Heritage ~

A History and Guide to a Denver Neighborhood

by
Alice Millett Bakemeier

FOREWORD BY BARBARA SUDLER HORNBY

Country Club Heritage

ISBN: 0-9659574-1-1

Library of Congress Catalogue Number:
00-91424

Cover design by Barbara Froula
Interior Design and Composition by Dianne Nelson, Shadow Canyon Graphics, Denver
Unless credited, photographs are taken by the author

Printed in the United States of America

First Edition
10 9 8 7 6 5 4 3 2 1

Country Club Heritage
A HISTORY AND GUIDE TO A DENVER NEIGHBORHOOD

By
Alice Millett Bakemeier

Published by the
Country Club Historic Neighborhood, Inc.

The project was partially funded by a State Historical Fund
grant award from the Colorado Historical Society

The following sponsors are gratefully acknowledged:
Boa Construction, Inc.
Cherry Creek Audio
The Cherry Creek Foundation
Eccentricity
Fuller and Associates, Architects
Guaranty Bank and Trust Company
Merrill Lynch
Paradise Cleaners
Perry & Co.
The Vineyard Wine Shop

Contents

This book is affectionately dedicated to

WILLIAM DICKSON "PETE" MILLETT

KATHERINE THAYER "KIM" MILLETT

ELIZABETH MILLETT COCHRAN

and

MARGARET "PEGGY" MILLETT ZEMACH

who spent their childhoods in the

Country Club Historic District

~ Foreword ~

By Barbara Sudler Hornby

One of the most stable and healthy neighborhoods in Denver is the Country Club Historic District. It is a residential area of nearly 400 homes. When founded at the beginning of the 20th century, it was known as the "Spanish Suburb," for not only its stucco walls and tile roofs, but also because it was away from the core city. Now, of course, it is considered "inner city."

There was a time when some thought its demise was in sight. In 1956 when we first bought a house here we went to the bank for a mortgage, only to be told that the neighborhood could not survive. "Those big old houses can't be maintained without servants." Our enthusiasm prevailed and we were still living in that house when the mortgage was paid off.

My interest in historic preservation began during a 32-year marriage to the late Jim Sudler, a prominent Denver architect who believed very strongly that we must save the past, as well as build in a contemporary mode worthy of the future. He and Helen Millett Arndt dreamed of a landmark commission for Denver, worked assiduously in that direction, and then jubilantly celebrated victory in 1967.

My association with the Country Club Historic District goes beyond that of a happy householder. I have been a resident within the district since 1956. At first I lived in the far western end in Park Club Place for 20 years, raising a family there, and now I have lived in Country Club Place, towards the middle of the District, for another 24 years.

When the District was first recognized, it was listed on the National Registry of Historic Places. I was, at that time, the State Historic Preservation Officer, who signed the recommendation to the Keeper of the Register for the listing. Within that same time frame, the Denver Country Club, and also Speer Boulevard itself, were listed on the National Register. The import of these listings is that federal funds cannot be used to alter or eliminate any of the pieces without comment from the State Preservation Officer, whose job it is to protect the integrity of places on the National Register.

The federal listing gives the neighborhood "bragging rights" and some protection, but in 1990 it was listed by the Denver City Council, on a favorable recommendation for the Denver Landmark Preservation, as a Denver Landmark District. All exterior changes that would require a building permit must be considered by that commission as to their appropriateness. As a member of the Commission for these ten years, it has been fascinating to see the District treasured by the city and flourishing in these affluent times. Historic designation maintains an admired look, and at the same time it gives owners access to certain monies and tax credits that are available to designated resources.

Beyond the area's historicity there are planning features that create an ambiance conducive to what the magazines call "gracious living:" mature planting with trees that arbor over serene gardens; parkways that lace through the district; fairly uniform setbacks that provide a setting for commodious homes.

Historian Alice Millett Bakemeier brings not only finely honed insights to this book but also her affectionate perceptions as a one time long-term resident of this neighborhood. When she left the Country Club District she moved to Hilltop, and her successful *Hilltop Heritage* was published in 1997.

Barbara Sudler Hornby

~

Acknowledgments

Special thanks go to: Edward D. White, Jr., A.I.A. for reviewing and revising the architectural details of each house. As a Denver native and member of the Denver Landmark Preservation Commission for 30 years, his historical perspective and editorial comments were invaluable.

Architect Philip Atchison for his helpful, professional comments on many of the houses.

Charles M. Moore, the Humboldt Historian, for sharing his vast memories and fascinating stories about people and places, taped in Charley's own inimitable style.

Charles A. Johnson, for reviewing parts of the manuscript, offering expert suggestions about maps and format, and lending photographs.

Emma J. and Charles L. Warren, for comprehensive review of the manuscript and knowledgeable comments about families.

Sharon Elfenbein, whose extensive inventory of the Country Club district for the nomination for the National Registry of Historic Places was a valuable resource.

Jedeane Macdonald for computer assistance and expert proofreading.

Rob Sontag, Historic Preservation Specialist at the State Historical Fund, for suggestions about architecture.

The staff of the Stephen Hart Library of the Colorado Historical Society.

The complete staff of the Denver Public Library Western History Department, under the direction of the late Eleanor Gehres. All willingly gave expert advice and suggestions.

For reviewing parts of the manuscript I would like to thank:

Gladys Barkalow Alexander
Karl Arndt, MD
Robert K. Fuller, II
Barbara Sudler Hornby
Charles M. Moore
William F. Wilbur

Most important were the indispensable support, comments, encouragement, and expert editing of my devoted husband, Richard F. Bakemeier, M.D., editor of the *Journal of Cancer Education*.

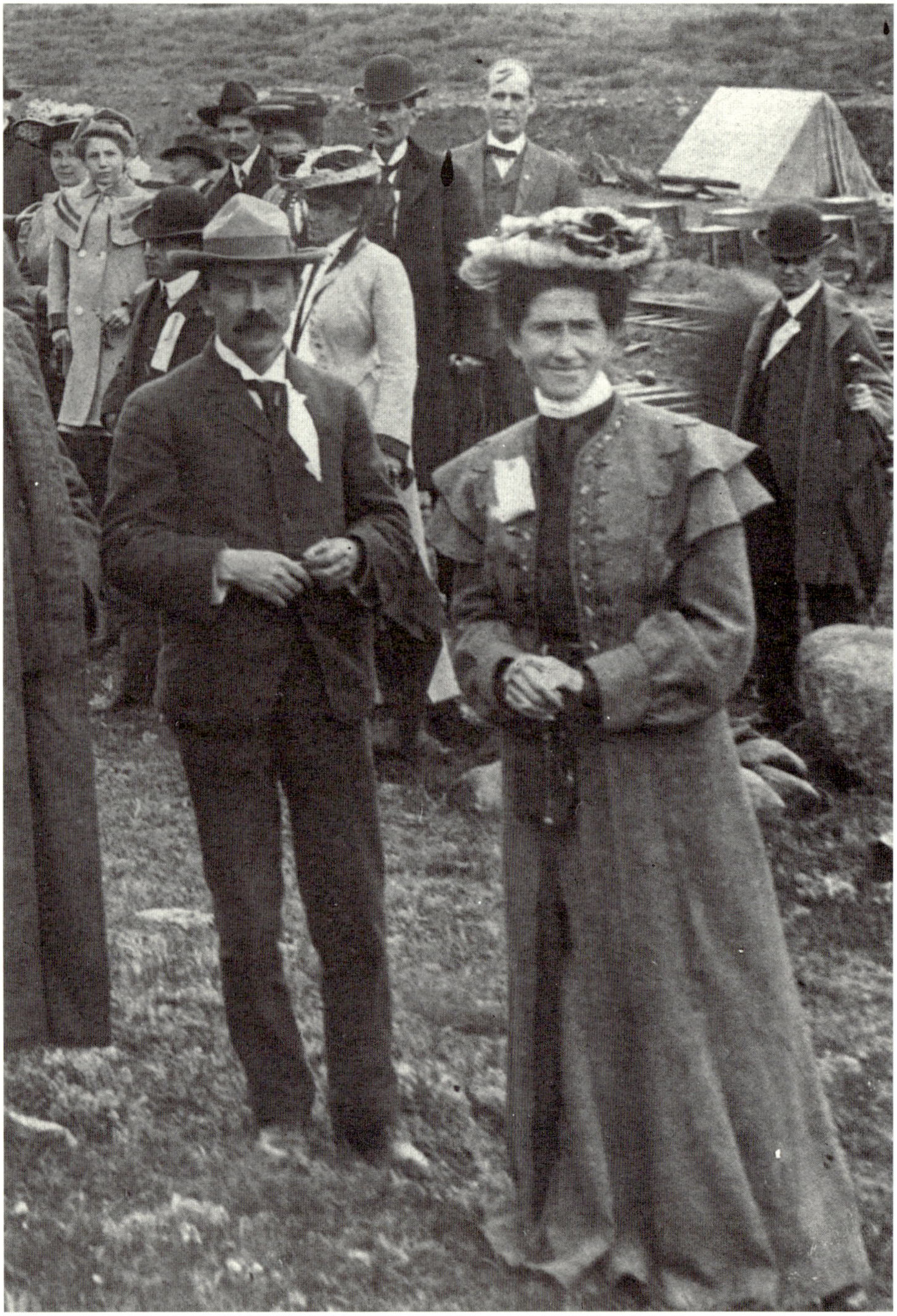

During the 1890s, Mr. and Mrs. Edwin S. Kassler enjoyed the "Last Days of Pompeii" and shooting the chutes at Chutes Park, just west of Downing Street. (Courtesy DPL Western History Department)

Mrs. Jeannine Gray
10200 W Asbury Ave
Lakewood CO 80227-2004

Mary
A big-Thanks for the very delicious, fun, lunch, recipe and the use of the book. Really Enjoyed all!
Use to baby sit at several places in the book and we use to go trick and treating in the area for Halloween.
Lots of childhood memories.

istory of the Country ~ storic Neighborhood

homes after bu... Denver Country Club to the south. For almost a century this venerable club has not only anchored the resulting prestigious residential district, but also has provided a center of gentility and a refreshing green oasis in the midst of a bustling city.

Until the turn of the twentieth century, this land remained a barren island, tucked between Capitol Hill on the north and the towns of South Denver (south of Alameda Avenue) and Harman (Cherry Creek North) on the east.

Two decades earlier, in 1880, this land was south of the city limits, then at Chamberlin (6th) Avenue and York Street (University Boulevard). By then, Denver, still a frontier town, had spent 22 years since the first gold discovery, displacing Indians and absorbing gold diggers of both genders, Civil War veterans, tuberculosis victims, and adventure seekers; and building its own dusty but thriving community.

"I can remember my father saying that when he was a boy [in the

The rows of wheat in Riethmann's fields gradually turned into roads of homes, such as these at 180 Humboldt and 181Franklin Streets. (Courtesy Denver Planning Office)

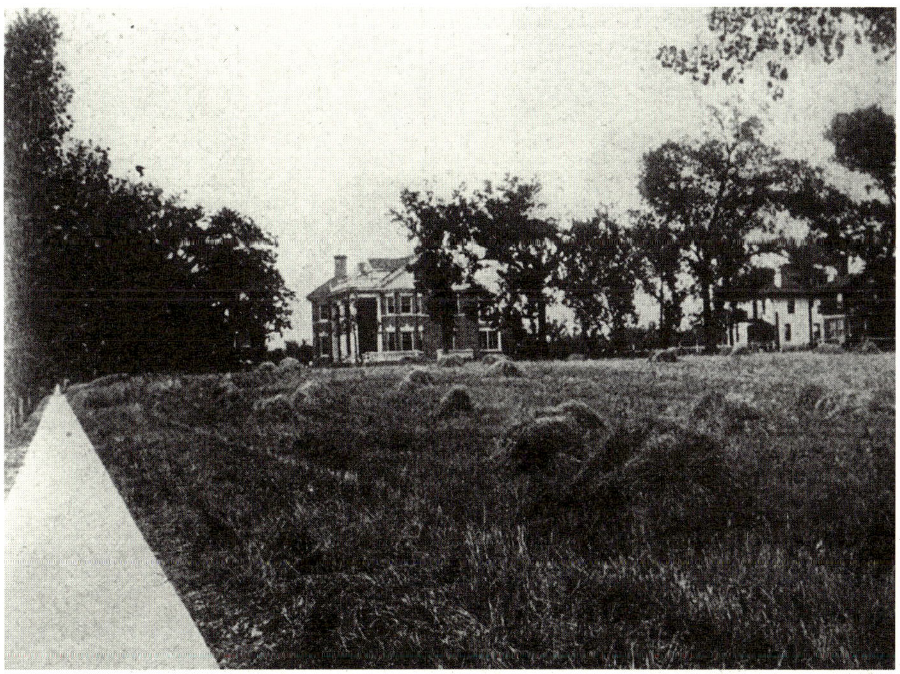

MAP OF EAST DENVER, 1885

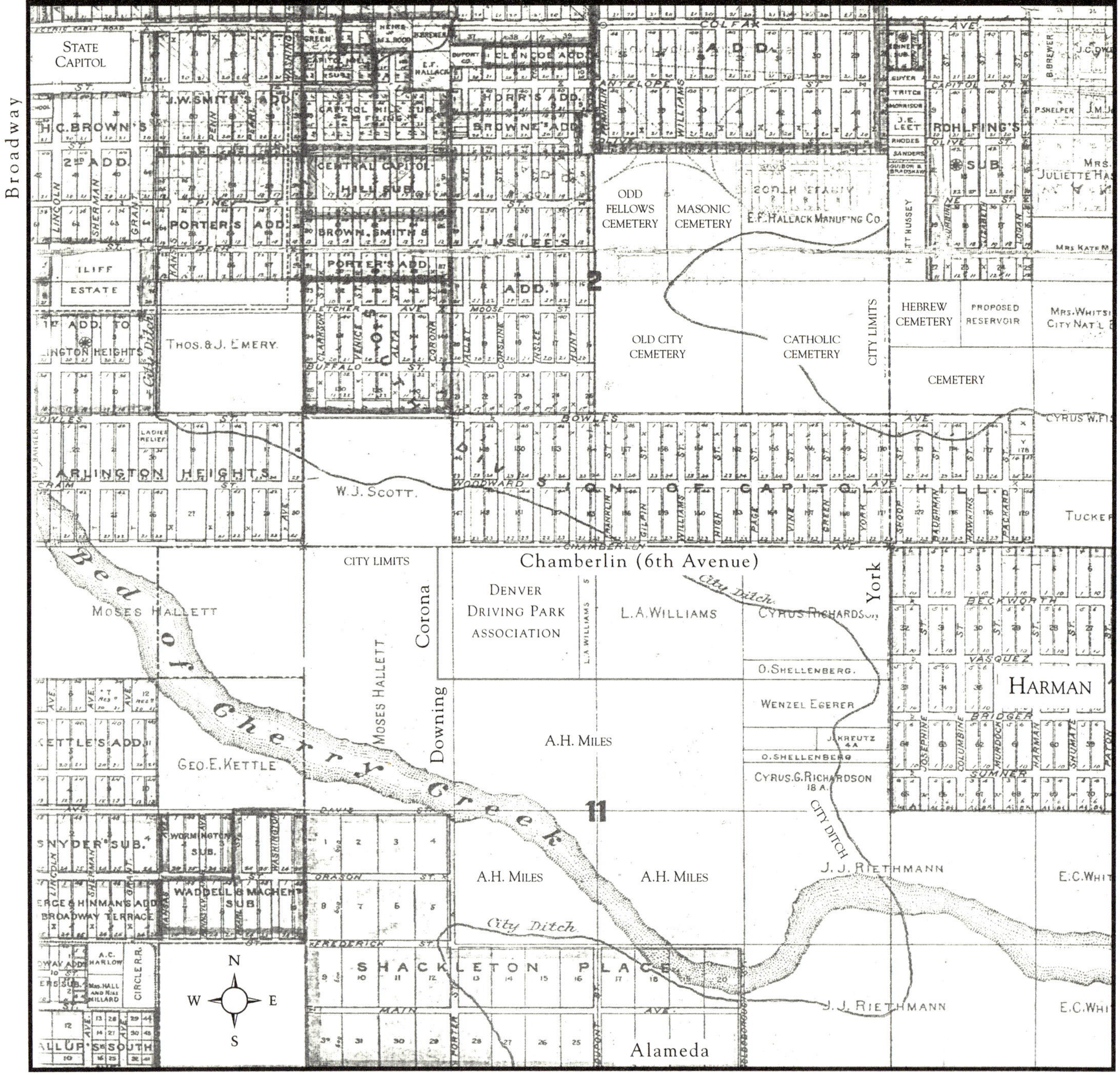

1870s] there were Indians—Utes and Arapahos I suppose—camped on the present site of the State Capitol," wrote early neighborhood resident Bethuel M. Webster, Jr., to his daughter, Eleanor. "Sanatoriums, with tents, sleeping porches, etc., were one of the principal industries."[1]

By 1880 the numerous railroads converging on Denver had swelled the population to over 35,000. Union Station, built in 1881, became the hub of the city with businesses, bars, and brothels clustered nearby. Denver was boasting such high-tech inventions as telephones and incandescent lights. Culture was promoted in 1881 by Horace Tabor's Grand Opera House at 16th and Curtis Streets, and the upscale Windsor Hotel opened in 1880 with 19-foot ceilings, English china, and hot and cold running water.[2]

As urban sprawl increased, home owners began building eastward from downtown, across Broadway, choosing Grant and Sherman Streets for their large stately mansions around the capitol, which was completed in 1886. The city cemeteries were located miles east of Capitol Hill at the current sites of Cheesman and Congress Parks.

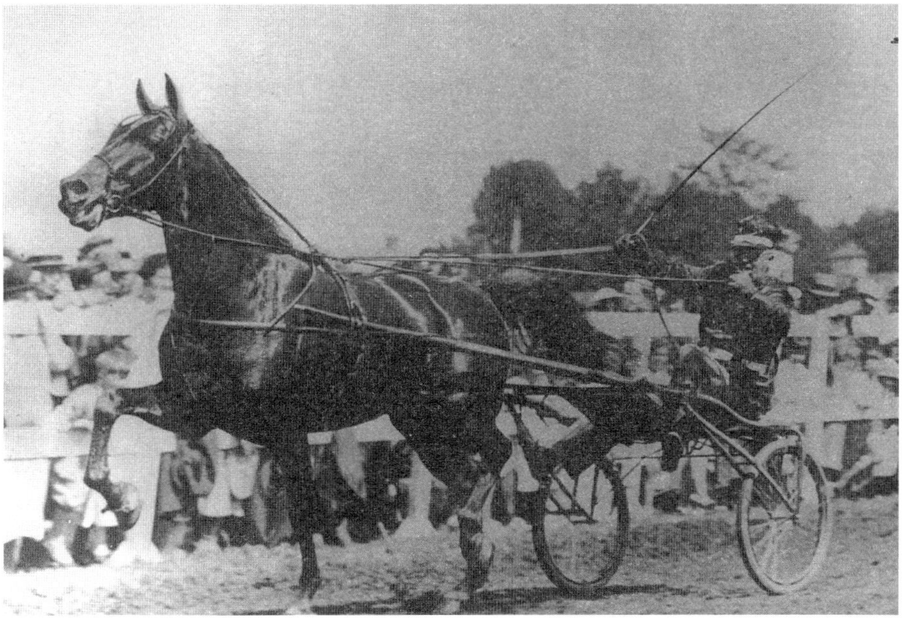

In the 1880s, harness racing was the sport of kings at the Gentlemen's Driving Association track at 4th Avenue and Corona Street. (Courtesy DPL Western History Department)

In 1880, some of the vacant prairie directly south of the city limits, at Chamberlin (6th) Avenue between Corona and Hunt (Humboldt) Streets, was used for a popular sporting event.

The Sport of Kings: Gentlemen's Driving Association

The dust began to stir at 4th Avenue and Corona Street when the Gentlemen's Driving Association was incorporated on March 18, 1880,[3] for the sport of kings: racing their harnessed horses. Just two months later the optimistic directors had "bought the ground, built the fastest and best track made in Colorado, laid out a second driveway, built stables, set out some 300 trees, bridged the City Ditch, and improved roads leading to their

[Opposite Page]
In 1885, the future site of the Denver Country Club was farm land, then owned by A. H. Miles, next to Cherry Creek. The Denver Driving Park Association, formerly called the Gentlemen's Driving Association, was in full swing at 4th Avenue and Corona Street. Cheesman and Congress Parks were city cemeteries, and the capitol building was near completion. (Courtesy DPL Western History Department)

grounds," reported the June 5, 1880, *Rocky Mountain News*. The city had objected when these influential leaders exercised their favorite sport up and down 14th Street in downtown Denver, kicking up mud and gravel, scattering frightened pedestrians into the gutters, and closing off the streets to more sedate carriage drivers and shoppers. The sportsmen then provided themselves with their own racecourse in this vacant tract south of the city limits (see 1885 map).

On Wednesdays and Saturdays crinolines rustled in the cool air. The wind tugged at bonnets and parasols, and clouds of dust covered top hats and knickers. As the crowds of gents and ladies cheered lustily, Denver's prominent citizens hopped into their two-wheeled carts, or sulkies, to drive their fastest trotters, like ancient Greek charioteers, around the new half-mile track at Corona Street and 4th Avenue.

These events were limited to harness racing. The Standardbreds, either trotters or pacers used for this sport, were the pride and status symbol of these socially prominent gentlemen. The mares (immortalized by Hiram Woodruff's folk song the "Old Gray Mare") were hitched to light sulkies, which were made with high wheels during the 1880s. When small bike wheels were introduced in 1892, high wheelers became history. The "bikes" were faster, negotiated the turns better, and reduced wind resistance.[4] The eminent drivers donned their individual bright-colored jackets and caps to be easily recognizable in the events.

The clubhouse of the Gentlemen's Driving Association at 1125 East 4th Avenue was condemned and demolished in 1931. (Courtesy DPL Western History Department)

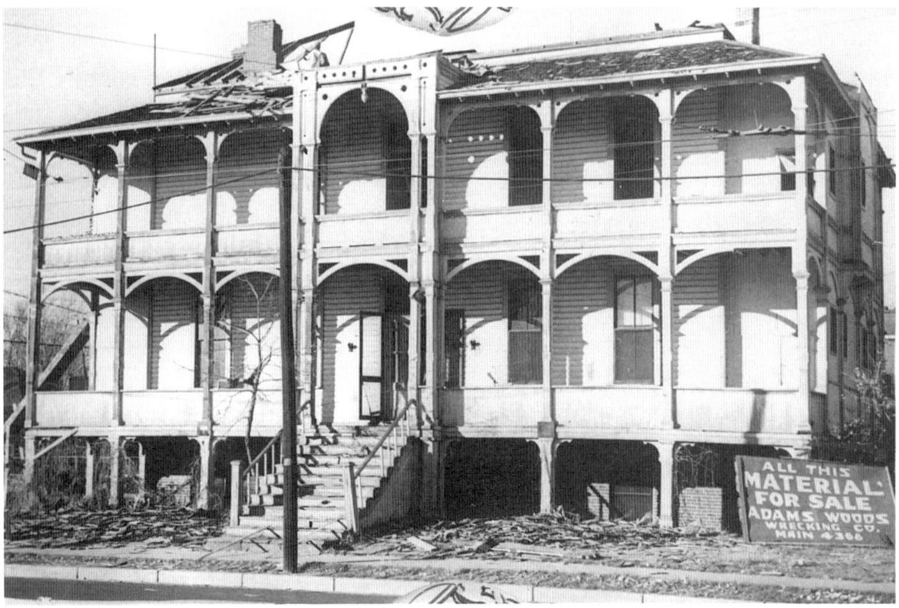

President of the organization was Gilbert B. Reed, judge of the Court of Appeals. Prominent members included Justice Moses Hallett of the Colorado Supreme Court; Charles B. Kountze, a founder of the Colorado National Bank; lawyer Henry Roger Wolcott; livery stable owner J. H. Estabrook; mining magnate H. A. W. Tabor; and railroad and real estate developer Walter S. Cheesman. Ninety-five other stockholders paid $100 each to enjoy "a driving park for pleasure driving and speed," as stated in the Articles of Incorporation.

Soon there was such a demand for races that the track was thrown open for public viewing and enlivened with a brass band. The Wednesday and Saturday matinees were so popular that the association voted to build a $9,000 clubhouse at 1125 East 4th Avenue. The June 19, 1880, *Rocky Mountain News* described the two-storied, 25-by-50-foot frame building surrounded by wide verandas at both levels: "It contained a ladies' and a gentlemen's parlor, dining room, reading room, billiard room, ball room, ladies' and gentlemen's dressing rooms with closets, and all the latest amenities of the time." Gala parties were frequent, where corseted ladies in their large picture hats, dust-catching skirts, and high-button shoes danced with their gentlemen in the ballroom while a banjo, Victrola, or player piano rang forth with "I Love You Truly" or "In the Good Old Summertime." "Gentlemen were beginning to wear colored shirt fronts with white collars and cuffs that were attached to the shirt, even in the evening with the dress coat and white tie," the *Daily News* wrote in 1895.[5]

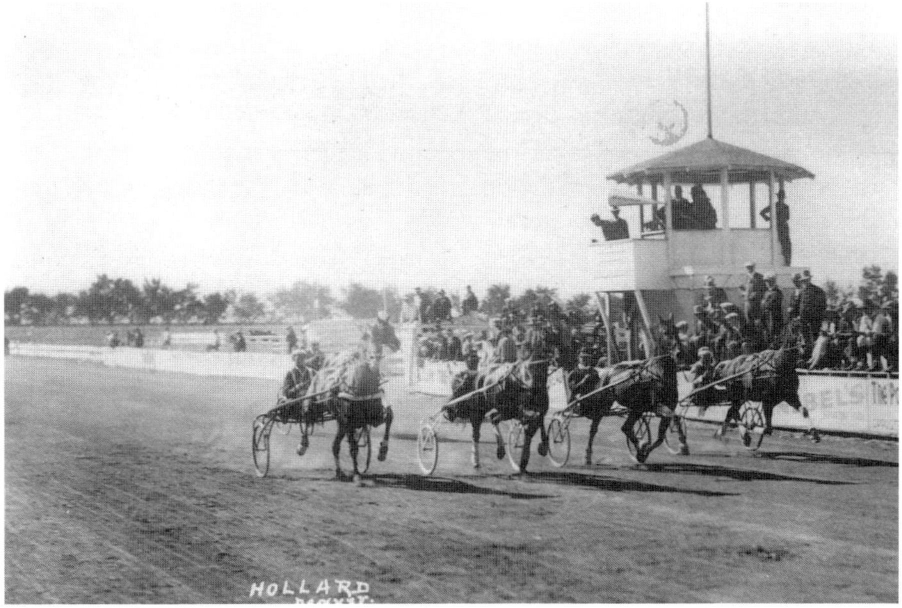

Twelve years after the Gentlemen's Driving Association closed, the Gentlemen's Driving and Riding Club was established, holding races at City Park. (Courtesy DPL Western History Department)

The club's popularity spread. The euphoric directors hired top-notch interior designer Louis Doll to furnish the clubhouse, despite their heavy debt to builders Halleck and Howard. Soon the bubble began to burst. An abstract of the area[6] records ominous trust deeds giving Halleck and Howard notes on the property. Doll had not been paid. By December of 1881 three firms had sued the association and the property was put up for public sale.

The sharply-honed business skills of these distinguished gentlemen became apparent. Newspaper reports in January 1882 revealed that the club, broke and auctioned off by the sheriff, was rebought by these same members of the Gentlemen's Driving Association for $8,700, about half the assessed value. For appearances they then incorporated a new organization in February named the Denver Driving Park Association, reported the Rocky Mountain News on February 5, 1882. They then asked $300 from each of 50 members and with this $6,300 surplus on their purchase, they built 17 additional stalls,[7] for a total of 40, and the same club rolled merrily along for six more years with boisterous matinees, billiard games, and splendid balls. Apparently the new association was in name only as the 1885, 1886, and 1887 city directories still list the Gentlemen's Driving Association, rather than the Denver Driving Park Association, at that address.

Meanwhile, Denver was spreading like a prairie fire southward from Capitol Hill, and land values skyrocketed. In May 1888, two years after completion of the capitol building, the association sold the land for $42,000 to Mr. H. C. Lowrie, who formed the Driving Park Land Company. The capital stock in the new real estate company was $150,000, over 17 times the $8,700 price paid in 1882, six years previously.

The Gentlemen's Driving Association, later the Denver Driving Park Association, at 4th and Corona, had ceased to exist by 1888. That organization is easily confused with the better-known Gentlemen's Driving and Riding Club, which was started 10 years later in 1898 and included races with saddled horses as well as harnessed trotters. This organization made a proposition to the City "that they would build a track at their own expense at City Park and transfer the same to the city if the city would provide for its maintenance."[8] For many years the club maintained stables and held an increasing number of matinees there. Besides their barns, grandstand, and race track at City Park, the club owned handsomely appointed quarters at 1525 Curtis Street. Although the number of members decreased over the next two decades, enthusiastic horse lovers continued to race at City Park until the grandstand was torn down in 1951.

Driving Park Place

Lowrie's Driving Park Land Company developed the well-fertilized residential subdivision Driving Park Place at 4th and Corona. Still south of the city limits, the land was platted between the scattered stables using streets named after prominent citizens. When the area was annexed to the city, the streets were renamed to correspond with those already north of 6th Avenue.

In 1890 the real estate advertisement boasted, "No Saloons or cheap buildings. These are by all odds the most desirable $600 residence lots in Denver! It joins Capitol Hill . . . has a plentiful supply of water . . . and the pure air is uncontaminated by proximity to any smelters or the smoke of manufactories. The walks will be paved and no dwelling of less than $2,000 value may be erected .. . . Electric lighting will come with the houses in a very short time."[9]

Two buildings survived on the original Gentlemen's Driving Association racetrack at 4th and Corona. One was a stable at 461 Humboldt Street that was made habitable in 1893 and became the home of the R. F. Lewises during the teens. Later the house was bought by psychologist Carla Swan, later Mrs. Albert J. Coleman, who lived there from 1941 until her death in 1991. She wrote proudly in a Fortnightly paper of 1959, "The elm trees on the front parking [space] are part of the original planting of the Gentlemen's Driving Park Association 79 years ago."[10] Her house, a small stable on lots 9 to 12 of Block 8, remains as the south section of this residence. The Colemans added a living room with a large-beamed ceiling, dining room, breakfast room, and kitchen, with a master bedroom, dressing room, study, and bath upstairs. Downstairs, the carriage house was converted into a large study for Mrs. Coleman. During her last years Mrs. Coleman turned her house into a nostalgic museum with family heirlooms. However, it was never maintained as a museum after her death.

The Association Clubhouse

The other building that survived was the large frame clubhouse at 1125 East 4th Avenue (between Corona and Downing Streets). In 1890 it was bought by pioneer lawyer Major Jacob Downing, who played an important part in developing Colorado, and for whom Downing Street was named. When Downing died in 1907, his widow turned the old clubhouse into the Downing Home for the Aged,[11] first listed in the city directory in 1914. In 1921 it was remodeled into the Park View, then Lake View, Apartments and was finally condemned and torn down in November 1931.[12] A gas station was built on the site.

Arlington/Chutes Park

The name Lake View Apartments seems unlikely at 4th and Corona. However, Arlington Park, the area west of Driving Park Place, hit its heyday in the 1890s, while the future Country Club district to the east remained a quiet farm.

Before the end of the "Gay 90s," Arlington Park was converted into a pleasure park with a lake, created by diverting Cherry Creek. As announced in the December 19, 1897, *Rocky Mountain News*, "There will be no difficulty in getting a lake of pure water, for the [Cherry] creek filters through the gravel and springs up as clear and crystal like as possible," said Police Commissioner Robert W. Speer, the owner of the property.

The next year, the pleasure park known as Chutes Park was opened. Wooden chutes, modeled after logging chutes, were constructed so that joyriders could slide down the long runways into the lake. "Boats plunged down the chute at such a speed that Mrs. Edwin S. Kassler, one of the two ladies selected to make the opening ride, 'lost the trinkets from her hair,'" wrote Louisa Ward Arps.[13] One Miss Sadie Boynton thrilled spectators by shooting the chutes on a bicycle, reported the *Denver Republican* on May 28, 1899: "Miss Boynton reached the base of the chutes and dove gracefully over the handle bars into the lake."

The most unique act was Professor Barnes's herd of elks, who dove into the water from 60 feet at the top of the chute at his command. "The elks seemed to enjoy the performance as much as [the spectators]. They trot contentedly to the top of the almost perpendicular runway, and, at a given signal, jump

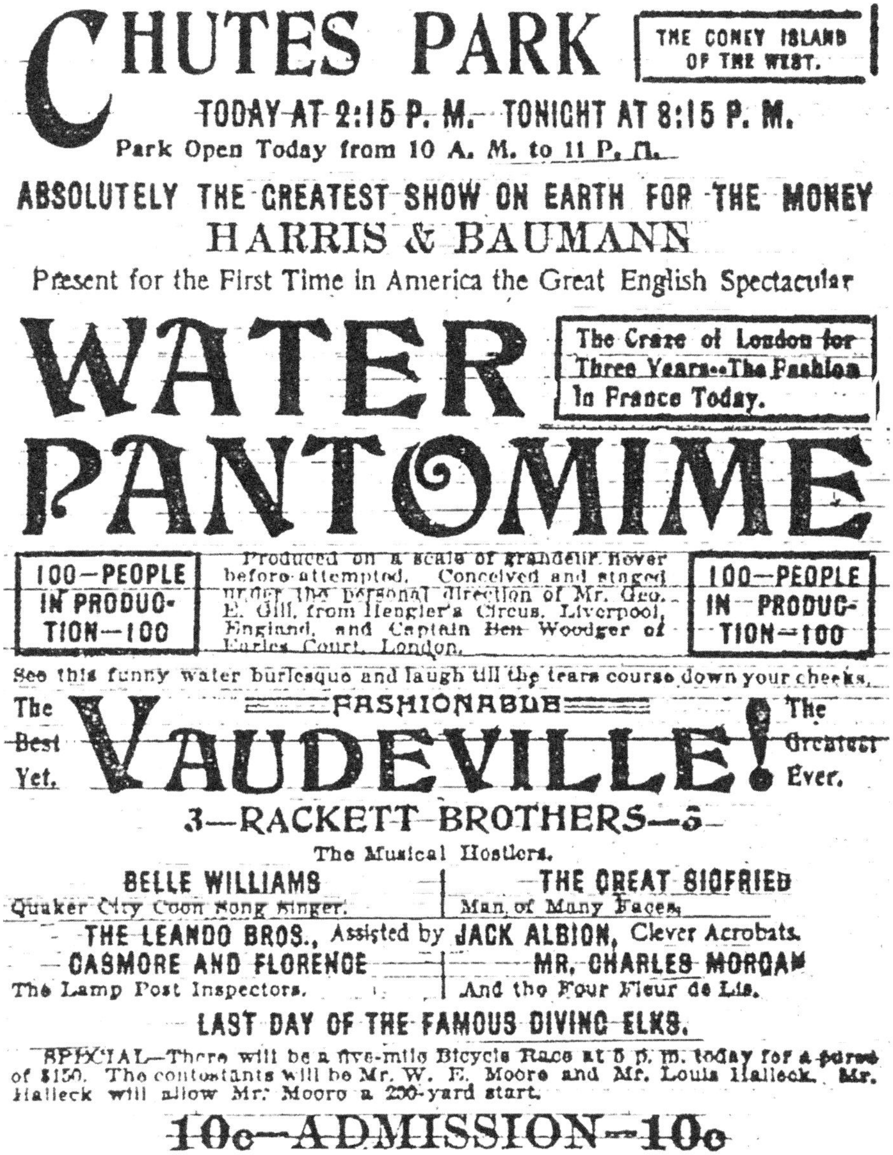

Late in the Gay '90s, Chutes Amusement Park opened just west of Downing Street. For 10 cents you could see the "greatest show on earth." (Courtesy DPL Western History Department)

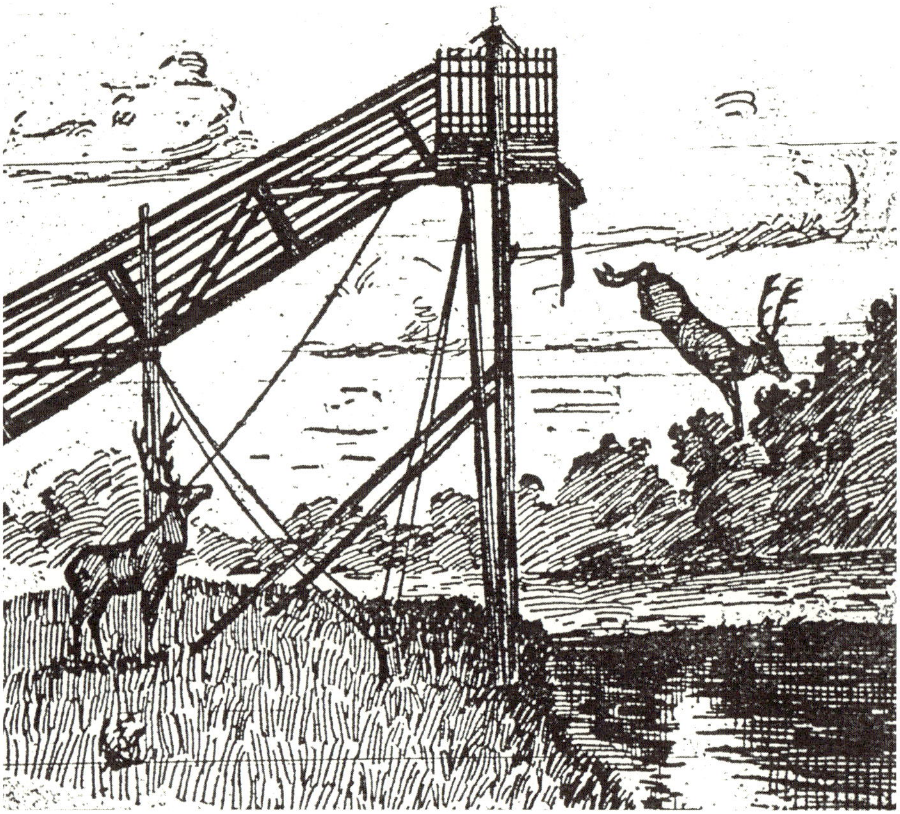

The main attraction at Chutes Park was Professor Barnes's diving elks, who climbed the logging chute and dove into the little lake below that is now Alamo Placita Park. (Courtesy DPL Western History Department)

head foremost into a tank of water 60 feet below," the article continued.

An advertisement in the June 11, 1899, *Denver Times* describes "Absolutely The Greatest Show On Earth For the Money: A scenic railway, two shows of Water Pantomimes, vaudeville, a bicycle race, and fireworks depicting the Battle of San Juan Hill and the Last Days of Pompeii, and the last day of the famous diving elks—all for 10 cents." Bands of musicians, bowers of flowers, and Passion Plays added to the entertainment. By then the Denver Tramway's electric streetcar conveniently ran up 6th Avenue beside the park.

Chutes Park was a howling success. However, fires, first in 1901, then another in 1902, demolished the chutes and grandstand owned by Speer. It was believed that both fires were started by tramps. The nearest fire hydrant was full of stones.[14] Restoration was impossible.

The park was torn apart and the land resurveyed in blocks for residential sale. The dried lakebed now fertilizes the lovely gardens of Alamo Placita Park.

Driving Park Place and Chutes Park were developed during the 1890s. Earlier, the suburbs of Harman, now Cherry Creek North, and South Denver, directly south of Alameda, had been incorporated as townships in 1886. However, the land along Cherry Creek between Downing and York had remained an island of wheat farms and barren fields. The final destination of the Denver Country Club was the farm of one of Denver's earliest pioneers, a '58er.

John Jacob Riethmann

John Jacob Riethmann was a typical young man who went West. After emigrating from Switzerland with his parents at the age of 10, he heeded the spreading news of William Russell's discovery of gold on the South Platte River in 1858. "I could scarcely wait a day before starting," declared the 20-year-old youth in an interview published in the April 1925 issue of *The Trail*.

He arrived in Denver with his brother, Louis, and "built a cabin near the present site of the Denver Union stock yards—the first house erected," reported the *Rocky Mountain News* on April 3, 1927: "The sight of [gold] was enough to electrify me. . . . I decided not only to locate here but to return to my home and bring my people out with me," the interview continued. While Louis remained in the cabin, John returned East on "a good tough Indian pony . . . and carried the first mail for the North and East ever taken from the region."

Riethmann returned to Council Bluffs, Iowa, but came back to Denver in March 1859 with his parents and a wagonload of supplies to start a cracker bakery. After making a success of this enterprise, he increased his fortune by starting a highly successful wholesale drug company. He founded the first German Bank in Denver and was respected as one of Denver's most successful and worthy citizens.

His parents, two brothers, and two sisters settled on a farm five miles north of Denver on the Platte River near Sand Creek. In 1887, a year after his father's sudden death, Riethmann increased his real estate holdings by investing in 391 acres along Cherry Creek that he bought for $24,000 from Alfred H. Miles.[15]

However, like many of his contemporaries who had amassed fortunes,

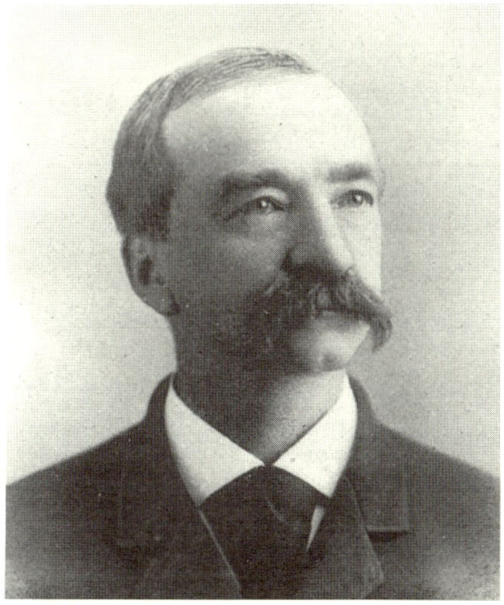

Pioneer John Jacob Riethmann sold his farm along Cherry Creek to the Fourth Avenue Realty Company that developed the Denver Country Club and the adjacent residential area, Country Club Place. (Courtesy DPL Western History Department)

Riethmann lost everything in the Silver Panic of 1893. The National Bank of Kansas City sued; the J. J. Riethmann Drug Company failed. The District Court dismissed the son, John J. Riethmann, Jr., as assignee of the property on June 20, 1895, and ruled that "all property, real and personal, be sold for the benefit of creditors."[16] The banks finally foreclosed on Riethmann's estate in 1901.

After his financial crisis, Riethmann lived at the family farm, then at various hotels and boardinghouses around Denver. Interviewed in his 87th, year Riethmann said, "I was long in the drug business, but I have not taken medicine for forty years, and I attribute my health to that fact. If asked for a recipe for long life I should say 'Drink plenty of water and let the medicine bottles alone.'"[17]

THE WESTERN SUBDIVISIONS

Fourth Avenue Realty Company

Meanwhile, at Denver's Overland Park at Santa Fe and Evans, owner-lawyer Henry Roger Wolcott had livened up the 1893 Silver Panic depression doldrums by introducing golf to Denver. He laid out a nine-hole course around the racetrack, and a number of prominent businessmen were so enthusiastic that they incorporated the Denver Country Club on December 5, 1901. They hoped to buy this property from Wolcott for their own club. However, the $150,000 asking price was too steep, not only for them but also for the Gentlemen's Driving and Riding Club, which finally built a track at City Park for their races.[18] In 1915 Wolcott finally sold the 165 acres for $150,000.

Denver Country Club

The Denver Country Club directors then turned to the Riethmann

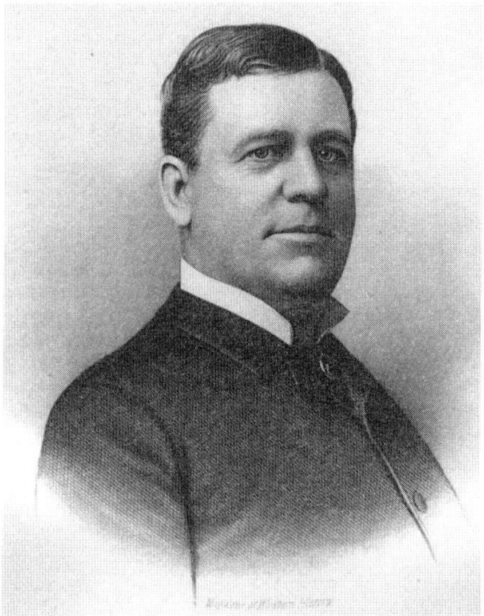

Henry Wolcott introduced golf to Denver at Overland Park where the Denver Country Club was organized in 1901. (Courtesy DPL Western History Department)

property on Cherry Creek. On August 4, 1902, the bid of John A. Ferguson for $49,000 secured 240 acres with appropriate water rights. This included the land south of 1st Avenue for a golf club and 40 acres directly north between Franklin and High Streets for residential development. The City Ditch ran through the east end of the property, crossing Cherry Creek at the current University Boulevard bridge. The next day, the Fourth Avenue Realty Company was incorporated with Ferguson as president and Gerald Hughes as vice-president.[19]

An agreement was received on March 10, 1903, between the Denver Country Club (Henry Treat Rogers, president) and the Fourth Avenue Realty Company (John A. Ferguson, president) stating that, "1st mortgage bonds to the amount of $42,800 issued by authority of said Club shall be given to the [Fourth Avenue Realty Company] and accepted as full payment for said land, water, etc." It also stated that "a street 30 ft. wide shall run E & W along N line of Club's property and Club shall have 15 ft. in width and [Fourth Avenue Realty Company] shall have 15 ft. in width across 40 acres owned by them." Also that "a street be laid out from 4th Ave through its property . . . not to place any stables or out buildings opposite any boulevard or park ways provided." Originally placed at Franklin Street, this entrance roadway was later changed to Gilpin Street.

The first order of the club's business was to lay out a golf course. James Foulis, Jr., was imported from St. Andrews, Scotland, to design a nine-hole course.

The clubhouse as originally designed by Theodore Boal was a T-shaped Shingle-style structure with a projecting gable entrance with columns and a wraparound porch facing east.[20]

The club house was completed for a "grand" opening on January 1, 1905. The opening was not gala: "The DCC will throw open its doors of the new club house to members on New Year's day. On account of the delay of a part of the furniture, only the cafe and the men's locker

The first clubhouse for the Denver Country Club, designed by Theodore Boal, was opened on New Years Day 1905. (Courtesy DPL Western History Department)

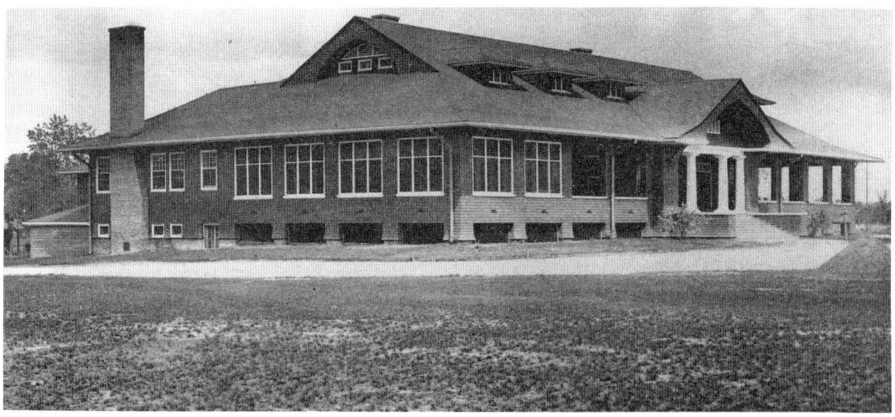

room will be available until further notice," the *Republican* reported.[21]

The west end of the property was converted to polo grounds on Thursdays and Sundays, and stables were added to the site. An article in *Denver Municipal Facts* on September 9, 1911, announced that "the public is cordially invited to attend all games of the annual polo tournament, there being no charge whatever for admission" An 8-by-75-foot frame grandstand was built in 1914.[22] Two clay tennis courts, built in 1903, were soon flooded in winter for skating.

Another event open to the public was the annual display of fireworks, started in 1910. In 1911 the Board of Directors voted to allot $100 for the celebration. The Denver Country Club board minutes reflect that the tab for the event in 1992 was $13,418 and drew hundreds of citizens to the north lawn with blankets and fried chicken to view the carefully orchestrated spectacle.

Country Club Place

By March 23, 1903, the 40-acre real estate development, Country Club Place, was platted by the Fourth Avenue Realty Company north of 1st Avenue between Franklin and High Streets. However, the officers of the realty company, who were also directors of the Denver Country Club, turned their attention to developing the golf course, clubhouse, and entrances to the club before promoting the sale of lots to home owners.

To plan the development of Country Club Place, the realtors retained architect William Ellsworth Fisher, who designed distinctive Spanish entrance gates at Franklin, Gilpin, and High streets along 4th Avenue. He planned each property to face a wide parkway with a landscaped median, making the area spacious and richly landscaped. To leave room for these large lots and parkways, Williams Street and 2nd Avenue were not platted in this subdivision.

Several restrictions were placed on buildings in Country Club Place. "On certain quarters deeds will not be given to the ground without the insertion of a condition that a home costing not less than $10,000 be built. . . . On Gilpin Street between Third and Fourth, houses must cost $7,000 and four lots must be used."[23] On Franklin Street requirements stated that no residence costing less than $4,500 shall be built, no industrial enterprise, no liquor sold, no fence over three feet, and the grantee agrees to begin construction within two months.[24]

Most of the first houses were located on corners with sweeping views of the Country Club. In 1906, Uriah and James Hollister built two of the first homes side by side on 1st Avenue at 103 and 109 Franklin Street, which was then the site of the Country Club entrance. Shortly thereafter, lawyer Arthur B. West built across the street at 100 Franklin, next to architect William Ellsworth Fisher's own home. Financier Raymond Sargeant moved into 181 Franklin, and soon a house to the south was built at 171 Franklin. The Edwin Scholtz house at 160 Franklin, the Edward Wilsons at 180 Franklin, and houses at 305 and 315 Franklin soon populated the southwest section of Country

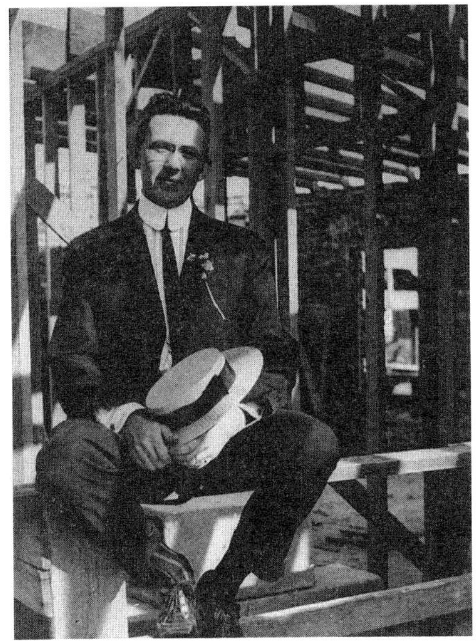

William Ellsworth Fisher was the chief architect of the Country Club Place subdivision. (Courtesy DPL Western History Department, Fisher papers)

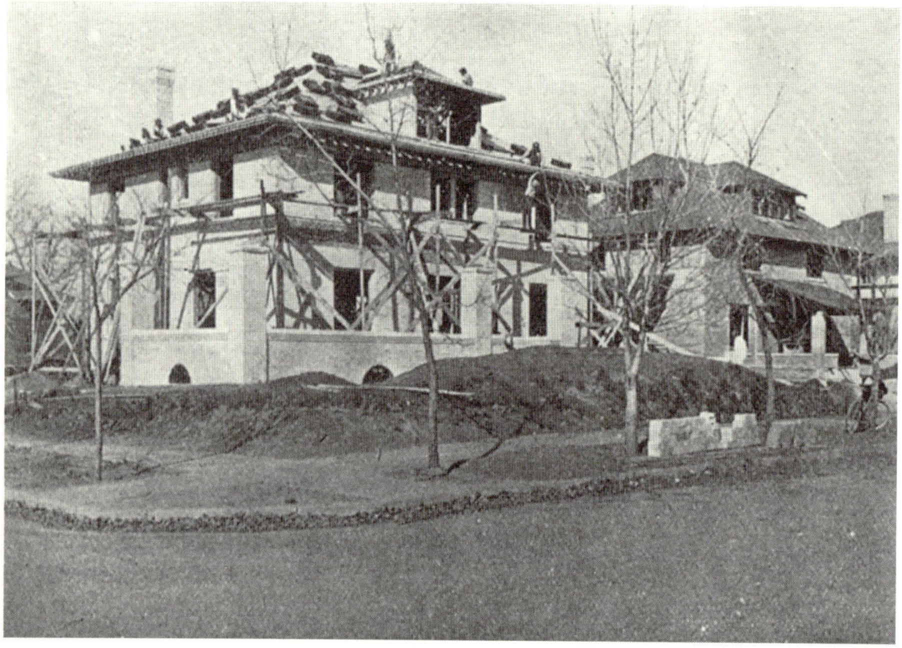

A 1909 issue of the city newsletter, Denver Municipal Facts, *showed these "new" houses at 305 and 315 Franklin Street. (Courtesy DPL Western History Department)*

Club Place. In 1909, Dr. Arnold Taussig built a Fisher-designed Tudor home at 305 Gilpin Street (later 1625 East 3rd Avenue) (See "Walking Tours" section for descriptions of these houses.)

Children in this area went to Corona (Dora Moore) Elementary School at 9th and Corona. Sixth Avenue was a quiet two-way street and children could easily run over to Charles A. Green's Country Club Pharmacy on Gilpin Street for penny licorice sticks and ice cream. "Mr Green became a neighborhood fixture," wrote Pat Lanagan Stearns, who discovered that if she brought in a bouquet of flower weeds from the vacant lot by the store, she would get a free ice cream cone.[25] Across 6th Avenue the Episcopal Church of the Ascension was maintained as Arlington Mission by St. John's Cathedral for five years before establishing its current parish building in 1909, designed by architect Arthur Fisher of 128 Gilpin Street.

Park Club Place

Another subdivision lay directly west, between Humboldt and Downing Streets. This development, Park Club Place, was adjacent to Chutes Park to the west and Driving Park Place to the north, areas that were thriving during the "Gay 90s." With both of these attractions the residential population had crept southeast across the old city limits at 6th Avenue. Although Country Club Place was platted earlier, Park Club Place was the first to be developed.

Neighborhood schools and stores were accessible. Corona (Dora Moore) Elementary School had been open at 9th and Corona since 1890. At the drugstore at 6th and Marion, children bought five-cent sodas from Tom Madden, and later Frank Mathis, after seeing Tom Mix at the Saturday matinee at the Hiawatha (Esquire) Theater.

Oliver's Meat Market is a five-generation store established in 1923 at 6th and Pearl Street by Edward Oliver with his son Richard. It moved to 6th and Marion in 1939 and is now run by Richard's son, Barry Oliver, and his three sons, Jim, Chris, and Rich. The fifth generation stops in after school to help, "just as we did," said Rich. The quality meat market has maintained this location, sharing space with nine different grocers from Piggly Wiggly to Grammone's Deli and Market. "Six months after we moved from Pearl Street, Bell Bakery followed us to this corner," said Barry Oliver.[26]

Arthur Bush Flower Shop and Pooh Corner Book Store were former tenants of the corner. 6th Avenue trolleys rumbled down Corona Street, turning at 4th Avenue where a small commercial strip of shops, such as Charlie's Grocery and Market, emerged near the rambling old clubhouse of the Gentlemen's Driving Club at 1125 East Fourth Avenue. That was demolished in 1931[27] to be replaced by a gas station. These small neighborhood stores later included a gift shop, The Lark, started by Pamela Macdonald Wulsin of 165 Franklin, Betty (Mrs. Moses) Taylor, Sheleigh (Mrs. Kenneth) Malo, and Katherine "Tinka" (Mrs. James B.) Kurtz. Joni Cary (Mrs. John) Vandeventer and Joan (Mrs. Robert) McKenna managed The Women's Exchange from 1976 to 1986. Sheleigh Malo opened an antique store, and Lenore Thomas (Mrs. John) Stoddart founded La Cache to benefit Children's Hospital.

The first houses built in Park Club Place were by the rather dashing Richard H. Malone and future Denver mayor Robert W. Speer, who had bought 40 "more or less"[28] acres from John Jacob Riethmann between Downing and Humboldt Streets on February 12, 1903, for $42,000. They immediately incorporated the Park Club Land Company, with Malone as president and Speer as secretary. Building restrictions were established: "dwelling for 1 family not to cost less than $3,500, no flat roof, no building to be erected on less ground than 50 by 125 ft." The northern five blocks, between 3rd and 4th Avenues, were platted on June 11, 1904, as the first filing. Along 4th Avenue at each of the streets, Marion, Lafayette, and Humboldt, the developers defined the area with red brick gateways with urns and etched street names.

Lots sold quickly on either side of Lafayette and Marion streets. Druggist Frank Quereau built at 379 Marion in 1905[29] and Richard Malone

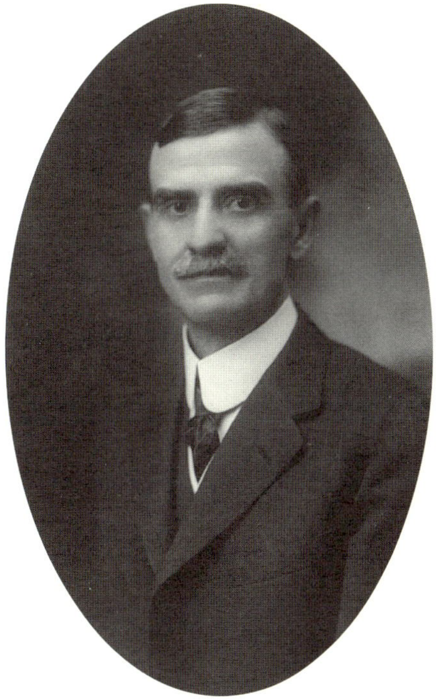

[Above]
Richard H. Malone was the president of the Park Club Place Land Company between Downing and Humboldt Streets and 1st and 4th Avenues.
(Courtesy DPL Western History Department)

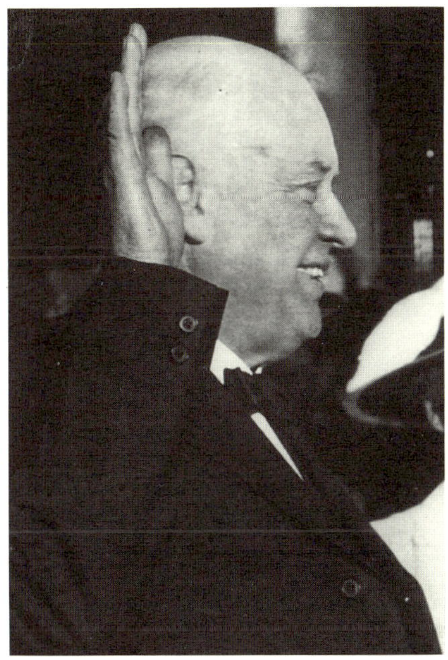

[Right]
Secretary and part owner of the Park Club Place Land Company was Robert W. Speer, who took his oath of office as the mayor of Denver in 1904, just as the realty company was starting.
(Courtesy DPL Western History Department)

built two houses at 301 and 315 Marion. In 1905, Lester Bridaham joined his partner, Frank Quereau, in Park Club Place, building at 350 Humboldt. Bethuel Webster placed his home at 370 Humboldt before he sold it to John M. Kennedy, Jr., then built one at 140 Humboldt. Twenty-six building permits were issued in Park Club Place by 1910.

Two years later, the second filing, consisting of the area south of 3rd Avenue, was sold with more spacious grounds. Houses, especially near 1st Avenue, were built on six to 12 lots with no wall or hedge separating their view of the Denver Country Club grounds to the south. Houses at 124 Lafayette and 135 Humboldt were built on 12 lots each by George B. Berger and his cousin, Lina Bell Kountze Ritter Brown. Houses at 100 and 180 Humboldt covered six to 10 lots.

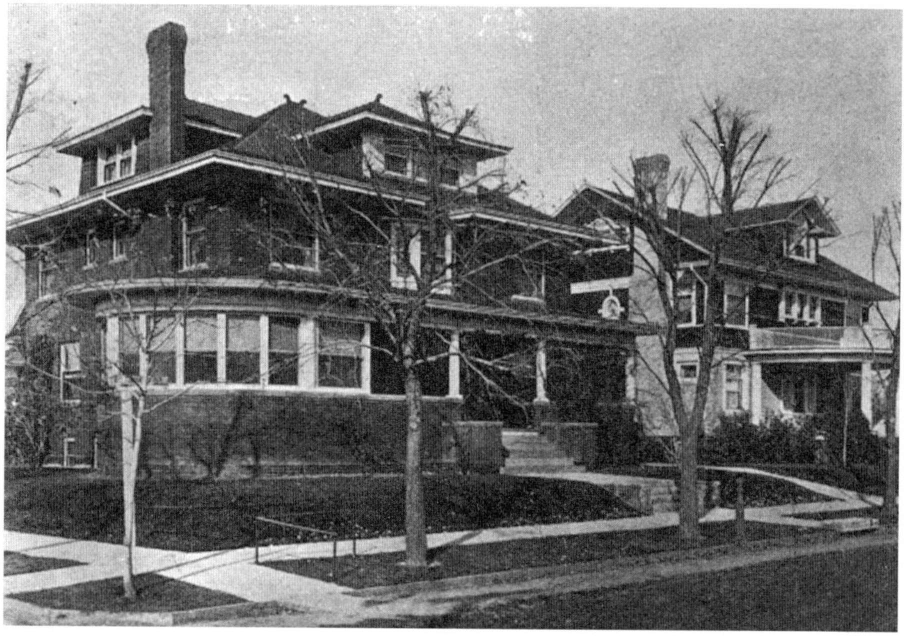

The residences of Richard H. Malone and Robert E. McCracken at 301 and 315 Marion Street were built in 1907. (Courtesy DPL Western History Department)

Many of the residents of the earliest houses in Park Club Place were instrumental in the growth of the Denver Country Club, using the facilities as extensions of their own homes. On Sundays and Thursdays, maids' nights out, they would abandon their vegetable gardens and chicken coops for family suppers at the club. Although men could slip across 1st Avenue for a game of cards, the Country Club restricted these on Sundays to the men's cafe or the card rooms in the basement. Liquid refreshment flowed until the 1915 Prohibition laws. Then, "no liquor shall be brought, distributed or consumed within the clubhouse or on the Club grounds" or the member would be suspended or expelled.[30] Ladies besieged their dressmakers for lace or satin gowns for the frequent dinner dances or the Crepe Paper Ball. However, in 1918, a ball in late December had to be "canceled due to rampant epidemic of Spanish influenza,"[31] which ravaged the country and Europe after World War I. The Country Club waived dues for members in military service for the duration of the war. About this time, there was a "substantial increase in nominated associate, that is, female"[32] members admitted to the Country Club.

Neighborhood members of these two subdivisions were dependent on the Country Club for recreational activities, especially when mobility was restricted before and during World War II. They had easy access to golf or croquet. By 1917 their children were racing around the new skating rink. After the swimming pool opened in 1934, they vied for the diving and swim teams, coached by Graland schoolteacher

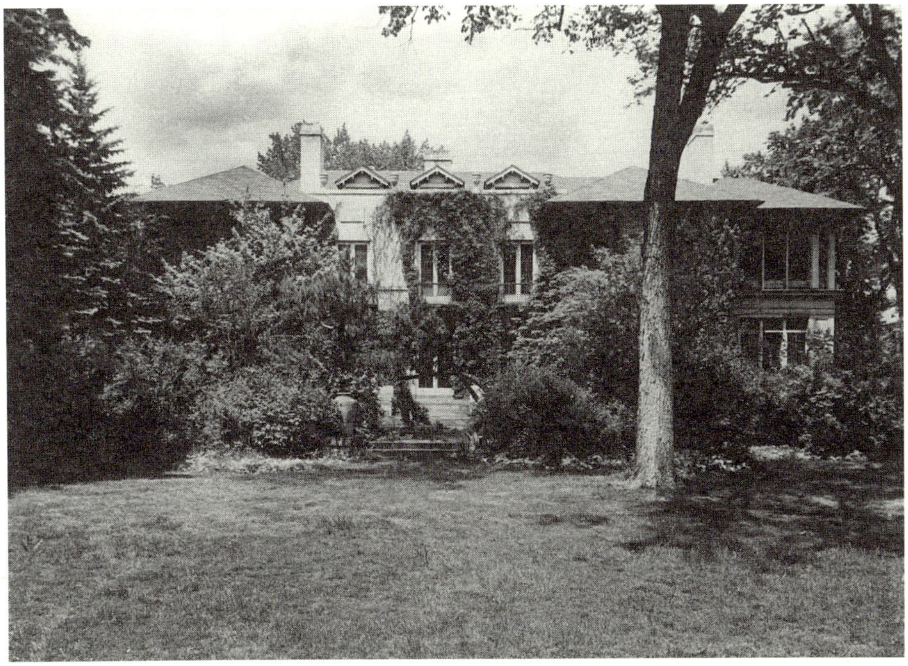

Chester Preisser. They could safely walk or bicycle across quiet, graveled, two-lane 1st Avenue to after-school and weekend activities. However, this road along Cherry Creek from downtown to Mayor Robert Speer's property was soon to drastically change the entrance to the area.

SPEER BOULEVARD

The route along Cherry Creek, once called the Cherokee Trail, had been a natural footpath for Indians and a well-traveled wagon road for gold-seekers since 1860 when caravans stopped at the Four Mile House (now a museum in the municipality

[Above]
The south garden of the George B. Berger, Sr., mansion at 124 Lafayette Street was a grand stand-seat for the Country Club polo matches.
(Courtesy W. Bart Berger)

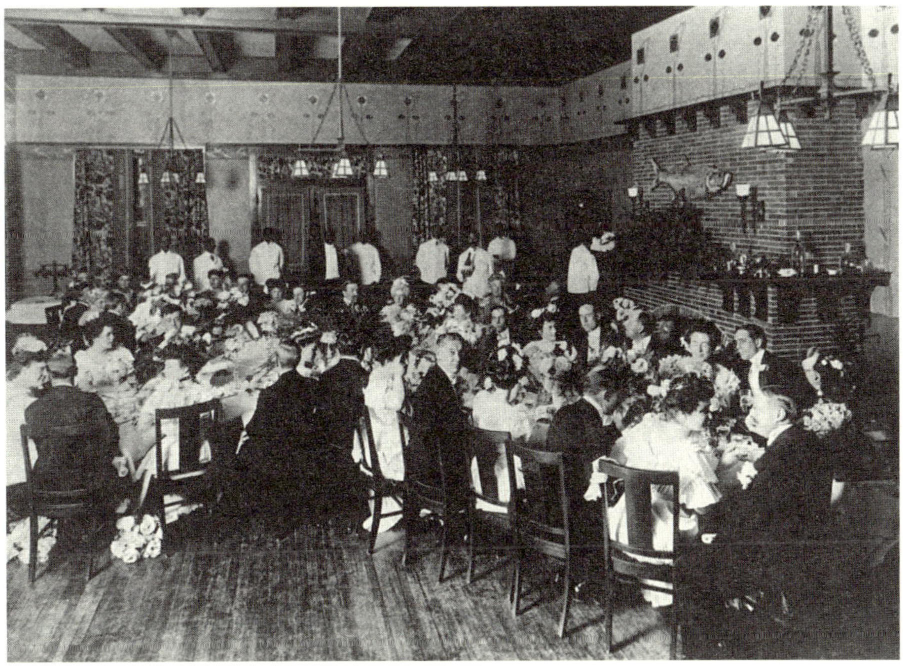

[Right]
The Denver Country Club sponsored parties such as this Crepe Paper Ball at which Mrs. George Berger is pictured with Maggie "Molly" (Mrs. James) Brown.
(Courtesy W. Bart Berger)

of Glendale) to freshen up before the long-awaited arrival in Auraria at the Platte River. The roadway had been named Cherry Creek Drive as it developed into a street for carriages and motorcars. In 1904, Robert W. Speer, who had spearheaded the development of Park Club Place and had chosen property at 300 Humboldt Street for his house, was elected mayor of Denver. With his agenda of remaking the town into a "City Beautiful," improving this entrance to his own property was a priority.

One of his first moves was to clean up the trashy sides of Cherry Creek and extend the road on the north bank east from the Platte River to Downing Street.[33,34] Over the years, travelers had camped, cooked, and tossed their garbage onto the banks, turning the whole waterway into a weedy junk heap. Upstream in Glendale, several dairies herded their cows beside the water. Near the current Cherry Creek Mall, tiny, boxy houses and outhouses huddled near the stream for bathing and drinking water.

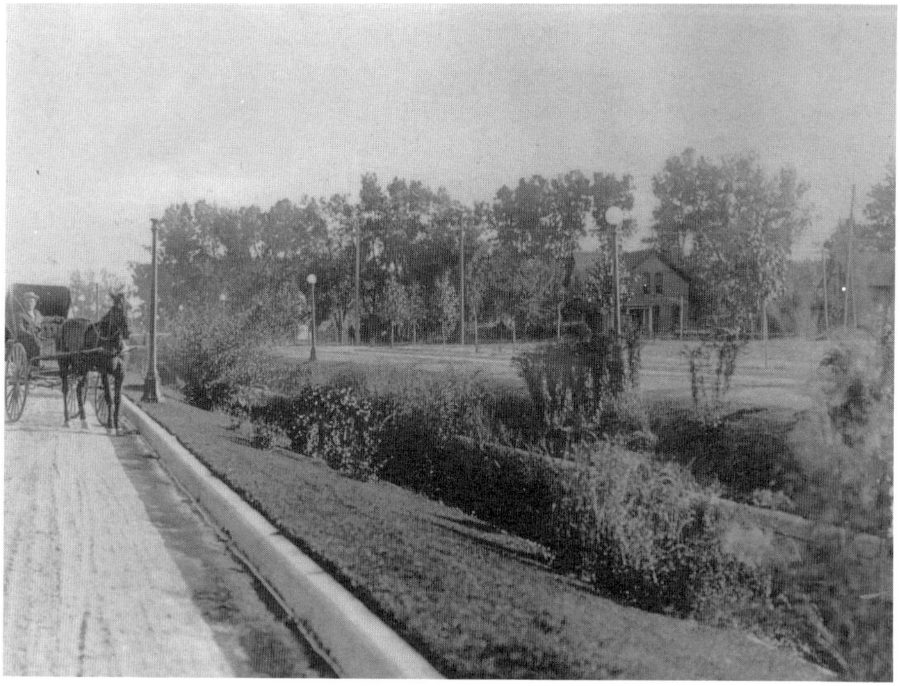

Marion Street Parkway is part of Mayor Robert W. Speer's plan for connecting all of Denver's parks with parkways. (Courtesy DPL Western History Department)

Saco DeBoer, Denver's foremost landscape architect, stated, "Cherry Creek was a three-mile-long dump right in the heart of the city and below the windows of the old City Hall."[35]

During his first two terms as mayor from 1904 to 1912, Speer cleaned up, paved, and planted three miles of Cherry Creek Drive east to Clarkson Street. High concrete walls were built to define and confine the creek, as flooding had been a frequent and disastrous problem since 1864. Elm trees were planted along the grassy banks, and a street lighting system was installed in 1910. A lawn was plowed from Broadway to Downing Street and small parks were planned along the roadway. The boulevard "will be continuous between 49th Avenue and Downing making a fine drive about seven miles in length. It will also connect up the north side boulevard system with the Denver system by way of the Marion Street parkway," which led to Washington Park. "The climax of the boulevard system will be the DCC grounds at Downing," reported *Denver Municipal Facts* in 1912.[36] Cheesman Park was connected to Speer Boulevard through a one-block landscaped median at Downing Street, the 3rd

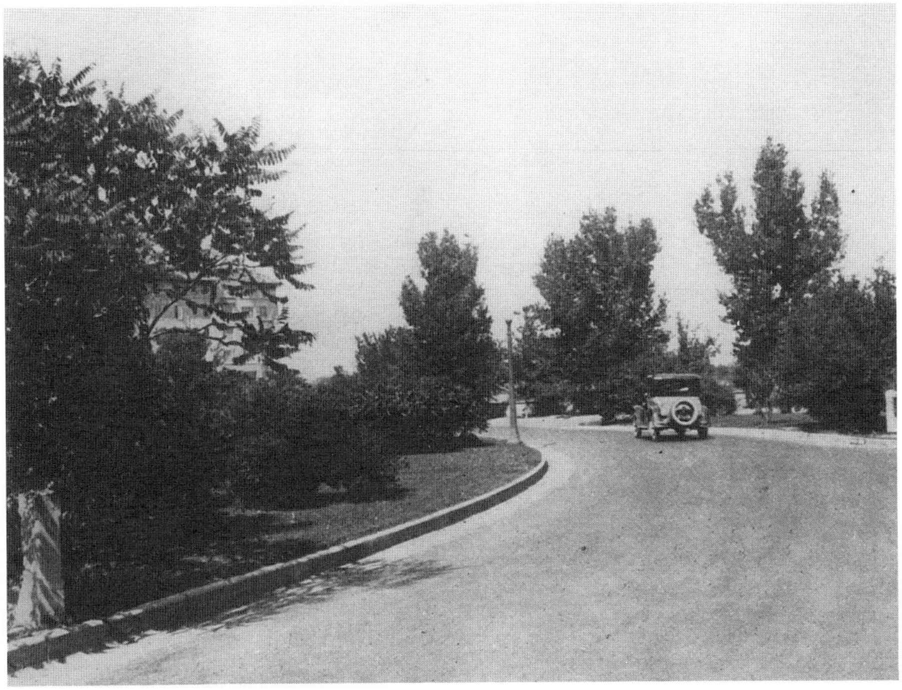

This one-block parkway on Downing Street between 1st and 3rd Avenue Parkway is a connecting link between Washington and Cheesman Parks. (Courtesy DPL Western History Department)

Avenue Parkway, Gilpin Street between 3rd and 4th Avenues, and the Williams Street Parkway, which was built in 1913.

Despite the concrete retainer walls, flooding continued to be a problem. On July 14, 1912, after the walls were completed, a flood resulted in torrents of water rushing down Cherry Creek, damaging the new walls. The next day, the *Rocky Mountain News* reported that "a cloudburst followed by a flood was unequalled for violence since the city was scourged in 1864. . . . the swirling waters overflowed four square miles of Denver. Hundreds of women and children fled to the roof of the houses for safety." The golf course of the Denver Country Club was flooded the day before the Trans America Tournament[37] and fairways and greens had to be rebuilt.

Although Mayor Speer is remembered for beautifying Denver, at the time he was known as the political and dictatorial "Boss Speer," and his terms in office were controversial. Landscape architect Saco DeBoer told of a conversation with a realtor at the Denver Country Club: "I had a blueprint in my hand and he asked if I were working on the Cherry Creek project. When I said that I was, he commented: 'Well, that's Speer for you. He lives right near Cherry Creek and 3rd Ave. And he's feathering his own nest.'"[38] Later the realtor was enthusiastically promoting monuments to commemorate Speer.

The *Denver Post* reported that "Dams in Cherry Creek put in by Speer for 'ornaments' [such as the lake in Chutes Park] were responsible for flooding and will be taken out."[39] The diversionary little lakes in the roadside parks were removed. The walls, bridges, mud damage, and planting were repaired and proposals made for flood control.

However, on August 3, 1933, a deluge again hit the area, bursting the Castlewood Dam near Franktown, and sending Country Club residents along Cherry Creek scrambling to higher ground.

Dorothy Moore Pate, who moved into 369 Humboldt with her husband, John C. Moore, in 1930, remembers the flood: "A policemen came around knocking at all the doors at 3:30 a.m. to warn us that water was rushing down the Creek at ten miles per hour. We all got ready to leave. John and I got dressed, and I found I had put on a yellow chiffon suit for the occasion," she said.

They took the two boys to John's parents' house at 1410 High. Some of the neighbors went to higher ground at Cheesman Park. "The next morning Mother Moore sent me up there to see if some of the people didn't want coffee."

The Robert L. Stearnses were living at 319 Lafayette. One of their daughters, Judith (Mrs. Ken Caughey), recalled the water rushing down Lafayette Street outside the house: "I remember the Knowles' maid next door to my grandmother's calling out, 'Miz Knowles. That Cherry Creek done just overflow.'"

People were alarmed at Gilpin Street. "'We'll all be killed,' yelled Victor Miller, running through the streets, ringing the alarm like Paul Revere," said Lenore (Mrs. John) Stoddart.

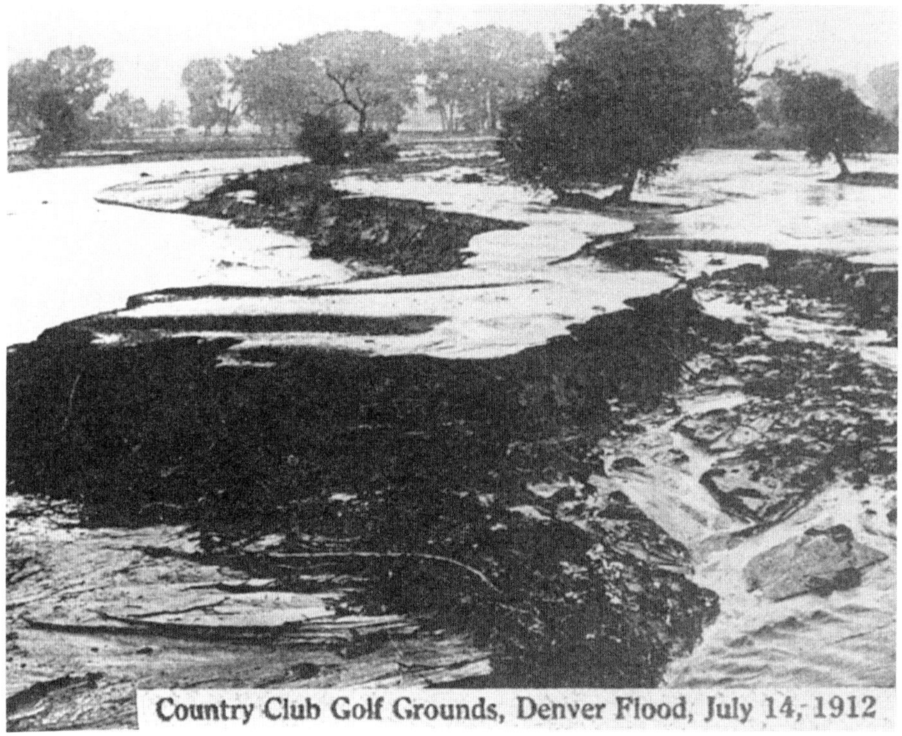

The 1912 flood ruined the Denver Country Club golf course the day before the Trans America Tournament. (Courtesy Constance Whiteley Smith)

Samuel Thomas of 321 Humboldt worked for Royal Crest Dairy, just north of Alameda at Colorado Boulevard. His daughter, Dorothy "Dody" (Mrs. William Phelps) said, "I remember the flood well. I can still see the dog houses floating down the street. I was only three and even now I can picture a cow rolling over helplessly in the torrents of water."

After the flood of 1933, city officials decided they should build a flood-control dam on Cherry Creek. They started in 1935 with Kenwood Dam,[40] but it was 1950 before work on the huge Cherry Creek Dam was concluded by the U.S. Army Corps of Engineers.

Speer Boulevard became one-way, going northwest to Larimer Street in 1957. The southwest side of the boulevard was once called Forest Drive because landscape architect Saco DeBoer's original blueprints called for a "forest of elms."[41] The traffic on the northeast side went in the opposite direction.

In 1978, ten-foot-wide maintenance roads beside the creek were built that doubled as refreshing scenic bike paths, bypassing the noise and heavy traffic to Confluence Park at the junction of Cherry Creek and the South Platte River. Further construction during the early 1990s at the bottleneck of Speer Boulevard at 6th Avenue resulted in a tunnel to disperse traffic.

Speer Boulevard technically ends at Downing Street but connects with 1st Avenue, which passes by the Denver Country Club. Early attention was focused solely on the boulevard, while the two-lane graveled 1st Avenue remained unimproved until residential development expanded eastward. Although the western residential areas, Park Club Place and Country Club Place, are often considered to be the oldest sections of the historic district, they were preceded by two subdivisions to the east.

THE EASTERN SUBDIVISIONS

During the late 1800s, while the gentlemen raced their harnessed horses at 4th Avenue and Corona Street, the Riethmanns harvested wheat from their farm, and the Denver Country Clubbers golfed at Overland Park, two subdivisions in the east of the present Country Club Historic District were platted and selling property, 15 years before the Country Club came to Cherry Creek. C. G. Richardson Place was platted in 1888 on the property of the present Park Lane Square (Circle Drive) area. Capitol Annex, platted in 1889, was developed just west of University Boulevard between 3rd and 4th Avenues. These two subdivisions preceded the other eastern subdivisions, Country Club Annex and Park Lane Square, by over three and a half decades.

Capitol Annex

In 1889, William Geddis (later William Geddes) "laid out and platted under the name of Capitol Annex in the County of Arapahoe"[42] the most historic existing section of the present Country Club Historic Neighborhood. This area, between Bridger (3rd) and Vasquez (4th) Avenues, and Vine and York Streets (University Boulevard) was south of the city limits and adjacent to Harman (Cherry Creek North), the township that was incorporated in 1886.

Geddis, born in 1850 in Northern Ireland, with a bit of Scotch blood, arrived in Denver at the age of 30, and started work as a contractor. While finishing the foundations for buildings such as the Brown Palace Hotel and the state capitol he turned to the manufacture of vitrified clay sewer pipe and in 1890 established Denver Sewer Pipe and Clay Company, "which became the leading business of its line in Colorado," historian Frank Hall wrote in 1895.[43]

The original houses of Capitol Annex were typically small on less than 37-foot lots. The building permit for a house at 320 Gaylord Street was issued in 1892.

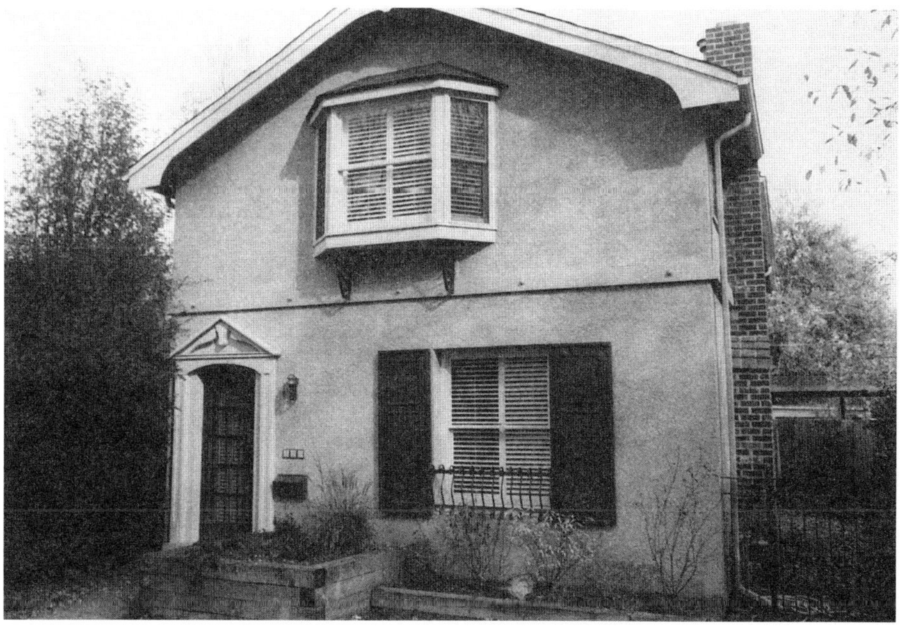

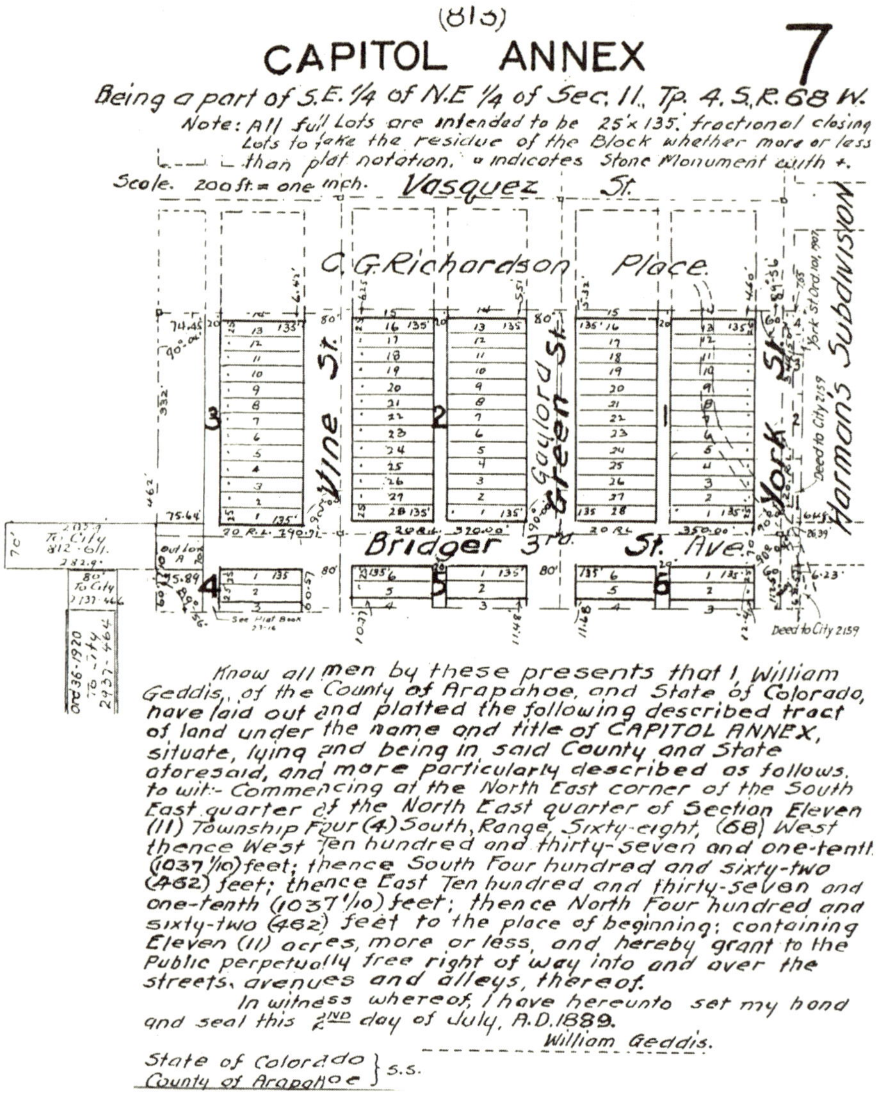

The small subdivision of Capitol Annex was platted between 3rd and 4th Avenues in 1889 by William Geddis (later Geddes), founder of Denver Sewer Pipe and Clay Company. (Courtesy Denver Engineer's Office)

Newspaper reports at the turn of the century list the president of the company as either William F. Geddes[44] or William Geddis,[45] with E. R. Ball as secretary and treasurer. His son, William John Geddes, later built a house at 2155 Hawthorne Drive in Park Lane Square (Circle Drive), while various family members lived nearby in Country Club Annex.

Both the streetcar winding up 4th, then 3rd Avenue, and the proximity of Bromwell Elementary School in Harman at 4th Avenue and Josephine Street helped popularize the area. The little town of Harman had started a nearby elementary school in a frame house on its present site at 4th Avenue and Josephine Street way back in 1867.[46]

The original houses in Capitol Annex were typically small on less than 37-foot lots. The first building permit was issued in Capitol Annex on March 14, 1892,[47] to build a 22-by-30-foot, one-and-a-half-story brick dwelling for $1,000 at 320 Gaylord Street. The 1893 Census revealed another house on the southeast corner of 3rd Avenue and Vine Street. There were three more houses on Gaylord and two on Vine in Capitol Annex by 1900.[48] It was a multiracial area and the owners of these houses were neither the aristocracy of Denver nor their servants. Most were middle-class workers, such as a carpenter, an electrician, and a paper-hanger.[49] In 1905, at the time the Denver Country Club and adjacent residential areas were just opening their doors, there were already nine homes in Capitol Annex.[50]

Capitol Annex does not lie between current streets because of private land holdings in the 1880s when it was platted.[51]

As the eastern area of the historic district developed, Capitol Annex was encroached upon from the south. In 1925, Lawrence C. Phipps, with Lawrence C. Phipps, Jr., as his lawyer, subdivided and replatted two of the three blocks of Capitol Annex on the south side of 3rd Avenue to add to the new Country Club Annex that extends south to 1st Avenue.[52] A tiny area 75 by 125 feet on 3rd between Gaylord and its alley remains in Capitol Annex. This area is the site of a row of six red brick townhouses that were built in 1910.

UNPLATTED LAND

The land between Country Club Annex and Country Club Place was, and remains, unplatted. This includes the west side of Race Street between 1st and 3rd Avenues.

Part of this land was owned by Elizabeth Iliff Warren, widow of Greeley cattle king John Wesley Iliff, who died in 1878. In 1913 she gave this piece to her daughter, Louise Iliff. Elizabeth had since married Methodist Bishop Henry White Warren, and the family founded Iliff Theological Seminary, fulfilling the cattle king's wish. "My grandfather owned land all over the place, east Denver as well as Weld County. I suppose my family sold these inherited lots whenever the seminary needed funds,"[53] said granddaughter Alberta Iliff Shattuck.

This unplatted land resulted in some unwieldy property descriptions. For instance, while the legal description of 300 Vine is "Capitol Annex Subdivision, Block 2, Lots 26 To 28,"[54] the description on the deed of 361 Race Street reads:

> Commencing at the point of intersection of the North line of 3rd Avenue as established by deed from Louise Iliff to City and County of Denver recorded in Book 3739 Page 535 and the West line of Race Street as established by deed from Louise Iliff to City and Country of Denver recorded in Book 4009 Page 549 thence North along the West line of said Race Street 120 feet; thence West and parallel to North line of 3rd Avenue to a point 30 feet East of the West line of the SE1/4 of NE1/4 Section 11, Township 4 South Range 68 West and 120 feet North of the North line of 3rd Avenue;thence South to a point on the North line of 3rd Avenue 30 feet East of the West line of the SE1/4 of NE1/4 Section 11 Township 4 South Range 68 West thence East along North line of 3rd Avenue to the place of beginning."[55]

In 1920 the original Race Street between 1st and 3rd Avenues, was vacated by Lawrence C. Phipps, Jr. and Louise Iliff, who dedicated land east of their property for the current Race Street, still part of the unplatted

Lawrence C. Phipps, Jr., added blocks of Capitol Annex along 3rd Avenue to the Country Club Annex subdivision. (Courtesy DPL Western History Department)

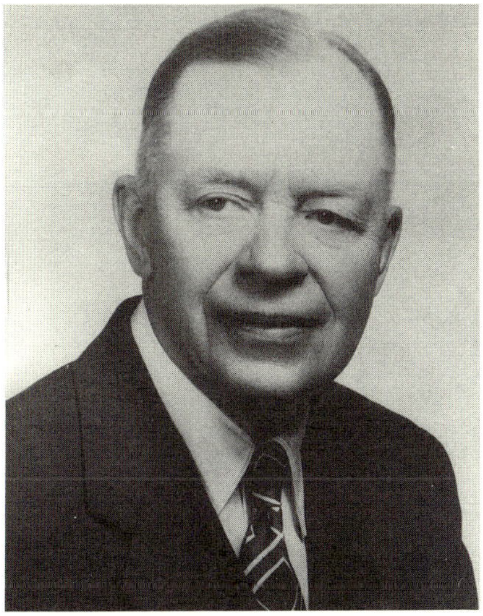

Baist Map, 1905

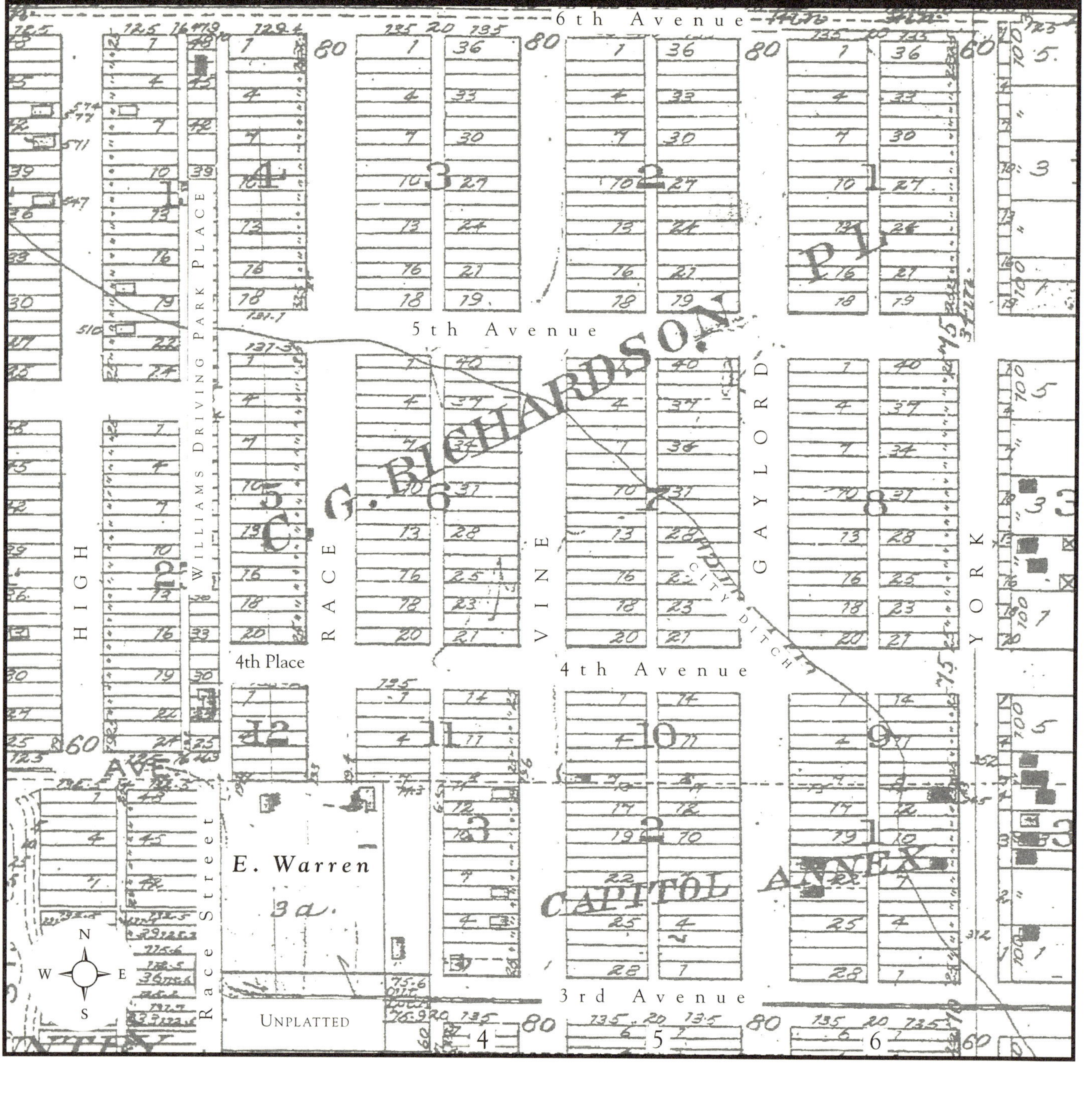

land. This vacated land "reverts severally to the owners of property abutting on said vacated street up to and as far as the center line,"[56] the ordinance states. (see Baist map, 1905)

This vacating of Race Street enlarged the unplatted Phipps' property at 161 Race Street. Also, the original alley between High and Race Streets had been vacated in 1909,[57] resulting in doubly-deep lots on east High Street. This allowed room for a tennis court at 360 High; a complex of three houses at 160, 170, and 180 High Street; and houses such as 200 and 310 High that were built back from the street, adjacent to the vacated alley. In 1984, Clayton Dorn sold off the back of his lot at 380 High and two new houses were built. The name Race Court was given to the access road, a section of the original Race Street.[58]

Mary Lee (Mrs. Martin) Anderson, who lives at 361 Race Street, found that the workers constructing these houses had trouble finding the correct address. "All these trucks came clanking up Race Street past our house trying to find the new houses, so Keith Brown [who was building one of them] went down to City Council and got the name changed to Race Court so they'd go to the right address."[59] The confusion continued, as the address of the house is officially 377 Race *Street*, not Race Court.[60] The other house, 1980 4th Avenue, was occupied by John and Vivian Sweeney, who had lived at 461 Race Street.

COUNTRY CLUB ANNEX

South of Capitol Annex is Country Club Annex, a subdivision that, as its name suggests, was an expansion of Country Club Place. It was bounded by Race Street and University Boulevard, and 1st and 3rd Avenues. Most of the houses were built between 1925 and 1950 and were often occupied by children of the early settlers in the western subdivisions where they were brought up. For instance, George Berger, Jr., raised at 124 Lafayette, lived at 230 Vine. William V. Hodges, Jr., settled his family at 261 Vine after a boyhood at 300 High Street. Lenore and John Stoddart built at 280 Race Street after her upbringing at 380 Gilpin Street. Mary Barkalow Holt, whose family lived at 319 Lafayette, and her husband, Marmaduke Holt, moved to 401 Westwood Drive, then 300 Race Street. Lawrence C. "Larry" Phipps, Jr., raised at 360 High Street, established the Country Club Annex subdivision and lived on 67,000 square feet of unplatted land at 161 Race Street.

By 1925, when the subdivision was completed, the Country Club had abandoned its polo field. Polo had moved east of University Boulevard and south of Alameda to land bought by Lafayette Hughes and Ira Humphreys from William Bart Berger, currently the exclusive Polo Grounds residential area. As a result of the move, the Country Club golf course was redesigned. The clubhouse was remodeled from Theodore Boal's original Shingle style into a Colonial Revival building designed by Arthur and William Fisher, retaining the ideal of "true hospitality in the atmosphere of a beautiful home."[61] The remodeling continued the tradition of a wide eastern porch sprinkled with comfortable wicker chairs facing the eighteenth hole. Long-term member Jane Bromfield Foster said, "The thing I really remember about the Club was the

[OPPOSITE PAGE]
This 1905 map shows land owned by E. Warren, the original Race Street bordering this land on the west, and the extra alley west of Race Street between 4th and 6th Avenues. The City Ditch runs through C. G. Richardson Place (the future Park Lane Square).
(Courtesy DPL Western History Department)

wonderful big porch that faced east. We could sit in the wicker chairs, chat with friends and watch the golfers come in."[62] Her father, Dr. Lawrence Bromfield, was a perennial golf champion.

The subdivision, Country Club Annex, grew rapidly during the late twenties and thirties. Even as late as the 1980s, the area between 1st and 3rd Avenues facing York Street was undeveloped. "We just had cars parked on the ground behind us, out my bedroom window. There wasn't even any alley then,"[63] said Diana Warren, who lived at 140 Gaylord during the sixties and seventies. In 1986 a sewer line was installed along the Gaylord-University alley from 3rd to 1st, and a line of stores with parking spaces filled the block.

C. G. RICHARDSON PLACE (CIRCLE DRIVE)

The other nineteenth-century subdivision was platted by Cyrus G. Richardson in 1888 on his seven-year holding of land in Arapahoe County. He laid out C. G. Richardson Place in a traditional grid,[64] using, of course, the original street names, since it was then south of the city limits. The property included Chamberlin (6th Avenue), Beckwith (5th Avenue), Vasquez (4th Avenue) and Bridger (3rd Avenue), then York (University Boulevard), Green (Gaylord), Vine, and Page (Race).[65]

After Julia Frances Richardson inherited this property from her deceased husband, she converted all the vacant land to the Richardson Investment Company, incorporated in 1917. This was sold in 1922 to Dean Realty and Investment Company with Mary (Mrs. Verner Z.) Reed, president, and Orville L. Dines, vice-president.

Park Lane Square (Circle Drive)

Few lots had been sold in C. G. Richardson Place, so Dean Realty bought up the remaining scattered properties during the early twenties. In 1926, C. G. Richardson Place was officially vacated[66] except for 12 lots on the west side of Race Street, south of 6th Avenue, which remain as C. G. Richardson Place. Mary Dean Reed, who had inherited two small lots of C. G. Richardson Place from a sister who died in 1909, claimed several of the large lots of Park Lane Square to build a castle on Circle Drive.

The rest of the subdivision was conveyed to the Park Lane Square Company, with S. N. Hicks as president; Ralph Antonides, vice-president; and Morton Herres, contractor.

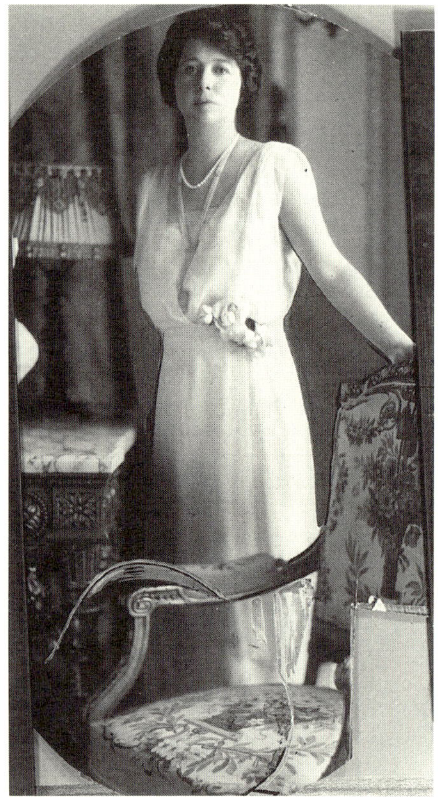

Mary Dean Reed was the president of Dean Realty Co. that sold land for Park Lane Square after she retained property to build her castle. (Courtesy DPL Western History Department)

[OPPOSITE PAGE]
The subdivision, Park Lane Square, at 6th Avenue and Race Street replaced the former 1888 subdivision C. G. Richardson Place. Note that Westwood Drive follows the old City Ditch.

PARK LANE SQUARE REPLACED C.G. RICHARDSON PLACE

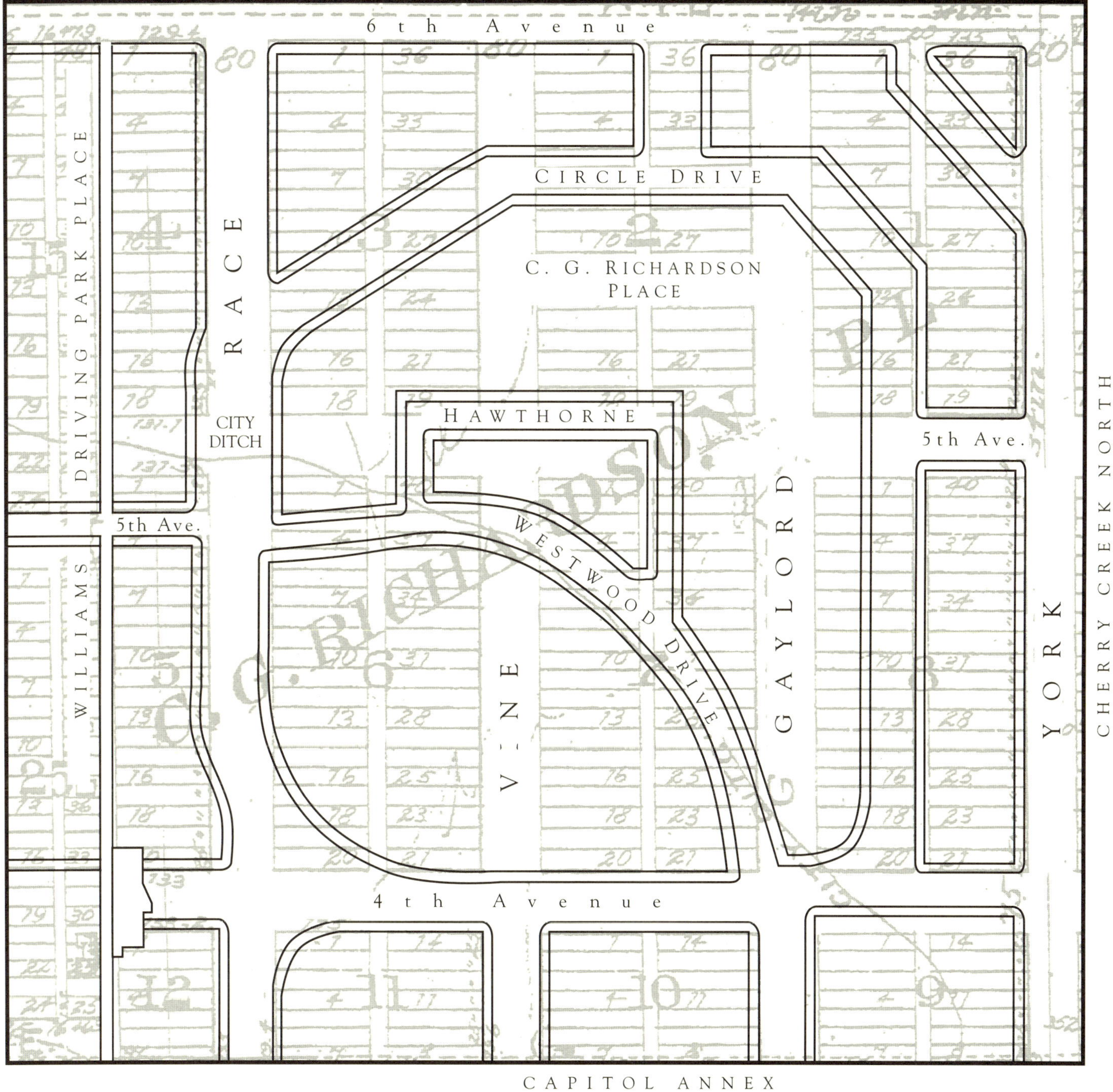

Designed by landscape architect Saco DeBoer, the area was replatted in a circular pattern with 58 large lots.

The covenants of the Park Lane Square Company, incorporated on March 22, 1926, required houses "to cost at least $15,000. All will be private family residences. There shall be no hotel or apartment, flat, terrace building, boarding and/or rooming house, industrial, commercial or business building, public garage, or stable in unsubdivided blocks.

"None of said lots . . . shall at any time, be used or occupied by, or be sold, leased, or given to any person or persons of any race, except the white race.

"These covenants shall be in effect until the first day of January, 1977, and the same shall continue hereafter until the first day of January, 2001, unless . . . the owners of 75% of the front footage of all said lots and blocks shall desire to cancel and amend any or all of said restrictions."[67]

A strange anomaly of this area was the existence of two alleys. The boundary line between C. G. Richardson Place and the subdivision to the west, Williams Driving Park Place, was a 10-foot-wide alley between Race and High Streets running between 4th and 6th Avenues. Parts of this alley were vacated at various times between 1934 and 1963.[68] The other wider alley already existed in Williams Driving Park Place. Although technically the 47.5-foot-wide properties between the alleys are in Williams Driving Park subdivision, this land is part of Park Lane Square and is included in the Country Club Historic District.

The directors of the Park Lane Square Land Company, most of whom were owners of these large lots, formed a home owners' association. The meetings of these dedicated neighbors to enforce the covenants, defend their turf, and address the threat of commercial development in Cherry Creek were the impetus for the Cherry Creek Improvement Association, later named the Country Club Historic Neighborhood, Inc. The organization added the other three subdivisions (Country Club Annex, including Capitol Annex, Country Club Place, and Park Club Place) as the threat of commercialism from the east became more imminent. Although the organization has grown to include 85 percent of the home owners, its beginning was tenuous.

COUNTRY CLUB HISTORIC NEIGHBORHOOD, INC. (nee Cherry Creek Improvement Association)

The original Park Lane Square Company, formed in 1927, specified that all home owners, their heirs and successive grantees shall keep the specified covenants. "That organization of home owners formed the core of our neighborhood Association," said Robert K. Fuller, II, of 2244 East 4th Avenue. Previously called the Cherry Creek Improvement Association (CCIA), the group is now named Country Club Historic Neighborhood, Inc. (CCHN).

The Park Lane Square or Circle Drive area was rural during its initial growth of the 1930s. Two-way 6th Avenue bordered the north, and the former small farming town of Harman lay to the east. As the Country Club residential area grew, the other subdivisions joined the CCIA.

DEVELOPMENT OF CHERRY CREEK SHOPPING AREA

The real threat to the residential neighborhood came after World War II with the City's attempt to widen East 6th Avenue during the sixties and the transformation of the former city dump into a large upscale shopping center.

In 1945 flamboyant architect Temple Hoyne "Sandy" Buell disclosed plans to develop an $11 million apartment and shopping project between University and Steele,1st Avenue and Cherry Creek.

Buell had held the property for 20 years. He had developed tuberculosis, and after he married Marjorie

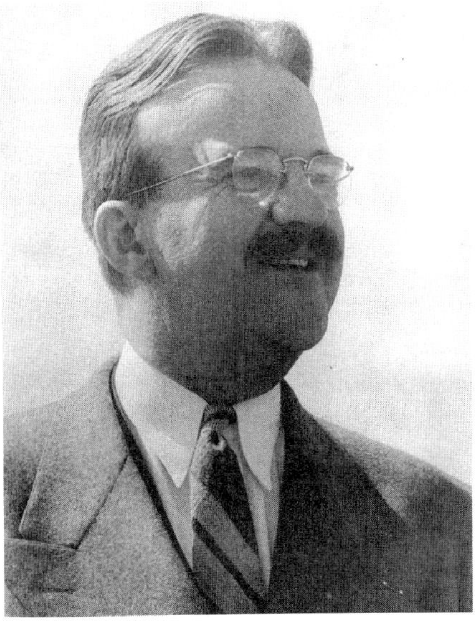

The Cherry Creek Shopping Center is the result of the determination and ingenuity of architect Temple Hoyne Buell. (Courtesy DPL Western History Department)

Macintosh in Chicago, they moved to high, sunny Denver for a cure. Their daughter, Callae Buell Gilman said, "My grandfather always had an eye for a good piece of property and owned real estate all over the country. In Denver he bought the land of the city dump and gave it to Daddy as a present."

This dump, at 1st Avenue, from University to Steele Street, a stone's throw from the Denver Country Club, was a colossal, soggy city-wide trash heap used by all nearby neighborhoods. "Treacherous water-filled pits were breeding grounds for polio," a 1946 newspaper pointed out. "The unsightly dumps spew smoke and refuse throughout adjoining neighborhoods. . . . The present dumps are breeding places for rats and disease." A picture of a sign at smoky 1st and Fillmore read, "NO DUMPING. Dump Closed. Go to Birch and Virginia."[69] In 1946 City Council voted to close the dump, and the property, owned and developed by Buell, became the foundation of his fortune.

Zinette Spore Moore Philipp recalled passing open burning trash heaps at 1st and University in the thirties as she travelled to her home in the Hilltop neighborhood. "We could see the smoke billowing up as we looked towards the mountains from our house on Cranmer Park."

Colodon Moor

After three years of negotiations, the Denver Zoning Board approved the plans for "Colodon Moor, the largest single private real estate

After World War II, Buell transformed his dump into a shopping center called Colodon Moor at University Boulevard and 1st Avenue.(Courtesy DPL Western History Department)

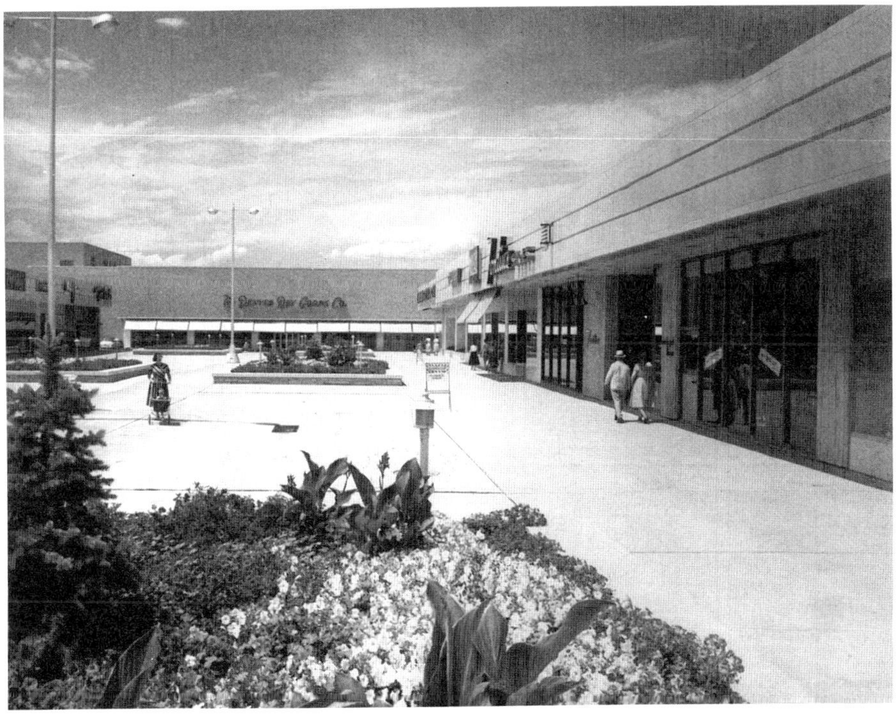

development in the history of the Rocky Mountain West," reported the *Rocky Mountain News*.[70] The proposal called for "1200 dwelling units in two apartment house areas, a 1500-seat motion picture theater and two modern store buildings. . . . providing space for up to 24 different shops."[71]

"The buildings . . . will be low and in a 'country club style' in keeping with the residential section in which it will be located," Buell promised in 1950.[72]

By 1955 a landscaped shopping mall was anchored by Denver Dry Goods at 1st and University with a Miller's Supermarket and two rows of little shops such as Anderson's Toyland, Fontius Shoes, F. W. Woolworth's, Vaughn Music, Squire Shop, Hummel's Delicatessen and Pooh Corner Book Store. A popular Baur's Restaurant was on the southwest corner. However, there were none of the garden-style apartments, promised in the presentation to City Council.

Meanwhile, in the old town of Harman (Cherry Creek North), small businesses were replacing farmhouses and small homes. In 1953 one of the first buildings was the prestigious interior decorating firm, (George) Bethune and (Richard M.) Moore, which moved into a building at 2412 3rd Avenue designed by Moore's brother, architect Thomas Edgar Moore. "It's a beautiful multi-leveled building with interesting spaces. It helped set a standard for unique retail stores in Cherry Creek North," said Zinette Moore Philipp, the widow of Richard Moore. The imaginative International-style building later housed a Persian rug outlet. The area grew into a community of friendly locally-run shops.

Cherry Creek North merchants organized "to create a Greenwich Village-type area of small art galleries, antiques, boutiques, and decorative arts, which they would promote with cultural and civic programs to draw attention to the area."[73]

Expansion

In 1968, not satisfied with his shopping center, Buell revealed extensive expansion plans. Despite the Cranmer Park Mountain View

After Colodon Moor was built at University Boulevard and 1st Avenue, the land to the east was cleared for the expansion of Cherry Creek Shopping center. (Courtesy DPL Western History Department)

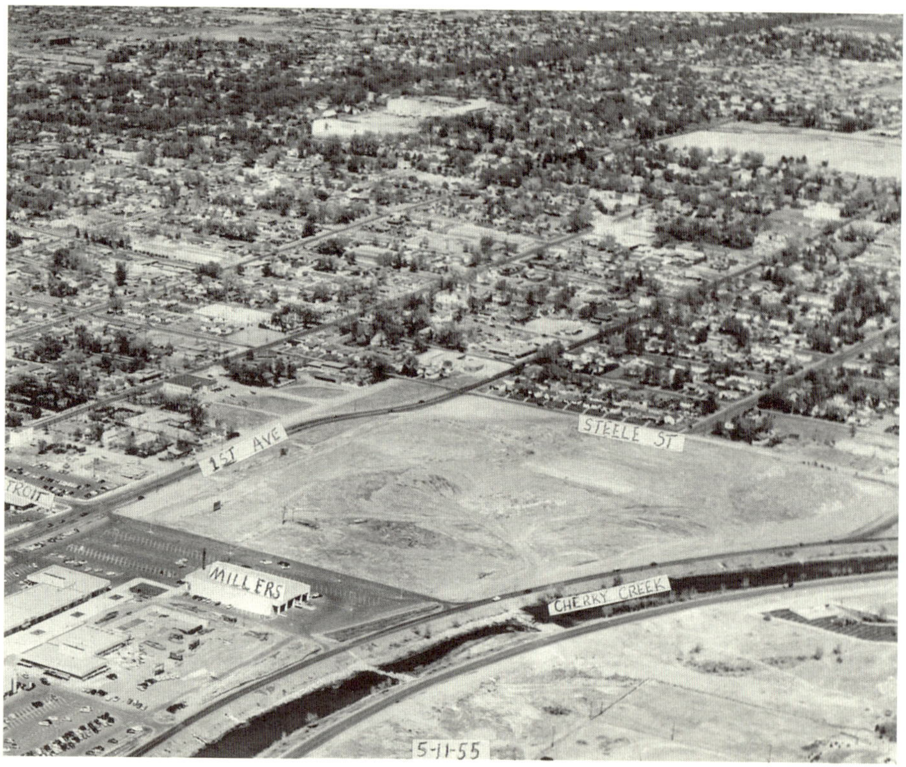

Preservation Ordinance limiting the height of buildings west of the park to 17 stories, Buell announced, "I'm going to build a 54-story office building in the middle of Cherry Creek Shopping Center, and nobody is going to stop me. . . . From the revolving restaurant on top there's a view they'd never see from Cranmer Park or Cheesman Park under any circumstances."[74] The dream met a rude awakening from neighborhood opposition.

The Cherry Creek Improvement Association (CCIA) sprang to life with the threat of a huge multi-million dollar Cherry Creek shopping center. To the east, nearest the commercial section, Park Lane Square home owners Julia "King" Dobbins, Robert K. Fuller, Joseph G. Hodges, Jr., Arthur Krill, Porter Nelson, F. George Robinson, Mary Alice Staub, Marie Vest, and Charles L. Warren monitored developments and battled business encroachment by signing petitions, attending hearings and City Council meetings, writing letters, and serving on relevant community committees.

"In 1975 the first neighborhood Master Plan for the Cherry Creek neighborhood was started," said architect, urban designer, and past association president Robert K. Fuller, II, who had moved to the Country Club area that year. The boundaries of the Plan were between Colorado and University Boulevards and 6th Avenue south to Cherry Creek.

In 1982 Buell and mall developers Jacobs/Kahan of Chicago announced further expansion—a gigantic $250 million plan with 3,800,000 square feet of construction, including office space, retail shops, and a 400-room hotel. Traffic would triple. "We don't need a second downtown in a neighborhood that has no major arterial highways feeding it," said Charles L. Warren, then president of the CCIA.[75]

Greater Cherry Creek Steering Committee

By 1981 neighbors had become alarmingly aware of the rapid changes in the whole Cherry Creek area, and a coalition of 12 neighborhood groups formed the Greater Cherry Creek Steering Committee to monitor and curb the plans. "Our traffic problems are escalating," said committee chair David Downs. Warren added, "It's not only the traffic congestion, it's the safety, noise and pollution that go along with it. . . . Now Cherry Creek is a low-key and personal area with sidewalk sales and a lot of fun. These guys want to build a monolith."[76] At this point, the Steering Committee asked the city for a Master Plan update.

By 1981 Jacobs/Kahan left, then went bankrupt. Buell collaborated with the Taubman Company of Troy, Michigan, as mall designer, and the city asked for an update of the Master Plan, inviting the Greater Cherry Creek Steering Committee to be part of a larger Master Plan team with representation from businesses and the developer. On August 17, 1987, ground breaking took place for a two-story shopping mall of May-D & F, Lord and Taylor, Saks Fifth Avenue, Nieman Marcus and 130 shops on one million square feet west of Steele Street. Twenty five new stores were added in 1998, including an exclusive Tiffany jewelry store and Rainforest Cafe. Thirty new stores were advertised in 1999 and Nordstrom's is hoping for space on the mall.

Taubman had agreed to tear down the 1950s center when the mall was completed and to replace it with a mixture of offices and housing with a few small stores. This had not happened by 2000. Rather than an empty, boarded-up eyesore, the old center was "temporarily" reopened in 1994 when Bed, Bath and Beyond came in. The future development on the west end is controlled by negotiations between the developers and the city.

Commercialism on University Boulevard

While maintaining a large profile in the Cherry Creek community, the CCIA found troubling commercial

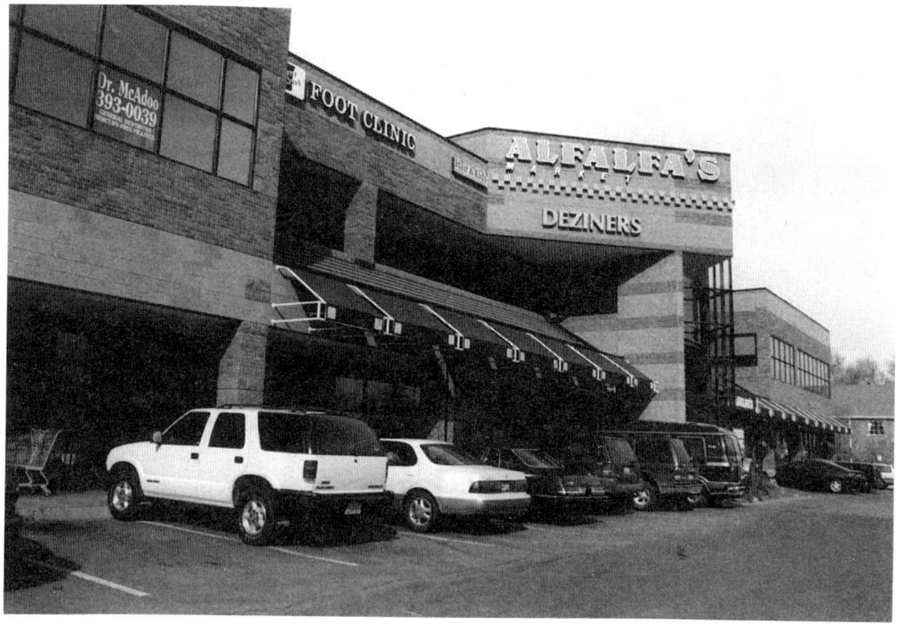

During the eighties, the neighborhood restaurant was replaced by a shopping strip anchored by Alfalfa's upscale grocery store.

issues on the east edge of the Country Club District.

During the early eighties the Blue Parrot, a small quiet neighborhood restaurant where customers were greeted with a cheery "hello" from a live parrot, was on the west side of University Boulevard, now a commercial shopping strip. When the site was vacated a large Oriental restaurant was proposed. Association president Charles Warren amassed 11 petitions with 157 names of residents in protest, and the restaurant application was withdrawn.

In 1987 the Cherry Creek Auto Service, grandfathered in as a business at 303 University, was sold. The corner, still a Planned Unit Development (PUD), now houses Homer Reed men's clothing store. The home owners were leery of an invasion of commercial properties on the west side of University Boulevard. "The Association settled on the dignified Homer Reed store, which later sublet space to the Turner Art Gallery," said close neighbor, Robert K. Fuller, II, of 2244 4th Avenue.

In 1989, Dikeou Realty proposed a four-story eclectic building at the corner of 1st and University. Unfortunately, during the fifties, neighbors had protested against a one-story clinic and pharmacy there because the sale of drugs might attract "undesirables." Instead, a much larger four-story office building for Perry and Butler Realty was built there.

Across Josephine, between 4th and 5th Avenues, the Association finally managed to defer a high-rise by negotiating for a group of two-story town houses, insisting on the pleasant hilly park (the grassed-over fill from the excavation) at the south end near Bromwell School. It was through the dogged determination of Marie Vest of 400 Circle Drive that this project was accomplished. "That should be named Marie Vest Park," said CCIA director Arthur Krill.

Another recent problem is the possibility of "grocery row," as Warren put it in 1999. "Whole Foods is moving from Boulder to the Sears Roebuck site at the northeast corner of 1st and University. The developer wants Safeway to move to the southeast corner, and Alfalfa's is already there [at University and 3rd Avenue]." There is concern that this will increase the traffic of frequent shoppers, making the intersection of 1st and University into a "grocery gridlock."

INTERIOR NEIGHBORHOOD PROBLEMS

Along with other neighborhood associations the CCIA tried in vain to exclude "unmarried couples living together" in an R-0 zone in the early eighties.

A median cut on 1st Avenue at Vine Street was eliminated to prevent traffic cutting through to 6th Avenue in order to avoid the clutter at 1st and University. "The traffic along Race had been terrible," said Mary Lee (Mrs. Martin) Anderson of 361 Race. The proliferation of stop signs, medians, islands and circles at this corner has mitigated this. Ruth (Mrs. George) Hopfenbeck lives at 450 Race Street. "The islands are great now, but I did wonder about having 36 signs at that intersection," she said. At the CCIA meeting on May 12, 1992, it was requested that 15 of the signs at 4th and Race be removed.[77] "That intersection was a huge wasteland of asphalt where kids played hockey and football," said architect Richard E. Henry, who remodeled the house at 344 Race Street.

In 1989 gates were installed on 1st Avenue that permitted only one-lane traffic in and out of the district. The "Save the Gates" committee replaces and repairs urns and columns on existing gates.

Other concerns were relocating homeless campers from under the

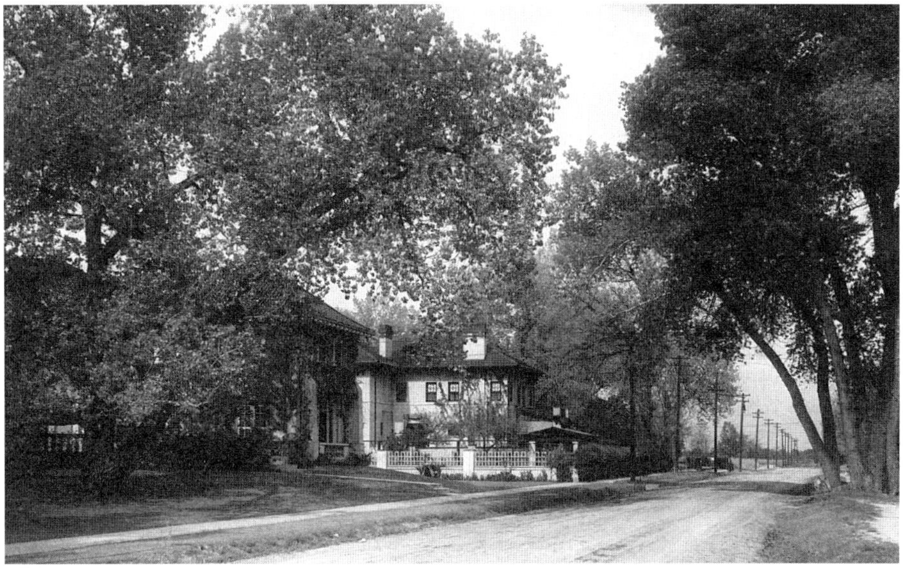

The houses at 100 Humboldt Street and 103 Franklin Street lay along quiet, unpaved, two-lane 1st Avenue during the thirties. (Courtesy DPL Western History Department)

bridges at Downing and Speer Boulevard and dealing with the loading trucks behind Alfalfa's at 1st and University. Clara L. L. Bebout has lived in the small townhouse next to the alley since 1948. "The area was quiet until nine years ago when the shopping strip came in," she said in 1999. "Being next to Alfalfa's, the alley is constantly blocked by trucks that are noisy and dangerous. One poked a hole in the side of the house and broke ten bricks out, and they're constantly bumping into the retaining wall," she said.

As Taubman proceeded with his gigantic plans for a shopping mall, the Association addressed protection of residents from traffic noise and disturbance from 1st Avenue. Taubman offered to build a solid wall along 1st Avenue, but this offer was rejected. "A solid wall would reduce the neighborhood to an affluent ghetto," said Robert Fuller. "There would be no interaction between the residents and outside world around them. They wouldn't be aware or care if the surrounding area were deteriorating."

An accommodation was included in a bond issue for home owners on 1st Avenue to be subsidized for "noise walls" of the owners' designs

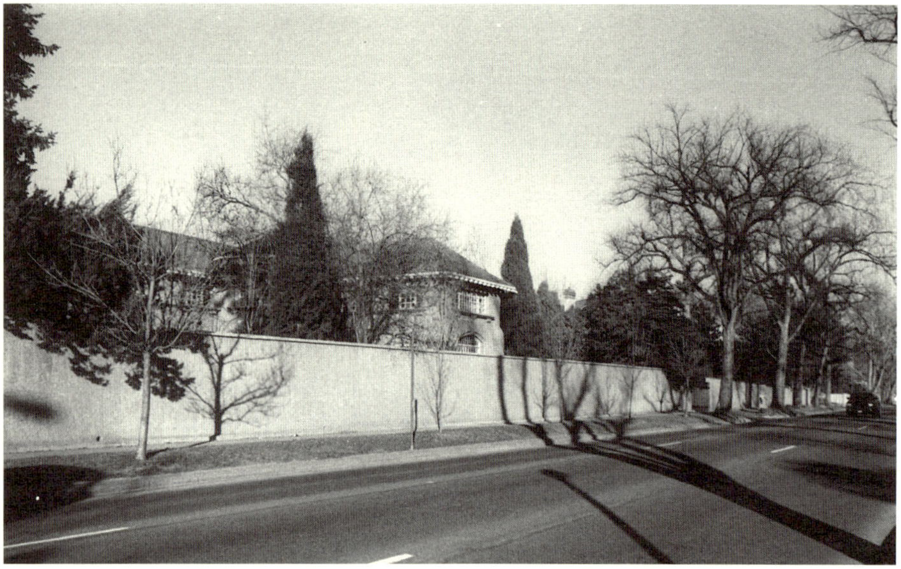

As the Cherry Creek Shopping Center attracted more and more traffic, the houses lining 1st Avenue at Humboldt put up high "noise walls" to protect them from the honking and screeching of automobiles.

along the south edge of their properties. 1st Avenue is lined with four to eight-feet walls to insulate residents from the increasing traffic noise.

HISTORIC DESIGNATION

During the seventies the CCIA applied to the National Registry for Historic Places for historic designation for the two western subdivisions that had the requisite percentage of 50-year-old surviving buildings. Through the expertise of Barbara Sudler (Mrs. William Hornby) of 180 High Street, president of the Colorado Historical Society, and the tireless research and comprehensive inventory drawn up by Sharon Elfenbein of 170 Lafayette, this was achieved in 1979.

Next was the more formidable local designation. The Denver Landmark Commission had been spearheaded by district resident Helen Millett Arndt of 170 High Street, who had become the first woman member of the Denver Planning Board in 1967. During the 1980s the association initiated Denver Landmark designation. This included the eastern subdivisions that were developed later and which, by then, were 50 years old. Although one application failed, a second application promoted by Allen Ferrel, was accepted by the Landmark Commission, then chaired by Professor of History at the University of Colorado at Denver Thomas J. Noel. This resulted in passage of an ordinance by City Council in August 1990, designating the whole area as a historic district, the largest one to yet attain that status. During the nineties the name of the neighborhood organization was appropriately changed to Country Club Historic Neighborhood, Inc.

To expedite the process of landmark designation for individual structures, the CCHN appointed a knowledgeable and dedicated Landmark Subcommittee, which, as current chairman Jeff Dohse said, "filters requests for building and remodeling to help the Landmark Commission in the decision process." The Committee often receives as many as four or five requests a month for approval of construction or exterior changes.

Mona Ferrugia, CCHN chairman during the nineties said, "We don't want to necessarily replicate the old traditional styles of architecture, but we would like to have good quality materials and design in the houses that are built. The development, designer-built, Highlands Ranch type of stucco house is not appropriate in this district."

Because the Country Club neighborhood has a unique character and beauty, one of the tasks of the CCHN Landmark Committee during the nineties was to draw up the booklet, *Design Guidelines for the Country Club Historic District*, for residents to use as a reference before considering any construction projects. Chairman for this project was Denver Landmark Commissioner Edward D. White, Jr. A.I.A., with help from Kathy Borgen, Dave Dutton, Kathleen Economos, Mona Ferrugia, Robert Fuller, Rosanne Hall, William Wenk, and a hired consultant. The Guidelines expand on existing Commission guidelines by addressing issues specific to the Country Club area. These special features of the district will become apparent as you hike through the history and architecture of the Country Club Historic Neighborhood.

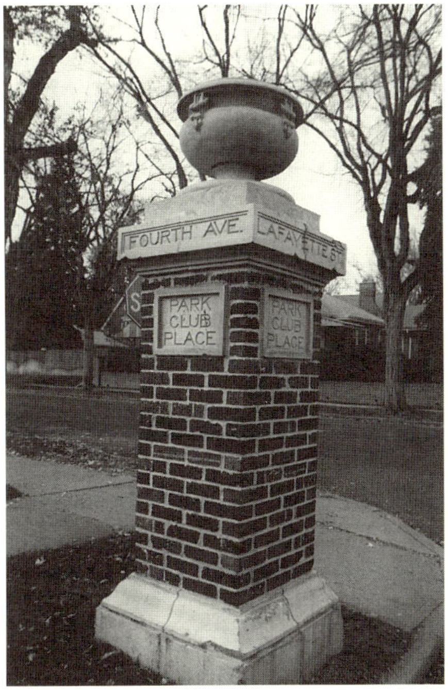

The gate marking Park Club Place.

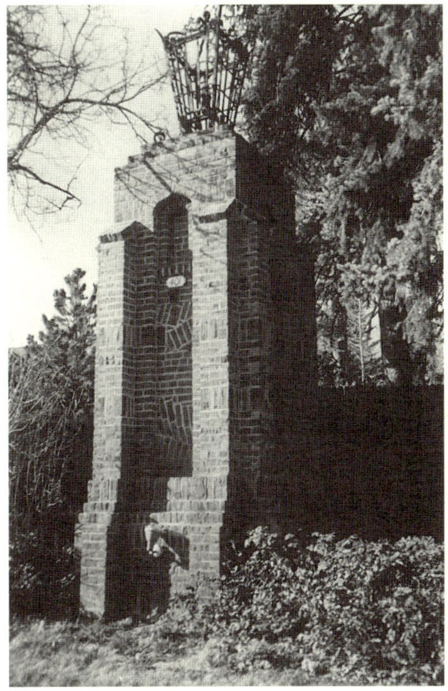

Stately English gates mark Park Lane Square (Circle Drive)

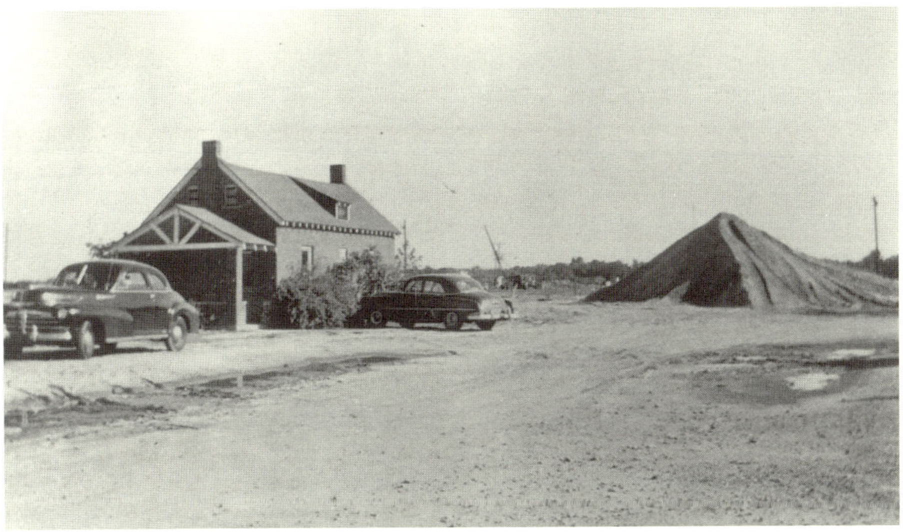

[Left]
The Shopping Center in Cherry Creek replaced the 1880s town of Harman. (Courtesy DPL Western History Department)

Introduction to Tours

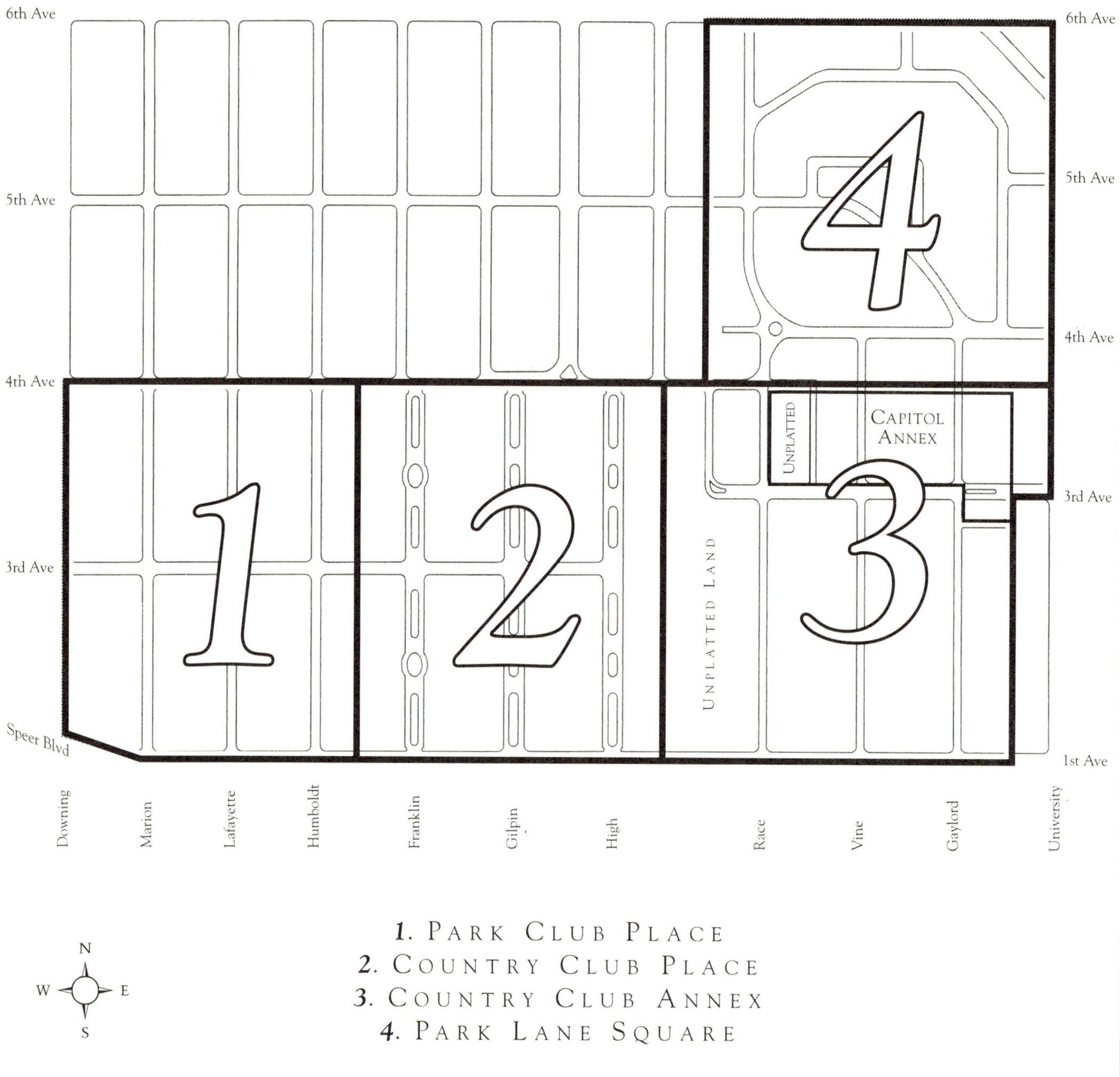

1. Park Club Place
2. Country Club Place
3. Country Club Annex
4. Park Lane Square

~ Introduction to Walking Tours ~

The Denver Country Club residential area was developed from west to east, starting in 1905 at Downing Street with Park Club Place and going to Park Lane Square at 6th Avenue and University Boulevard two decades later. The homes radiate a quiet elegance and are generally smaller than the more pretentious mansions of Capitol Hill. Few can be categorized by "style." Most are Revivals or eclectic, containing elements of several styles. General characteristics of architectural styles are described in Appendix II. Many have changed character through additions or remodeling. Whenever possible historic photographs of the houses have been used so that changes can be detected while walking by. Special features of the neighborhood are defined by the CCHN Landmark Committee's *Design Guidelines*.

The homes are usually at least one and a half to two stories high, rectangular in shape, and built of brick, stone, or stucco. Roofs are steeply pitched, gabled, or hipped, with long lines broken by dormer windows or tall chimneys. Windows are vertical and deep set. Flat roofs, A-frames, or large picture windows would be out of place.[1]

Outstanding are the architectural styles of the houses, many of which were custom built between 1905 and 1940. The area offers examples of the designs of Denver's most distinguished pre–World War II architects. Several residences each were designed by the firms of Frederick Harnois, Frederick Sterner and George Williamson, Maurice Biscoe, Willis Marean and Albert Norton, Jean Jacques Benois Benedict and Merrill and Burnham Hoyt. William E. and Arthur A. Fisher designed the Spanish entrance gates and parkways as well as 18 houses in the District. (For biographies of these architects, see *Denver: The City Beautiful* by Noel and Norton, and Appendix I).

The 1907 house at 370 Humboldt Street was built with a front driveway entered over a curb cut. (Courtesy DPL Western History Department)

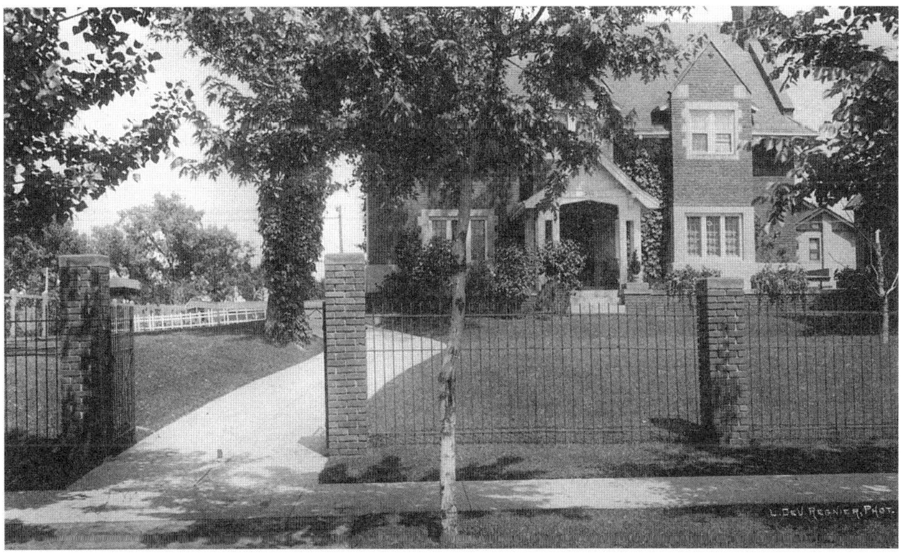

[Opposite Page]
Four 40-minute walking tours cover each of the major subdivisions of the Country Club Historic District.

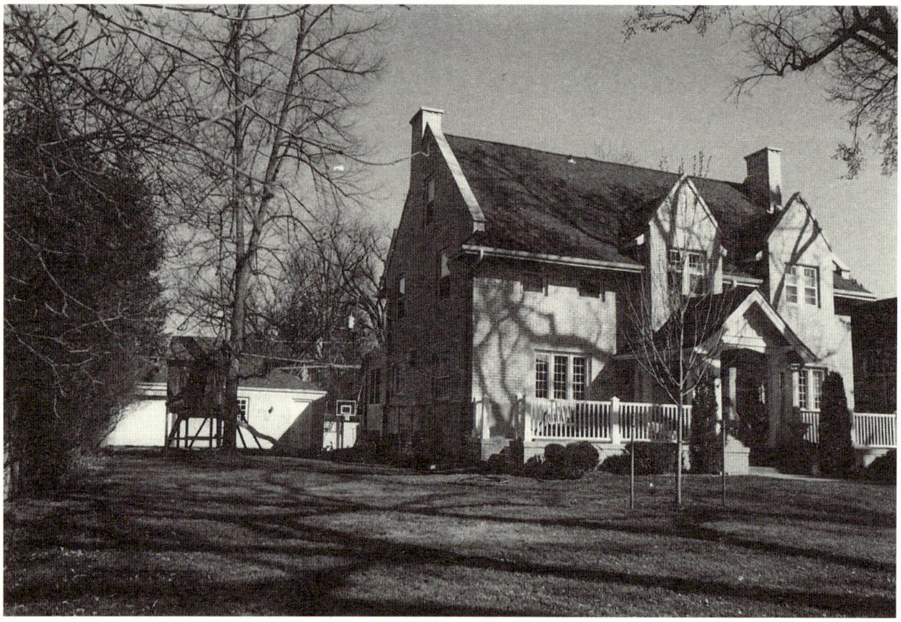

[LEFT]
In 1998 the curb cut and front driveway at 370 Humboldt were filled in and grassed over. A new garage was built off the alley.

Typical is the quiet, open well-kept front yard raised above the street, grassed and punctuated by a few deciduous trees.The artificial turf and plastic flamingos found in other areas are not appropriate here.

The Guidelines encourage detached garages with an alley entrance rather than curb cuts, driveways crossing the lawn or front garages. For instance, Judith and Bryan Tonton, owners of one of the earliest houses at 370 Humboldt, have replaced the former front driveway with fill and grass and built a garage on the alley. Alterations of front facades must be reviewed by the Landmark Committee.

The four major subdivisions were each planned as a cohesive unit with financial and lot-size building restrictions imposed by each developer. Each has its own individuality. Because this historic district has an overwhelming wealth of both architectural excellence and history of influential families, only about a third of the houses are described.

PARK CLUB PLACE

Because Park Club Place was the first subdivision to be developed, the architecture reflects Victorian characteristics such as wide front or wrap porches, converted carriage houses with second floor haylofts, and abandoned ashpits still visible on many alleys. Hitching posts for horses can still be found. The architecture of many of the houses is Foursquare. Some are Bungalows. Houses are built on the minimum requirement of two lots (50 by 125 feet), so there is limited space between homes, especially in the first filing of Park Club Place between 3rd and 4th Avenues.

Two years later the second filing, consisting of the area south of 3rd Avenue, was sold with more spacious grounds. Houses, especially near 1st Avenue, were built on six to twelve lots with no wall or hedge separating their view of the Denver Country Club grounds. Houses at 124 Lafayette and 135 Humboldt were built on twelve lots each. Homes at 100, 177, and 180 Humboldt covered six to ten lots.

The first walking tour starts at the west end of Park Club Place on Downing Street at 1st Avenue and winds back and forth between the brick gates at 4th and 1st Avenues at the intersections of Marion, Lafayette, and Humboldt streets.

COUNTRY CLUB PLACE

The second tour ambles through Country Club Place, starting at the signature Spanish Gate at 4th Avenue and Franklin Street. This subdivision, developed slightly later than Park Club Place, was planned by the Fourth Avenue Realty Company that hired architect William Ellsworth Fisher as its chief overall designer. Although the same size as Park Club Place, Fisher planned wide parkways with landscaped medians and tree lawns, resulting in one less street than the earlier subdivision. Widest is Franklin Street where lush circular islands herald the original entrance to the Denver Country Club.

Homes are separated by wide side lawns and cover less than a third of the property. Front yards are left open or have low or see-through wrought iron fences to preserve a park-like feeling. Most spacious in feeling is High Street where, before the seventies, only seven houses were built on the east side.[2] Many of these estates, once vibrant with children playing in the parkways, have recently given away to quiet gated transient properties, sometimes owned by corporations.[3] Because the alley between High and Race streets was vacated in 1909,[4] and the original Race Street was vacated in 1920,[5] these lots are doubly deep as well as wide. A 1933 ordinance closed 3rd Avenue between High and Race,[6] virtually cutting off access to the eastern subdivisions.

This walking tour covers Franklin, Gilpin, and High streets, ending at the eastern Spanish gate at 4th Avenue.

The signature Spanish Gate at 4th Avenue and Franklin Street marks the original entrance to the Denver Country Club. (Courtesy DPL Western History Department)

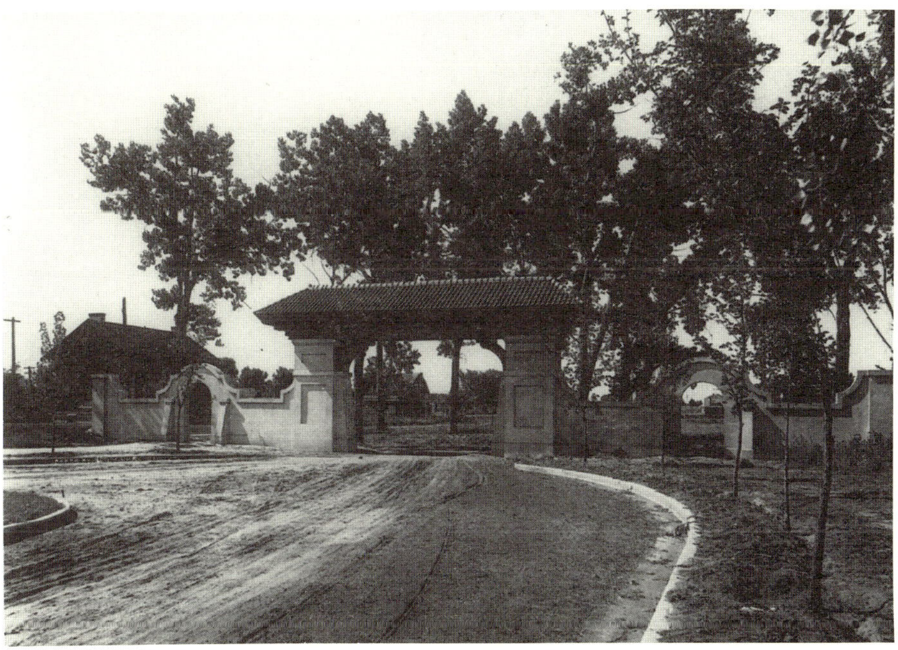

COUNTRY CLUB ANNEX

The eastern subdivisions were developed more than twenty years after the western ones. Country Club Annex, the subdivision between Race Street and University Boulevard, is the most accessible of the four residential sections. There are no defining gates to deter entrance. Cutting through from 1st to 6th Avenues is possible, though discouraged by the insertion of islands and medians. The architectural styles are mixed because this subdivision borders, not only on the commercial strip of University Boulevard, but on the former blue-collar subdivision, Capitol Annex, that was platted in 1889. Country Club Annex grew in spurts as Lawrence C. Phipps, Jr. added pieces

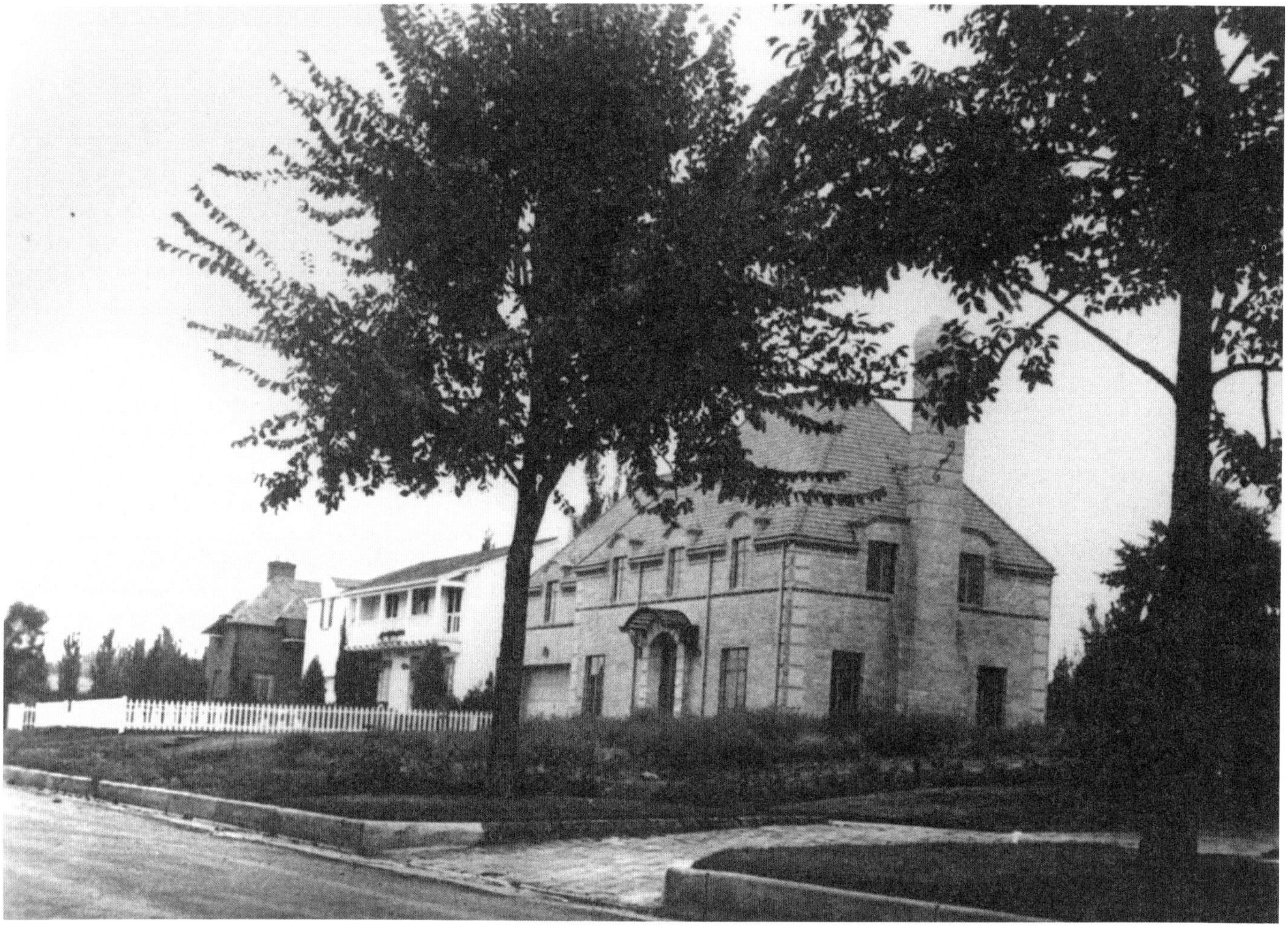

The architecture of Country Club Annex is similar to these houses at 230 and 250 Vine. The house at 230 Vine was built by developer Elton S. Boerstler. (Courtesy Charles A. Johnson)

of Capitol Annex and unplatted land to carry the subdivision from 1st to 3rd Avenues and from University Boulevard west to Race Street.

Country Club Annex runs from the east side of Race Street to the alley between Gaylord and University. Although there is no Second Avenue, 200 numbers are included in addresses. This area, largely developed between 1925 and 1940, was an extension of the western subdivisions of the Country Club district. The architecture is similar to its neighbor, Country Club Place, with wide lots, large rectilinear houses raised from the streets, sidewalks, and tree lawns. However, it has no parkways. Rather than a preponderance of Mediterranean style there are more Tudor-inspired houses in this area. Although many houses are custom-designed by architects, some are built for speculation by developers, such as the Writers Brothers or Elton S. Boerstler.

Both the unplatted land on Race Street and the northern subdivision, Capitol Annex, are adjacent to, so are included in this walking tour of Country Club Annex. Race, Vine, and Gaylord Streets are included in this tour.

Anchoring the subdivision Park Lane Square is the 1931 castle built by Mrs. Verner Z. Reed at 475 Circle Drive. (Courtesy DPL Western History Department)

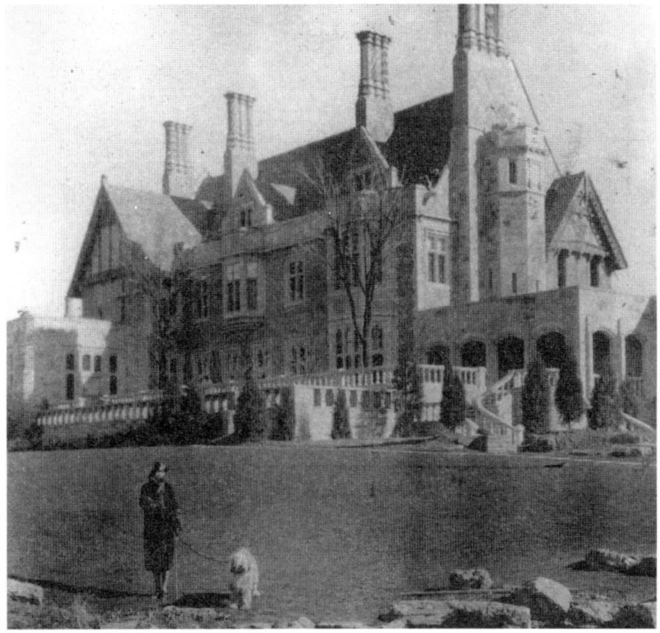

PARK LANE SQUARE (CIRCLE DRIVE)

The fourth tour continues along Gaylord Street to Park Lane Square, the former C. G. Richardson Place, which was bought from Dean Realty by a group of home owners and redesigned in a circular pattern by landscape architect Saco DeBoer in 1926. Intended as a large country estate—a piece of suburbia in the city—the curved narrow streets, lack of sidewalks, and 58 large lots (average 18,000 square feet each) without alleys form its own private community. Stately English gates mark the entrances. There are wide front lawns with few separating hedges or fences.

Anchoring the neighborhood on two and a fourth acres is a castle completed in 1931 at 475 Circle Drive by Mary Dean (Mrs. Verner Z.) Reed, president of Dean Realty. Charles A. Johnson, Jr., who later lived at 230 Vine, remembers the mansion when it was first built during the late twenties: "Here was this huge house sitting in the middle of a prairie," he said. "There were no trees around it, and it looked out of place against the bare landscape."

This subdivision includes the south side of 4th Avenue and eastern blocks of Williams Driving Club Place. Twelve small lots with turn-of-the-century houses and sidewalks, are all that remain in C. G. Richardson Place, south of 6th Avenue on the west side of Race.

These tours are designed as a vehicle to absorb the architecture, history, culture, and growth of this residential community that was developed north of the Denver Country Club. They trace how the area broadened into a cohesive neighborhood that maintained stability, elegance, and dignity throughout the fast-moving twentieth century.

TOUR 1: PARK CLUB PLACE

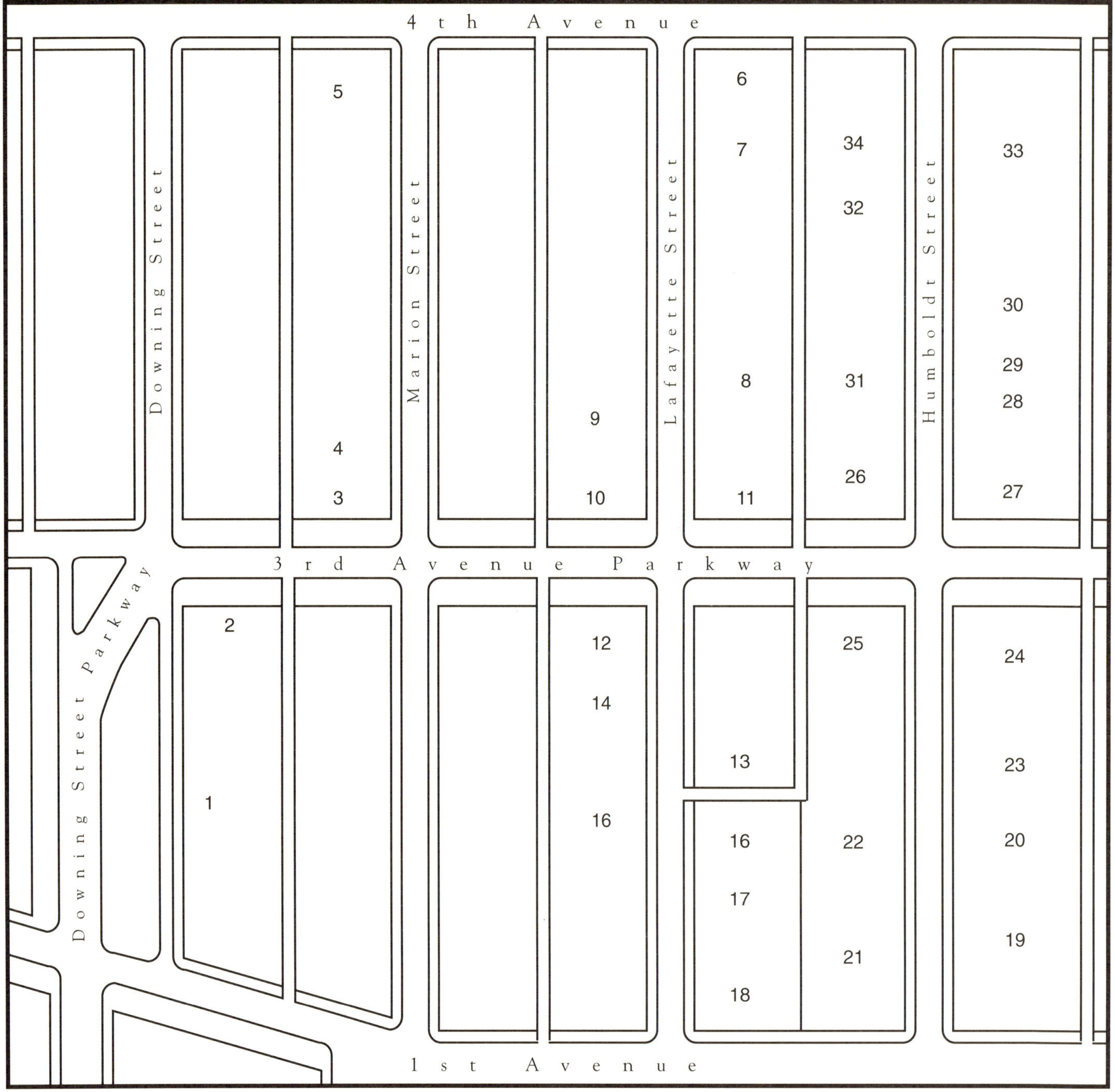

TOUR #1

1 144 Downing Street*
2 1200 East Third Avenue*
3 301 Marion Street*
4 315 Marion Street*
5 379 Marion Street*
(410 Marion Street)
6 1410 East 4th Avenue*
7 378 Lafayette Street*
8 330 Lafayette Street*
9 319 Lafayette Street*
10 1333 East 3rd Avenue*
11 300 Lafayette Street*
12 199 Lafayette Street*
13 170 Lafayette Street*
14 167 Lafayette Street*
15 145 Lafayette Street*
16 140 Lafayette Street†
17 130 Lafayette Street†
18 100 Lafayette Street†
19 120 Humboldt Street*
20 140 Humboldt Street*
21 135 Humboldt Street*
22 145 Humboldt Street
23 160 Humboldt Street†
24 180 Humboldt Street*
25 177 Humboldt Street*
26 301 Humboldt Street*
27 300 Humboldt Street*
28 320 Humboldt Street*
29 330 Humboldt Street*
30 350 Humboldt Street*
31 335 Humboldt Street*
32 369 Humboldt Street*
33 370 Humboldt Street*
34 375 Humboldt Street*

* Buildings which contributed to the character of the neighborhood, resulting in listing as a Historic District in the National Register of Historic Places in 1979.

† Modern buildings compatible with the character of the District.

[Opposite Page]
The walking tour of Park Club Place starts at Downing Street and goes along Marion, Lafayette, and Humboldt Streets, ending at 4th Avenue and Humboldt.

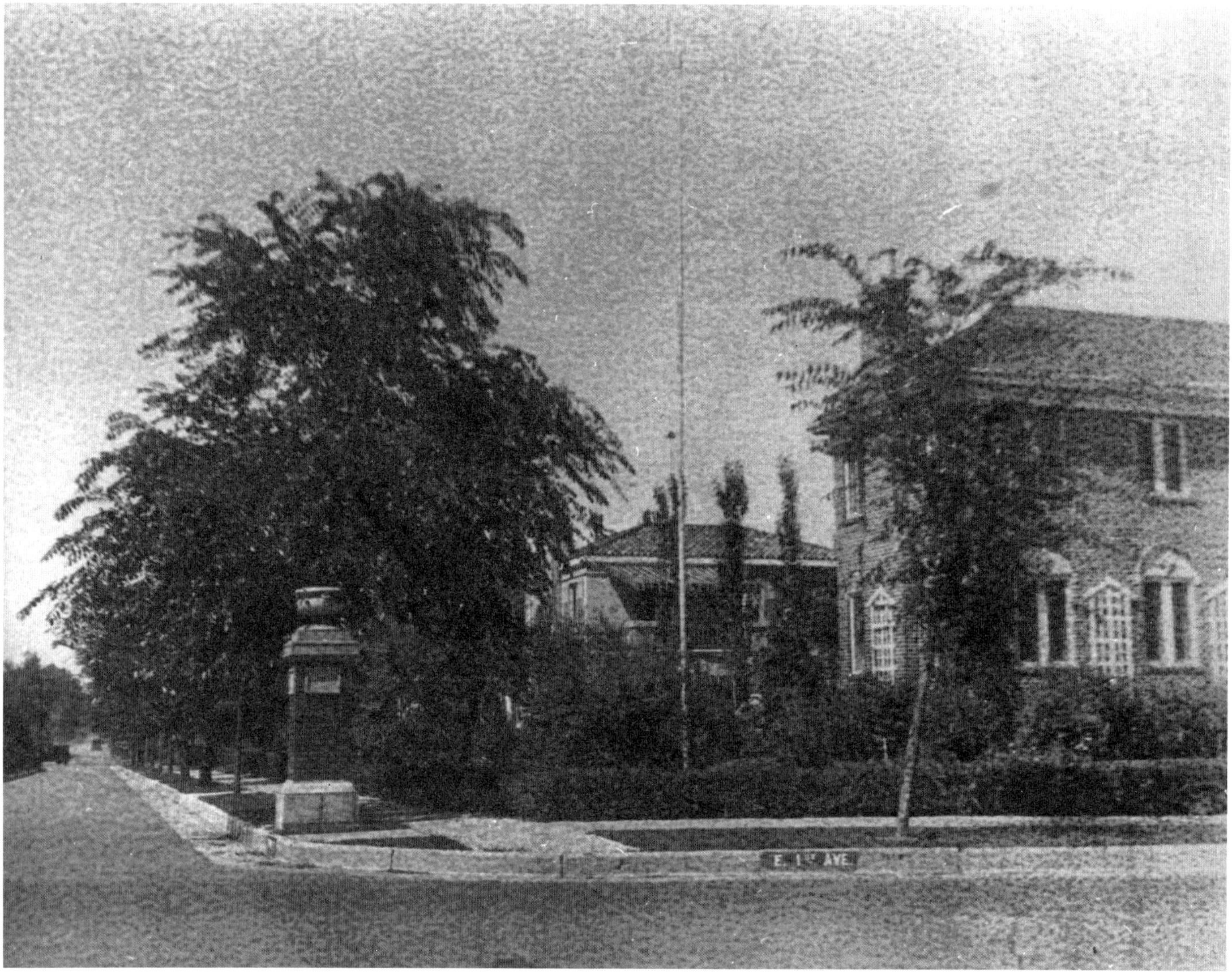

The Park Club Place Land Company marked their territory at 1st and 4th Avenues with brick columns like this one at "little Downing Street." (Courtesy DPL Western History Department)

~ Tour 1 ~

1
144 DOWNING STREET
Built: 1923
Architect: Frank W. Frewen

This excellent example of a Georgian Revival house was built by the architect for himself. Denverite Frank Walter Frewen, Jr., designed churches, hospitals, and more than 80 schools in Colorado and Wyoming.

Frewen designed his own red brick house with a low-pitched, end-gable roof trimmed with dentils. The recessed, central six-paneled door surround has fluted pilasters and a triangular pediment. Multi-pane wood and double-hung sash windows flanked by dark green shutters provide balanced fenestration on either side of the doorway.

The house is located on "little Downing Street," a narrow road dividing the residential row of houses from a lush green median. This landscaped island is part of Mayor Speer's City Beautiful plan to connect all parks with parkways. Washington Park connects with Cheesman Park via the Marion Street Parkway, this Downing Street Parkway, through 3rd Avenue Parkway, Gilpin Street, and the Williams Street Parkway.

In 1937 at the tender age of 50, while serving as president of the Colorado chapter of the American Institute of Architects, Frewen died of pneumonia as a complication of influenza. His widow, Jessie, continued living in this red brick house after his death.

In 1950, Betty (Brodhead) Nicola and her lawyer husband, Charles, moved into the house and lived there for the next four decades. Architect James S. Sudler, II, designed a rear addition of three levels, with a recreation room, a garden room, and a master bedroom. The living and garden rooms open onto a terrace which leads down two steps to a loggia, which is covered with a flat roof supported by two brick pillars. The single-car detached garage, built in 1923, was used for storage, and a carport was built on the alley north of the loggia.

Architect Frank W. Frewen built this Georgian Revival house for himself in 1923 on "little Downing Street."

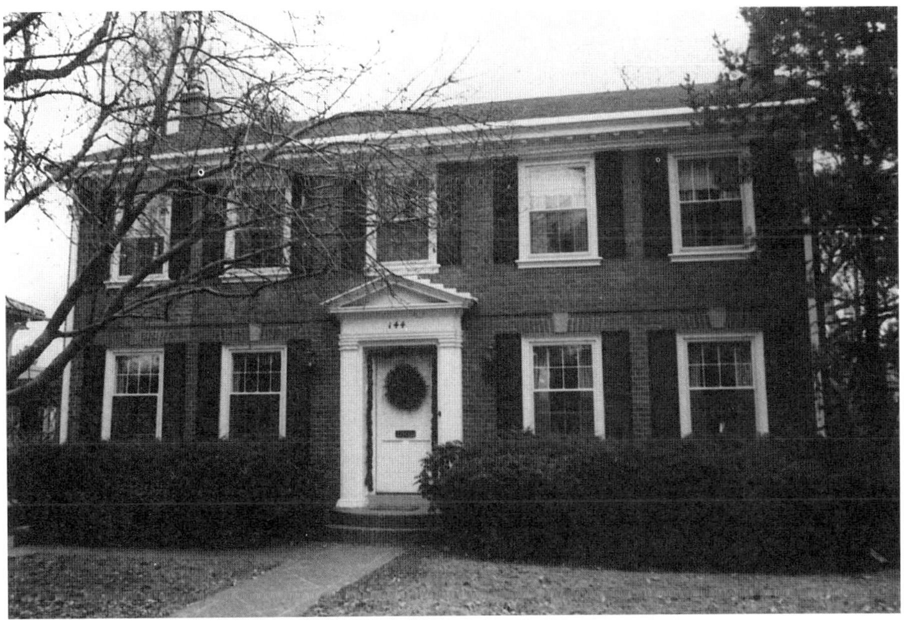

The owner since 1992, William J. Grier, Jr., added a fountain to the south garden and plans to renovate the garage into a hobby room to harmonize with the house. "We have lots of privacy here as we are well protected from 1st Avenue by the very mature trees," Grier said.

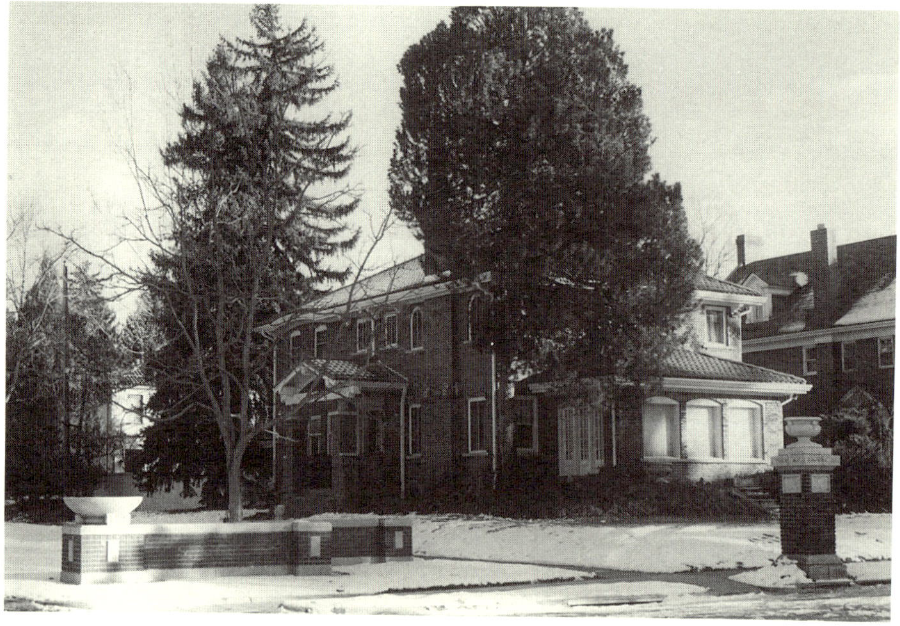

The house at 1200 East 3rd Avenue lies just inside the red brick gates that mark the west entrance to Park Club Place.

2
1200 EAST 3RD AVENUE
Built: 1926
Architect: unknown

Heralding the west entrance of Park Club Place is a two-story Mediterranean house just inside the recently built three-foot red brick entry gates at Downing and 3rd Avenue. The medium-pitched hipped tile roof is repeated on the west sunroom that overlooks the "little Downing Street" parkway. The triangular pedimented porch, featuring an open gable with exposed tie beam and roof framing, is supported by square brick columns made of the same projecting (or weeping) mortar joints as the house. East of the entry, three windows are trimmed with a wide, patterned keystone arch. Fenestration patterns vary throughout the house.

The home was built for Henry F. Evans, a partner of Charles Cashman of 149 High Street. In 1952, just after they were married, Barbara and architect James S. Sudler, II, moved to the house for 23 years.

The house was later owned by attorney William Brayshaw who was chairman of Country Club Historic Neighborhood, Inc. from 1999 to 2000.

3
301 MARION STREET
Built: 1905
Architect: James B. Hyder

Richard Harwell Malone, founder of the first subdivision to be developed in the Country Club Historic Neighborhood, chose this site for his own home. The Tennessean moved to Chicago when he was six years old, then to Denver in 1873. He ran a successful biscuit company, sold it, then turned to real estate in 1899. Malone initiated a Colorado chapter of the youth group Demolay. The *Denver Post*[1] dubbed him "The Daddy of the Colorado Demolay."

In 1901 Malone and Robert W. Speer purchased 40 acres of the John Jacob Riethmann property bounded by Downing and Humboldt Streets, 1st and 4th Avenues. Malone then incorporated the Park Club Place Land Company with

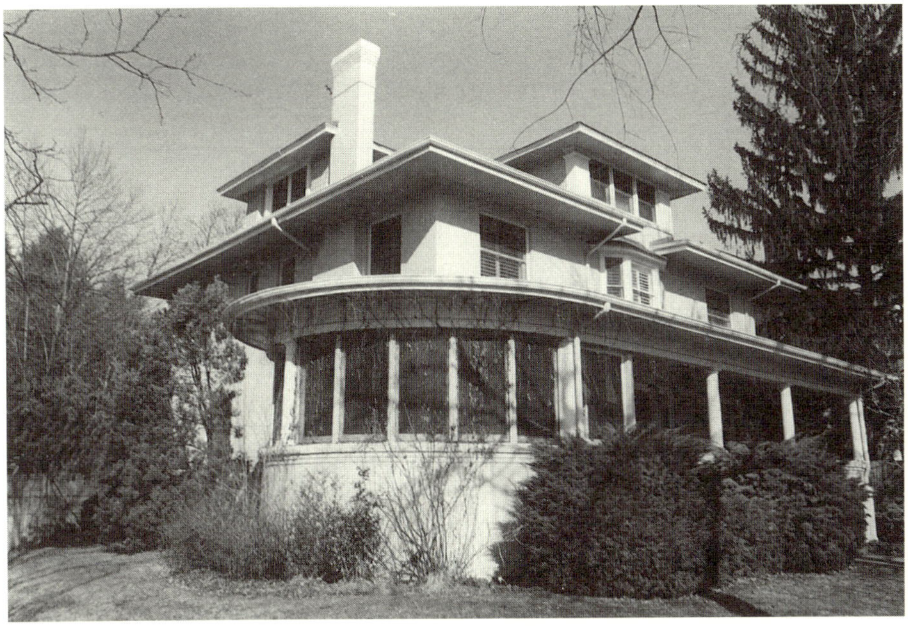

One of the first houses in the neighborhood was built In 1905 at 301 Marion Street by the developer of Park Club Place, Richard H. Malone.

Fisher lived there with her pioneer mother, Louise Perrenoud (Mrs. Redwood) Fisher, and the society columns duly reported meetings of these illustrious, righteous groups at the house of their president at 301 Marion Street.

A subsequent owner of the house was Richard L. Deane, owner of Deane Buick-Saab and a community leader. He served on the boards of the Boys Clubs of Denver, the Chamber of Commerce, Mile High United Way, and was appointed to the Denver Planning Board by Mayor Frederico Pena.

Courtney and Reid Godbolt bought the property in 1991 and generously showed it for the 1998 Dora Moore School House Tour.

himself as president and Speer as secretary. The land was platted in 1903, and the two immediately picked out choice plots for themselves. Malone chose this corner of 3rd and Marion, and Speer chose the corner of 3rd and Humboldt Street.

Malone hired architect James B. Hyder to build a three-story brick residence at 301 Marion Street. Although the Assessor's Office lists the year of construction as 1901, the building permit wasn't issued until April 1, 1905. This large house, in the popular turn-of-the-twentieth-century Foursquare, or Denver Square style, has a wide wrap porch, the southern end of which is rounded and glassed in for a bright sunroom. Symmetrical dormers break the low-pitched roofline, and double-hung sash windows are used throughout the house. The center hall floor plan is dominated by a magnificent staircase leading to the four bedrooms of the second floor. The large third floor holds a playroom and two more children's bedrooms with bath.

In 1922 the house was bought by a staunch moralistic Daughter of the Colorado Territory and pillar of the Ladies Relief Society. Louise A.

4
315 MARION STREET
Built: 1907
Architect: unknown

When Richard H. Malone built his own house at 301 Marion, he bought three lots next door for his partner in promoting Park Club Place, real estate investor Robert E. McCracken. McCracken, who came to Denver in 1872, was a director of Denver's first Festival of Mountain and Plain, a recently revived event that attracts thousands to the down-town Civic Center.

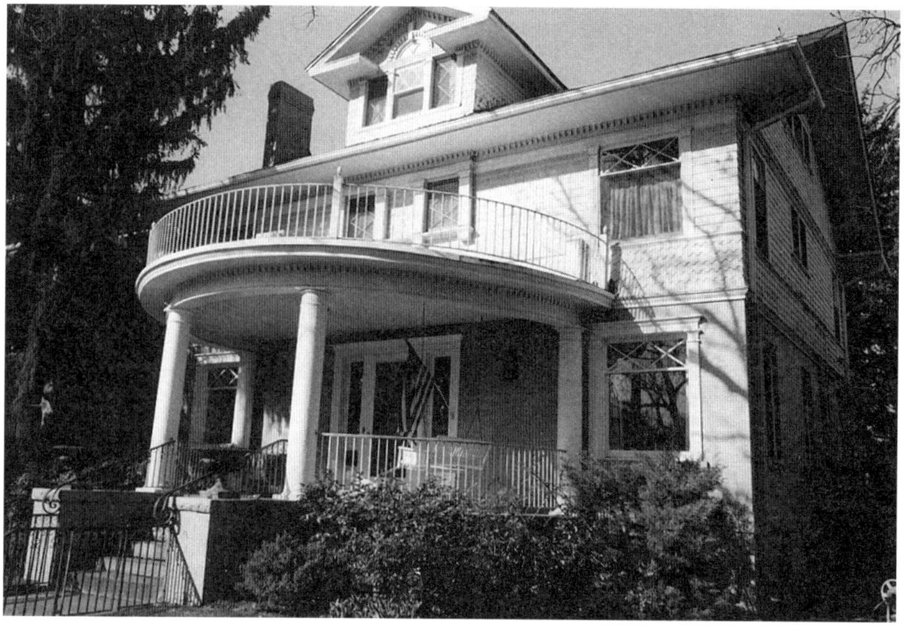

Malone's partner in developing Park Club Place was Robert E. McCracken, who built this house next to Malone in 1907.

McCracken's three-story symmetrical brick house has a low-pitched roof with wide, overhanging eaves. Decorative dentils emphasize the cornices, and shaped shingles are used for the second-floor siding. A dramatic, semicircular front porch and balcony, supported by Tuscan wood columns and frieze, distinguish the entry. Both upper and lower levels feature metal balustrades painted to match the wood trim. The front door is framed by lead-pane sidelights. "The furnace in the house is still the original one, dated 1905!," said owner Ursula Works in 2000.

The house was eventually bought by John and Ursula Ronnebeck Moore. Ursula was the daughter of Arnold and Louise (Emerson) Ronnebeck, both distinguished Colorado artists. Ronnebeck, a Prussian who had been a member of the Kaiser's personal guard, came to Denver as the first director of the Denver Art Museum. Emerson painted murals and the reredos at the Church of the Holy Redeemer in Denver.

After Moore died, Ursula married John Works. They do not really use the graceful semicircular front balcony: "There are no doors opening out on it, just two little windows. If the kids get an airplane stuck there, they have to crawl out the window to retrieve it. It's too bad because it would be a great place to watch the Country Club fireworks on the Fourth of July," Ursula said.

5
379 MARION STREET
Built: 1906
Architects: Sterner and Williamson

This Sterner and Williamson designed Dutch Colonial house was one of the first homes to appear in Park Club Place. The symmetrical house is remarkable for its gambreled gable with a covered balcony over the wide front porch. The white picket porch railings are repeated on the front and back balconies. The first story is now yellow-painted brick; the second floor has clapboard siding. Six Tuscan columns support the front porch. The entrance door is flanked by paneled sidelights that reflect the exterior window pattern.

On April 6, 1906, the Park Club Land Company transferred the property to Frank J. Quereau. Two months later he signed a contract to "build a complete residence on SW corner of 4th and Marion St., except plumbing and heating for $5,023."[2] Although the Assessor's Office dates the year of construction as 1900,

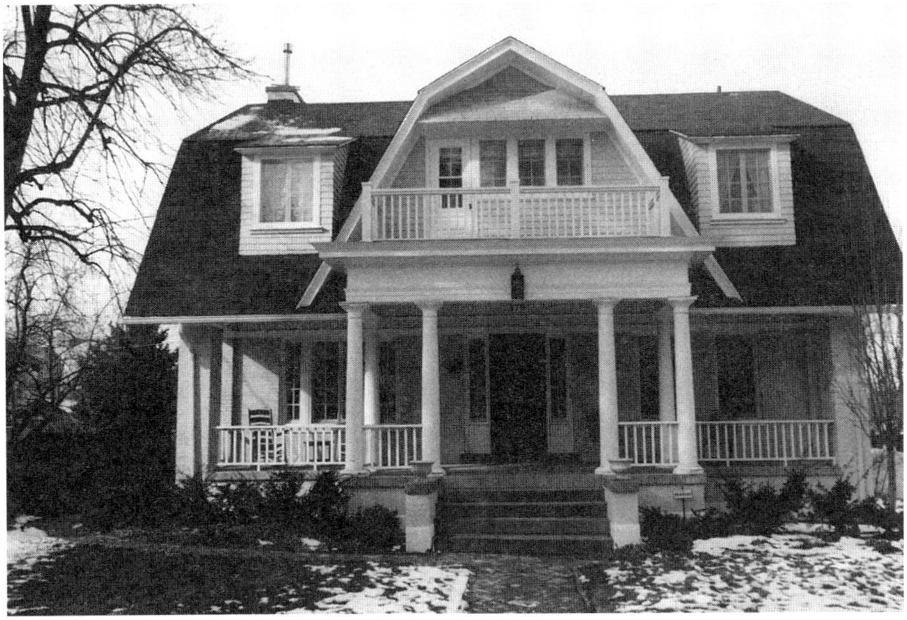

The Dutch Colonial Revival house at 379 Marion Street was built in 1906, one of the earliest in the Country Club Historic District.

this seems unlikely as the Park Club Land Company was not yet organized. The only nearby house was catercorner at 410 Marion, built in 1890 as one of the first houses in Driving Club Place.

Quereau had a varied career. He first ran a commercial travel company, C. H. Howe and Co. In 1893 he changed businesses and formed a new partnership with his friend, Lester Bridaham. "I remember well our entering into business in 1893—the year of the panic. Bridaham had had much experience in the drug business, so with but little money we decided to start a wholesale drug house. . . . By hard work we built up our little business that later became the largest wholesale drug house between the Missouri River and the ocean," Quereau said in the October 19, 1912, *Denver Republican*.

In 1910 he sold the house to Allan B. Bowen, a stockbroker at the Century Building. After living a couple of years on Pennsylvania Street, Quereau came back to the Country Club area and built a house at 141 Gilpin Street.

A prominent Denver resident lived at 379 Marion during the 1920s and 1930s. British-born Stephen A. Ionides was an Oxford-educated mining engineer. He worked in Cripple Creek when he came to Colorado and served in the Canadian army during World War I before settling in Denver in 1920. Ionides was an esteemed astronomer and combined this knowledge with his engineering abilities to build the landmark Chinese sundial in Cranmer Park in the Hilltop neighborhood in east Denver.

After Ionides died in 1943, Hugh B. Terry lived in the house while he was manager of KLZ radio. When the station expanded into television, the forerunner of Channel 7, Terry masterminded the transition.

The current owners, Matthew and Gigi Dalton, bought the house in 1996, "and are never going to move again," Gigi said. A door from the guest room opens onto a semicircular balcony. The Daltons find it a marvelous place to grow plants. "There is no deck or patio at the back of the house, and we just love to sit on the front porch," Gigi said. "We rock and see the neighbors and activity of the street, just like people did a century ago."

(across the street)
410 MARION STREET
Built: 1890
Architect: unknown

Because this house is across 4th Avenue, it is technically not part of the Country Club Historic District.

This eclectic home, with its varied and decoratively rich use of forms, textures, and materials, characterizes the turn-of-the-twentieth-century Queen Anne style and is one of the oldest buildings in the area. As Denver moved south of the city limits, this house was built in 1890 when the Driving Park Land Company purchased the property from the Gentlemen's Driving Association. The house has undergone dramatic changes.

During the fifties the old farmhouse was bought by prominent surgeon Dr. Henry Swan, II, and his wife, Fletcher. After a divorce she stayed there with her second husband, Dr. Charles Gaylord.

A complete three-year remodeling and renovation occurred in the early 1990s before the house was included on a Dora Moore School House Tour.

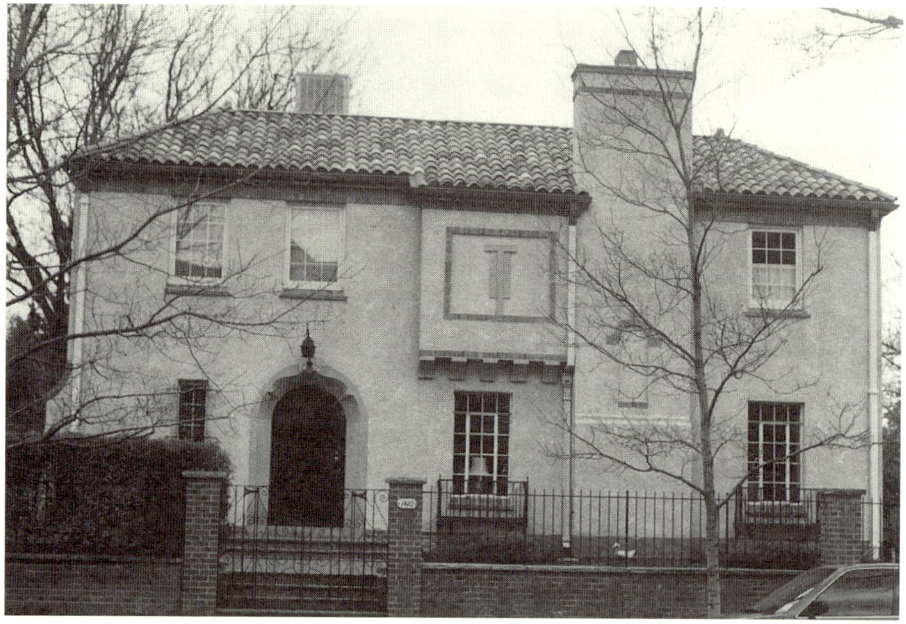

This house at 4th Avenue and Lafayette Street was the home of Brian Priestman, conductor of the Denver (later Colorado) Symphony Orchestra from 1969 until 1978.

6
1410 EAST 4TH AVENUE
Built: 1922
Architect: unknown

Brian Priestman, the flamboyant British conductor of the Denver Symphony Orchestra (now the Colorado Symphony) from 1969 to 1978, lived in this house during his brief marriage to Mary-Ford "Fordie" McClave. The 45-year-old bachelor fell in love with the 22-year-old musical comedy player just after her graduation from the University of Colorado, where she starred in such musicals as *Finian's Rainbow* and *Kismet*. Apparently "Fordie" was singing in the chorus of Beethoven's Ninth Symphony when she caught the eye of the dashing conductor. Though popular in musical circles, Priestman was discouraged with the small size of the orchestra and the lack of support for recordings. He left Denver just before the Boettcher Concert Hall was opened to take a similar post with the Greater Miami Philharmonic.

The beige stucco, two-story, rectilinear Mediterranean house has a red tile low-pitched, hipped roof. Beside the north-facing entrance is a tall chimney with a red brick band and ornamental inset in the wall. The door surround is of rust-colored stucco, matching the red brick trim. The wrought-iron fence and gate design is echoed in the iron balconets at the windows.

The house was built in 1922 by Baptist Kentuckian Elmer L. Brock, who had graduated from the University of Denver Law School in 1909. Brock served as assistant attorney general of Colorado in 1911 and was president of the Denver Bar Association in 1931 and 1932. He married Nora Linden, who continued to live in the house after his death in 1949. The Brocks were a popular couple and belonged to such social clubs as the University and Denver Country Clubs.

7
378 LAFAYETTE STREET
Built: 1908
Architect: unknown

"This house was originally a Denver Square or Foursquare style with a big front wrap porch," said architect Philip Atchison, who remodeled the house during the eighties.

The two-story, painted brick home was bought during the depressed thirties for $5,000 by manufacturers' agent Samuel J. Carson, who lived there for six decades. It has a hipped roof with wide eaves supported by paired brackets. Atchison designed a new gracious entrance approached by graduated steps with graceful curved railings. The entrance portico with arched pediment is supported by paired columns and flanked with small side windows. Atchison also extended the south end of the living room and added a family room on the back.

While remodeling the house Atchison was fitting conspicuous copper pipes. However, Denver was not humid or dirty enough to form a soft patina on the pipes naturally. His father, architect Paul Atchison, had a special method: "The foreman sent a workman out back, who soon returned with a bottle of yellow liquid that worked magic on the pipes."

A subsequent owner added a room over the living room extension that opens onto a second-floor balustraded balcony.

8
330 LAFAYETTE STREET
Built: 1909
Architect: unknown

Most of the district's oldest homes built in Park Club Place, the first Country Club subdivision to be developed, are on 50-foot lots along the 300 block of Lafayette Street. Thirteen shot up between 1904 and 1908.

This house is an example of the popular turn-of-the-twentieth-century efficient Foursquare, or Denver Square, design. This home, built for Homer A. Handy, a bookkeeper at the Broadway Bank, was a typical two-story box with a wide front porch and four symmetrically placed openings (a door and large double-hung window on the first floor with two similar windows upstairs) on the front facade. The roof is hipped, usually with a central attic dormer, and the overhanging eaves are bracketed. The single-car detached garage was built in that era for the newfangled "horseless carriage."

The Foursquare style occurs with many variations, enlargements, adornments, and additions. The usual late-twentieth-century addition is a two-story family room and master bedroom, bath, and dressing room on the rear of the house. Other examples of Foursquares are at 389 and 341 Lafayette.

During the early 1980s, Dan Warner was jogging down Lafayette Street. "I saw this Open House sign, ran in to take a look at it, and bought it in 1983," he said. He remodeled, installing passive solar windows and custom-designed stained-glass windows, both inside and out, including the oval window on the paneled front door. He also extended the rear of the house by 15 feet for a family room off the kitchen, a hot tub, and a circular stairway to a bright upstairs sitting room, adding a contemporary touch to the 90-year-old home.

9
319 LAFAYETTE STREET
Built: 1910
Architect: unknown

Lafayette Street was something of a family enclave for the Barkalow-Stearns family. Robert V. Barkalow

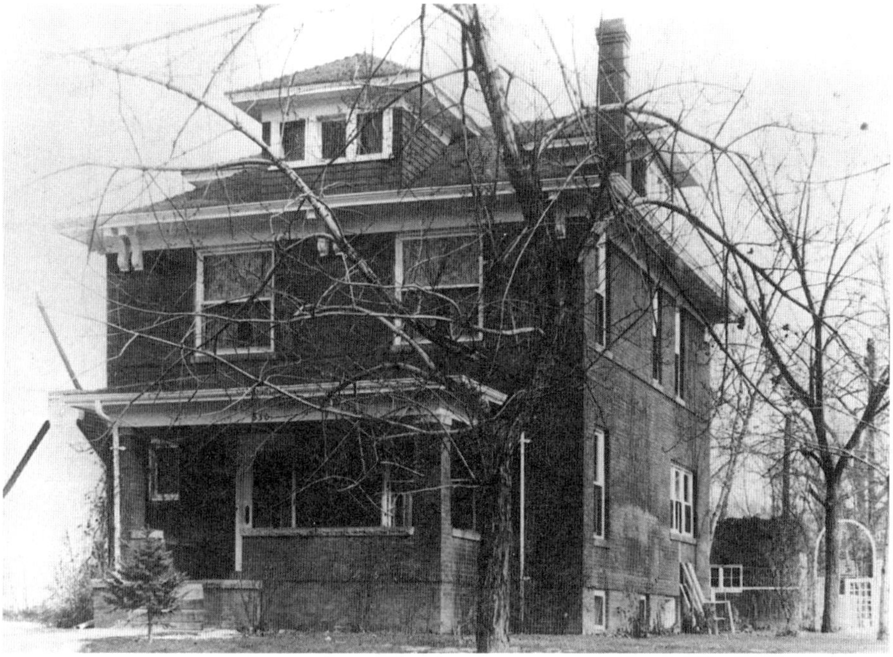

This house at 330 Lafayette Street was originally a typical Foursquare style with a door and three windows symmetrically placed on the front.
(Courtesy Dan Warner)

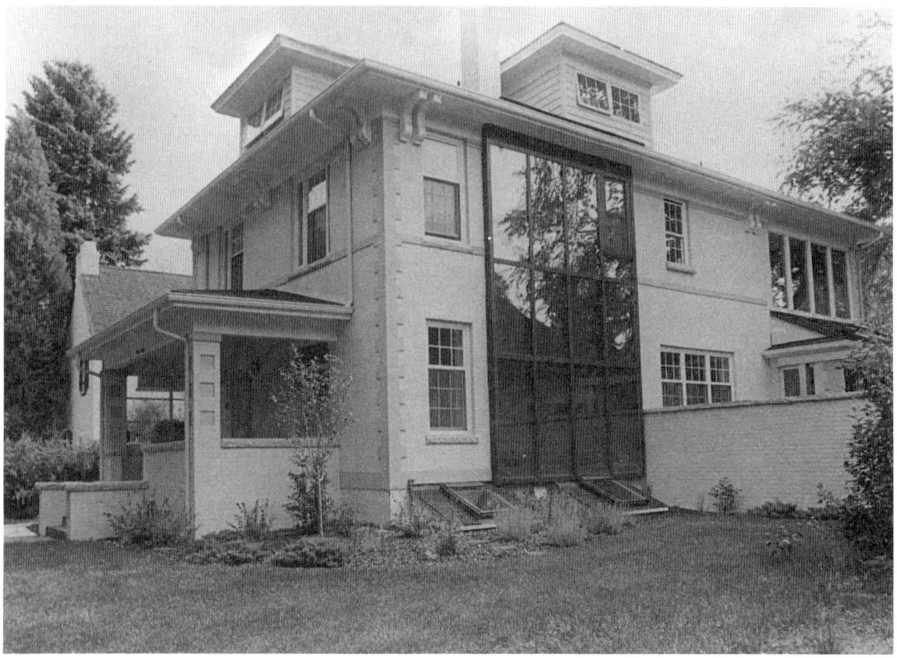

During the 1980s it was remodelled into a contemporary design with passive solar windows, a garden room, and a hot tub.

and his wife, the former Mary Stearns, lived at 319 Lafayette Street, one block north of both of their widowed mothers. Kate (Mrs. Derrick V.) Barkalow was at 170 Lafayette and Ella (Mrs. John L.) Stearns lived across the street at 167 Lafayette.

Four Barkalow brothers had started a railroad news agency in Omaha, Nebraska, in 1865. The business was so successful that they opened branches in several other cities. Of the brothers, only Derrick brought the company to Denver, setting up agencies in the Brown Palace and Albany Hotels, as well as the brand new Union Station. The store sold apples and snacks, cigarettes and cigars, as well as news items. "Tobacco was a big thing in those days," said grandniece Gladys Barkalow (Mrs. Philip, Jr.) Alexander. "The Barkalow brothers proudly rolled their own cigars."

Robert V. Barkalow entered the family agency in Denver for a short time, then became vice-president of Chemical Production Company, a business he developed with Lafayette and Varian Hughes. His and Mary's two daughters, Jean and Mary (Barkalow Holt Joyce) were brought up in this house and went to Corona (Dora Moore) Elementary School. "I saw lots of my grandmothers," said Mary Joyce. "My father always saw to it that his mother was well taken care of."

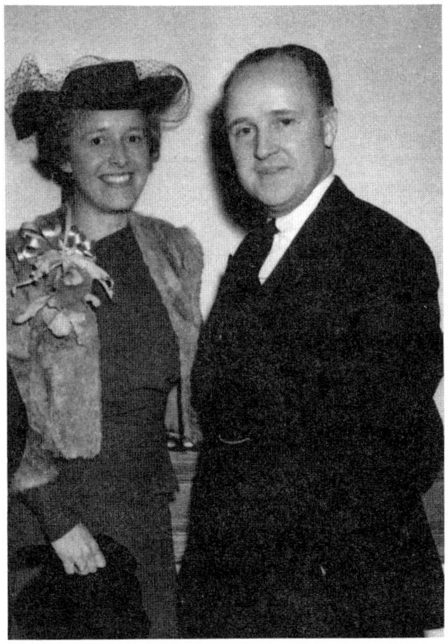

During the twenties and thirties the house at 319 Lafayette was occupied by Amy and Robert L. Stearns and their four daughters. Later, Stearns became the president of the University of Colorado. (Courtesy DPL Western History Department)

This white brick house has a Georgian-style pedimented entry door framed by pilasters and flanked by two narrow sidelights. Above the front entry are two small square windows. Throughout the house are double-hung sash windows. The low-pitched gable roof is lined with a white, molded wood cornice. The house was originally built for assistant secretary of North American Accident Insurance Company Frank J. Forest.

It is like many houses on the west side of Lafayette that have two-stories, and are symmetrical rectangles with a center hall floor plan. They have a living room on one side of the entrance and a dining room with a kitchen behind on the other. Upstairs are three small bedrooms, and the house was served by one small bathroom, a luxury after plumbing allowed outhouses to move in. "On the west side of the street there are at least five houses with the same floor plan by the same builder," said Eunice (Mrs. John) Sneed, who has lived at 357 Lafayette for over 50 years.

In 1926, Mary (Mrs. Robert) Barkalow's brother, Robert L. Stearns, took over the house, bringing with him his wife, the former Amy Pitkin, daughter of Governor Frederick W. Pitkin, and four daughters: Marion (Mrs. Byron White), Amy (Mrs. Robert Goodell), Judith (Mrs. Ken Caughey), and Barbara (Mrs. Rike Wooten).

Later, Robert Stearns became president of the University of Colorado. "We moved to Boulder when Dad was appointed temporary dean of the law school," said Judy Caughey. "The dean, James Grafton Rogers, had left to go to Washington for a two-year term in the State Department. He didn't come back, so Dad became acting law dean in

1931, then permanent dean. He resigned in 1939 to become president of the university." Stearns served as president of the University of Colorado from 1939 until 1953. He was much respected and acclaimed as one of the nation's leading educators. During this period he fulfilled several government assignments dealing with education and received numerous honorary degrees. He resigned at 59 to take over the helm of the Boettcher Foundation for 11 years before his retirement.

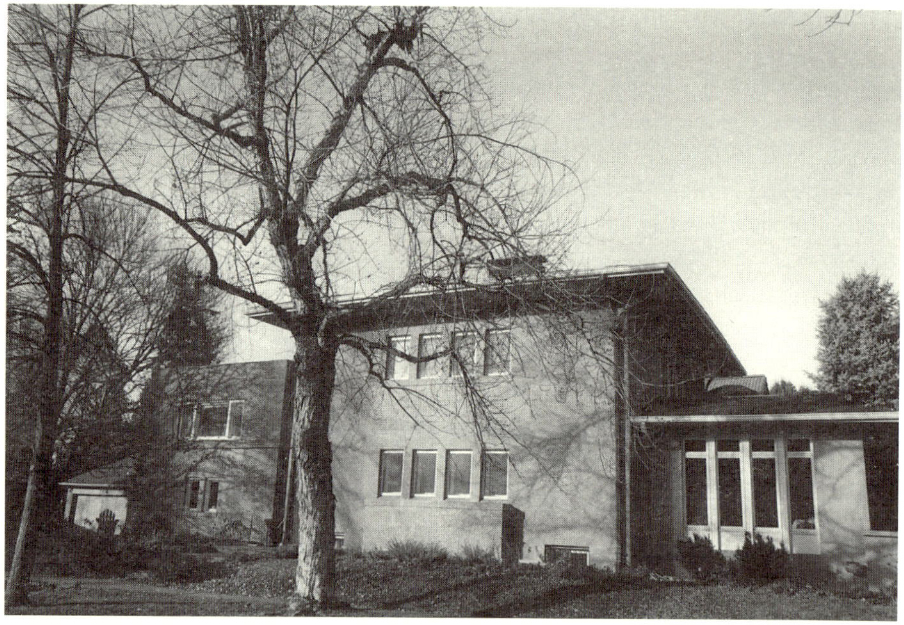

This Prairie style house at 1333 East 3rd Avenue was originally square with all four walls identical. Wings were added on both the west and east.

10
1333 EAST 3RD AVENUE
Built: 1913
Architect: Office of Frank Lloyd Wright

At the turn of the twentieth century it was common practice to buy pre-designed house plans sold in books or described in magazines. William H. Sharpley sent to Frank Lloyd Wright in Oak Park, Illinois, for the mail-order plans for this Prairie School design, described in the April 1907 *Ladies' Home Journal.* Wright would send plans, specifications, details, and complete service for 10 percent of the cost of the $5,000 house.

The article points out that "reenforced concrete is now affordable and is warmer than a wooden house in winter and cooler in summer. The walls, floors, and flat roof are a monolithic casting with the chimney in the center carrying the central load of floor and roof construction. The house was designed with four sides alike so that forms made for one side may serve for all four." No attic, butler's pantry, or back stairway was planned for this 30-by-30-foot house, "as they would be unnecessarily cumbersome in this efficient scheme," states the article. The house was not built until 1914.[3]

During the twenties, Vulcan Iron Works owner Rudolph H. Fox and his wife, Karen, moved in, staying for over 40 years. Barbara (Mrs. James) Sudler (now Mrs. William Hornby) lived across the street from Karen Fox. "She was a lovely person. She had a daughter, Phyllis, who was a brilliant mathematician, but she lived in Chicago. Mrs. Fox became more and more depressed and debilitated with lupus before passing away."

A garage, a master bedroom, and later a family room were added. The

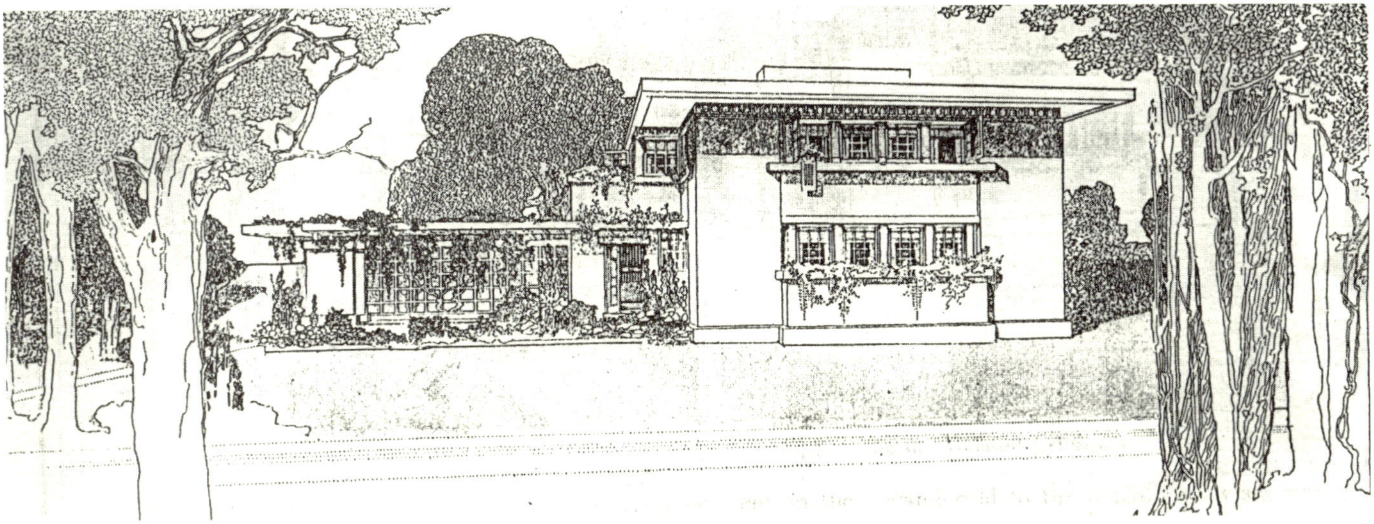

The plans for the house at 1333 3rd Avenue appeared in the April 1907 Ladies' Home Journal *and were purchased from the office of Frank Lloyd Wright.*

kitchen was extended to the north to add light and a breakfast nook. The stucco door surround is trimmed with red tile insets over the door.

"Those tiles were original with the house," said Sally (Mrs. Herbert) Koether, who lived there during the seventies. Their son, who was studying architecture, built a sunroom on the east with a Prairie-style, flat, overhanging roof; ribbon windows; and an unadorned exterior.

Current owners Carol Ganz and Timothy Singer knew the Koethers and bought the house when they returned from Washington, D.C., in 1992. "The only difference in the original plans for the house is that one of the upstairs bedrooms has a cupboard instead of the center fireplace," Ganz said. Architects Philip Atchison and Edward D. White, Jr., agree that "it used to look more Wrightian than it does now."[4]

11
300 LAFAYETTE STREET
Built: 1916
Architects: Marean and Norton

This was a honeymoon house, built in 1916 for $9,000 by the Hugh John Alexanders for their son, Philip Knox, and his prospective bride, Ruth Kassler, daughter of Edwin S. Kassler. The lot was catercorner to his own house at 199 Lafayette (there being no 2nd Avenue at that point).

The *Denver Post* reported on March 16, 1916, "The house is built in a modified English style with broad, low eaves. The first story is of tapestry brick of dark maroon color. The second story is smooth-finish cement, much like the English residences of the sixteenth and seventeenth centuries. The house contains seven rooms and two baths. It is finished throughout in mahogany and plaster. There are two immense sleeping porches and the whole structure is thoroly [sic] modern and convenient in its appointments." The center of the west facade is dominated by a wide chimney with three chimney pots towering over a low-pitched, hipped roof. The inconspicuous entrance is recessed up a straight walkway on the north. The two additions have flat roofs with wide eaves and ribbon casement windows facing the sunny south.

After the Alexanders moved out in 1924, Frank and Lelia Chamberlain bought the house. Lelia stayed after her husband's death. The Kassler ties to the house were renewed when Lelia married Ruth Alexander's father, Edwin S. Kassler, who lived in the house until his death in 1962.

Kassler was a much respected citizen of Denver from a pioneer family. His father, George Washington Kassler, had left New York at 15 and worked his way west to Omaha before embarking on a 24-day wagon trip to Denver in 1860.[5] He started the firm of G. W. Kassler and Co., which boldly displayed the sign "Wholesale and Retail Dealers in Fine Tobaccos, Segars, Pipes, Books, Stationery, Newspapers, Periodicals, etc."[6]

Like many pioneers, Kassler kept a diary of his life in early Denver and recorded the devastating flooding of Cherry Creek on May 19, 1864. Kassler was sleeping in a room over the southwest corner of his store. "Before I got undressed I heard the noise in the street of people running. I put on my vest and coat and went down to the banks of the creek . . . through water that was deep enough to [flow] nearly to over my boots. I took everything on the floor of the store and put it on counters and shelves. The water came up to the door sill."[7] At least eight people died in this flood. The damage was estimated at $350,000.[8]

Edwin Kassler grew up in his father's stationery store, carrying tobacco to the Indian encampments strung out along the Platte River. His father traded the tobacco for leather work, pelts, and handiwork. In 1970 his son, Edwin, while living at 300 Lafayette at the age of 93, described the old family store. It "stood on the corner of Blake and F (15th) Streets, the heart of the bustling town of Denver, then a little more than a decade old. Across the street, the Elephant Corral was clogged with wagons, schooners, and saddle horses, standing in the rain. To reach the Kassler store, the skinners, carters, and horsemen had to wade through the mire of Blake Street. They stopped at the stoop of the little store, kicked as much of Blake Street off their boots as they could, and entered. Most of them came for the long twists of tobacco . . . . the chawin' sort."[9]

In 1892, Edwin Kassler married one of the city's most eligible women, Olivia Cooper, the daughter of Governor Job A. Cooper. Olivia was lively and full of fun. It was said of her that she was "vivid, vital, alert, active, eager; she lived the life abundant."[10] This was born out by the fact that she would gaily shoot the water chutes at nearby Chute's Park, "her hair flying to the wind."[11]

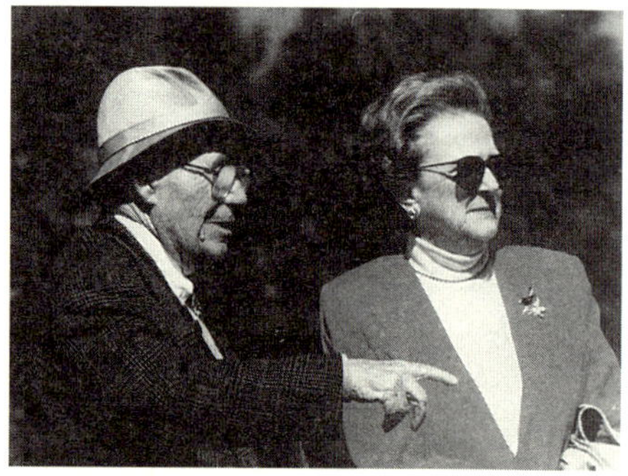

During the seventies and eighties 300 Lafayette was occupied by the Robert C. Blacks, III. (Courtesy Robert C. Blacks, III)

The couple had three children: Ruth, who married Philip K. Alexander; Genevieve, who married Sidney D. Brock and lived at 130 Gaylord Street; and Edwin S., Jr, who built at 369 Humboldt Street. It was after Olivia died that Kassler married Lelia Chamberlain, moving into her house at 300 Lafayette, where he lived for over 20 years.

George K. Hayden, vice-president of Van Schaack Realty Company, then lived in the house with his wife, Barbara "Bookie" Buchtel Hayden.

In 1968, Colorado historian Robert C. Black, III, brought his wife, Regina, back to this house in her native Denver after he had been teaching at Trinity College in Hartford, Connecticut. Although the

Philip K. Alexanders had found this home too small for three children, the Blacks had six children. They retained architect Edward D. White, Jr., to enclose the downstairs terrace and add a dressing room above. He designed a retaining wall with a metal fence to surround the backyard. "At that time the children were older, and we only had two or three actively living there," Black said. "I was teaching at Colorado Women's College and the house was convenient."

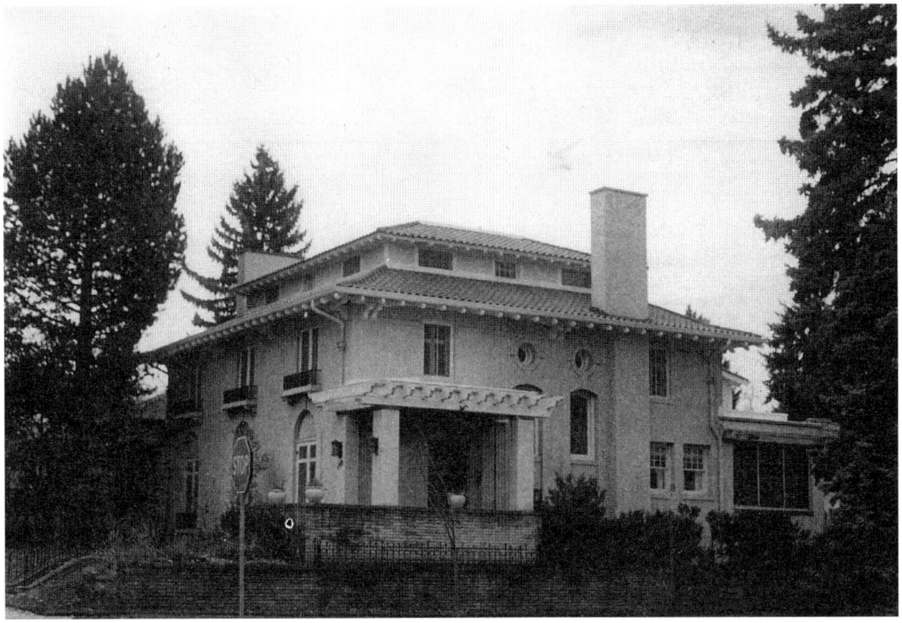

Hugh J. Alexander, president of the First National Bank, built this house at 199 Lafayette Street for his own family in 1913.

12
199 LAFAYETTE STREET
Built: 1913
Architect: Henry H. Hewitt

Hugh John Alexander was an early settler of the Country Club district. After 30 years in Colorado, he arrived in Denver in 1902 from Trinidad, Silverton, Lake City and Iowa, where he had been born in 1851. Banking was his training, and by 1914 he was president of the First National Bank, becoming the patriarch of a prominent banking family.

Alexander retained architect Henry Harwood Hewitt to build a two and a half story stucco Mediterranean house in 1913. The half third story is really full-sized with two bedrooms, a bath, and a large sitting area, said the current owner. The low-pitched, red-tile, hipped roof is carried on exposed rafters under wide, overhanging eaves. The entry portico with trellis design faces 3rd Avenue and is supported by square brick columns. Facing east, three arched casement window surrounds of low-relief stucco were later painted grey for contrast with the beige stucco house.

The family historian, Hugh Alexander's grandson, Philip K. "Pete" Alexander, Jr., recorded the early days when motorcars chugged down the gravelly lanes: "Hugh owned an Electric Car with handles to steer with. . . . Occasionally the power would drop down to a point when the car would come to a dead stop. Then followed a long, patient wait in the middle of a dirt road until the batteries recharged sufficiently to move along."[12]

Hugh Alexander was much respected in business as well as social circles. When death ended his 37-year banking career on December 8, 1928, "the members of the Denver Clearing House closed at 2 o'clock for his services."[13]

For his widow, Jennie, a house was purchased at 310 Humboldt, just a block away from her son,

Philip "P.K" and Ruth, who had moved to 140 Humboldt because "their 'bungalow' across the intersection at 300 Lafayette had proved too small for themselves and their three growing sons."

The next owners, the Hudson Moores, sold it in 1954 to Audrey (Mrs. Harold F.) Klock, who continued to live there after she married Paul Baxter Lanius, president of Glen Rock Coal Co.

Libby and Benjamin Trevor, who had wanted the house for a long time, bought it in 1996. "I liked the east windows, not only because of the arch, but because they went all the way to the floor," said Libby, an interior designer who has served five years on the board of Historic Denver, Inc.

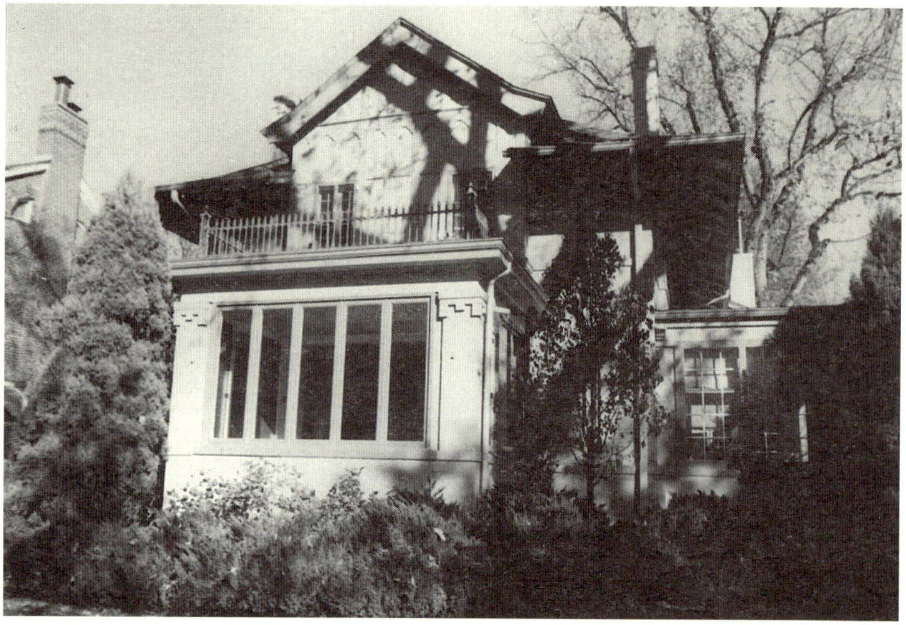

The Dell Van Gilder family of the Van Gilder Insurance Company lived in this house from the mid-1930s until the mid-1970s.

13
170 LAFAYETTE STREET
Built: 1907
Architect: Frederick Harnois

Frederick Harnois was the architect of the two-story square house at 170 Lafayette Street. Along with Theodore Boal, he also designed the first Denver Country Club clubhouse, the Grant-Humphreys Mansion, and Henry Wolcott's palatial home, Wolhurst, as well as his own house at 164 Lafayette. The painted brick house with a low-pitched flared hipped roof was built by Charles Rettig in 1907. Subsequent modifications were a brick garage in 1920 and a brick rear addition in 1925.

Of the four Barkalow brothers who founded the Barkalow Brothers News Agency in Omaha, only Derrick came to Denver to run a branch of the family business. When he died, his widow, Kate, moved to 170 Lafayette to be near their son, Robert, vice-president of Chemical Production Company, who lived at 319 Lafayette. The house is associated with the Dell Van Gilder family, who lived there from the mid-1930s until the mid-1970s.

Dell Van Gilder, Jr., was born there in 1940. "I remember the coal furnace in the basement. My father had to shovel coal into it every morning," he said. "Then there were the Cherry Creek floods. Rivers were flowing down Lafayette at the bottom of our steps. My father had fits because the water seeped into the basement and the plaster came off the walls." The successful insurance company has been maintained by the family since 1905.

While Sharon and William Elfenbein lived there from 1974 to 1997, they first glassed in the front porch to make a sunroom. Over this is a balcony with a wrought-iron balustrade under a half-timbered gable. On the back they added a family room with a little breakfast room.

Sharon, who had studied architecture at the University of Colorado at Denver, spent four years producing a detailed and comprehensive inventory of 167 houses in the Country Club district (Downing to High, 1st to 4th). Architect "Alan Fisher drove me around the neighborhood and told me who lived in the houses," she said. This monumental document, which records the year of construction, original owner, and detailed architectural descriptions of each house, resulted in historic designation by the National Registry of Historic Places in 1979. The complete district (including Race Street to University Boulevard) was designated by the Denver Landmark Commission and the Denver City Council as the Country Club Historic District in 1990.

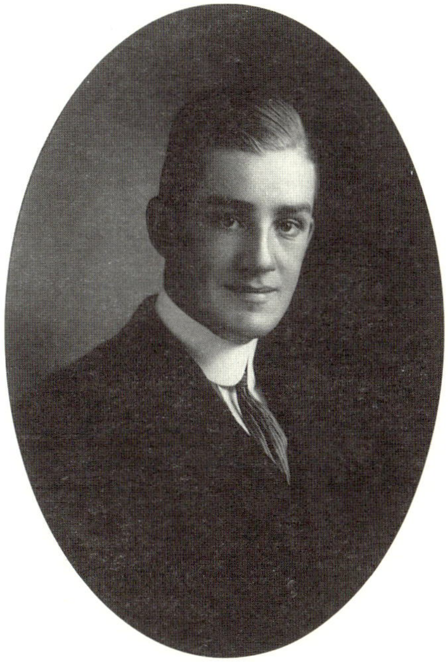

Henry Van Schaack, founder of the prominent real estate company, Van Schaack & Company, built two houses on Lafayette Street in 1912. His widowed mother lived at 167 Lafayette. (Courtesy DPL Western History Department)

14 and 15
167 LAFAYETTE STREET
145 LAFAYETTE STREET
Built: 1912
Architect: George L. Bettcher

Realtor Henry C. Van Schaack built two, two-lot houses on Lafayette Street in 1912. Restrictions for building residences in Park Club Place were not so stringent as Country Club Place, which required houses at a minimum cost of $5,000.

The two-story, 25-by-34-foot house at 167 was built for $4,000 by Van Schaack for his widowed mother, Renetta Van Schaack. At the same time he built a $3,000 one-and-a-half story house at 145 Lafayette for himself and his new bride, Clara Mitchell, sister of Clark Goodell Mitchell of 1640 East 3rd Avenue. Both of the Lafayette Street houses were designed by George L. Bettcher, a New Jersey native who came to Denver in 1895.

Van Schaack had just formed the promising real estate company, Van Schaack and Company. His house at 145 Lafayette is two stories, and is of painted brick with a deep gable that covers the front porch. Within four years the Van Schaacks built a larger, more elaborate home at 323 High Street.

In the late teens both Van Schaack families left and Mrs. John L. (Ella) Stearns took possession of 167 Lafayette, making a few changes

Van Schaack built the house at 145 Lafayette Street for himself and his new bride, Clara Mitchell, the sister of Clark Goodell Mitchell. (Courtesy of the DPL Western History Department)

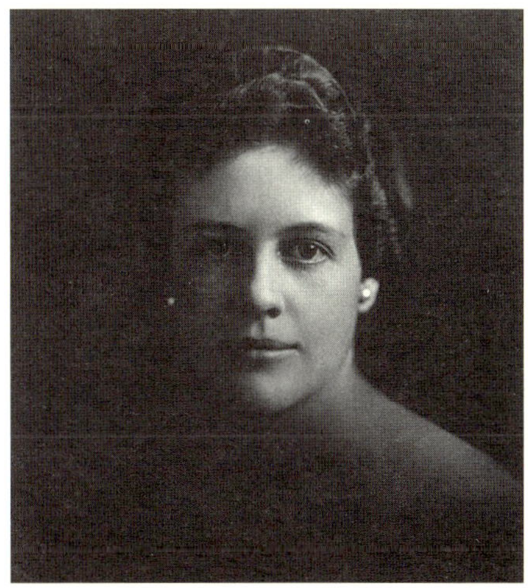

in 1918. The house was right across the street from 170 Lafayette, where Kate (Mrs. D. V.) Barkalow lived. When their children, lawyer Robert L. Stearns and Mary Barkalow, married, the newlyweds moved down the street to 319 Lafayette in a house owned by Mary's brother, Robert V. Barkalow. Thus, Lafayette Street became something of a family compound.

The small, dark, brown brick square house at 167 Lafayette still maintains its Victorian air with a wide front porch, dentil-lined, flat, hipped roof, and large front chimney.

When Barbara Stearns Wooten visited her grandmother while living in Boulder, she stayed in a little room at the back of the house. "I could hear the milkman rumbling down the alley in his horse and wagon to deliver the milk," she said.

The Walter W. Grahams occupied the house at 167 Lafayette from 1956 to 1989. Jean and Michael L. Churchman lived at 145 Lafayette during the sixties when he was headmaster of Kent School for Girls.

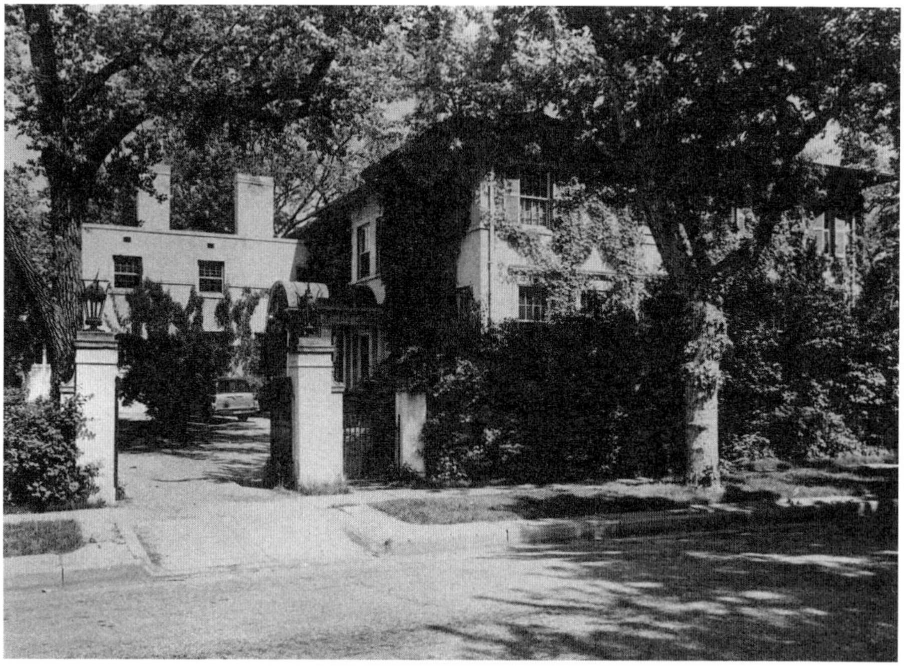

The old mansion built by George B. Berger, Sr., at 1st and Lafayette in 1914, was replaced by four houses in 1964. Developer William S. Falkenberg managed to save the old elm tree by the entrance. (Courtesy W. Bart Berger)

16, 17, and 18
140, 130, AND 100
LAFAYETTE STREET
Built: 1964
Designer: William S. Falkenberg

"The gracious, historic old mansion [of George Bart Berger, Sr.] was in bad repair when we bought it," said architect-builder William S. Falkenberg, of the Falkenberg Construction Company. He was describing the mansion at 124 Lafayette that was built in 1914 on 12 lots. Even grandson William M. B. "Bill" Berger said, "It was getting to be too difficult to keep up the big house." In 1964, Falkenberg purchased the property at 1st and Lafayette for $50,000.

The old mansion was built on land George Berger, Sr., had bought from his cousin and next-door neighbor at 135 Humboldt Street, Lina Bell Kountze (Mrs. Samuel) Ritter Brown, and represented a historic era of the grand parties and gracious life of a large prominent Denver family that occupied no less than 12 houses in the Country Club Historic Neighborhood at various times.

The home had many very elegant features. "While planning the four new custom-designed houses we invited the new owners to visit the old mansion and incorporate any items available," Falkenberg said. "Some shutters, a mantlepiece, and solid brass hardware and stone urns from the garden will be included in the new construction," reported the *Denver Post* on May 25, 1964.

Falkenberg was able to save some of the old trees from the former estate and landscaped his new three-lot homes with lush planting of evergreens and bushes. An original elm tree from the old estate still stands by the front garage of the two-story, four-bedroom house at 130 Lafayette. The square, low-pitched, hipped-roof house was custom-built for Jean Williams after her husband, Ford, died. They had raised their family at 360 Franklin Street. Her current husband, Hugh Catherwood, served as city budget director under Mayor J. Quigg Newton in 1947 and has subsequently

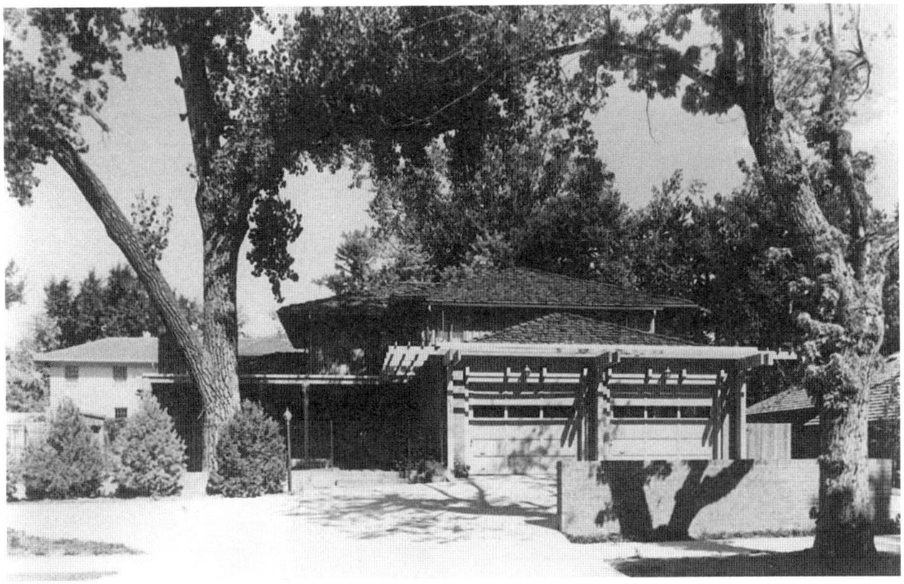

Jean and Hugh Catherwood live in this contemporary house at 130 Lafayette Street. The tree by the driveway was saved from the old Berger mansion. (Courtesy William S. Falkenberg)

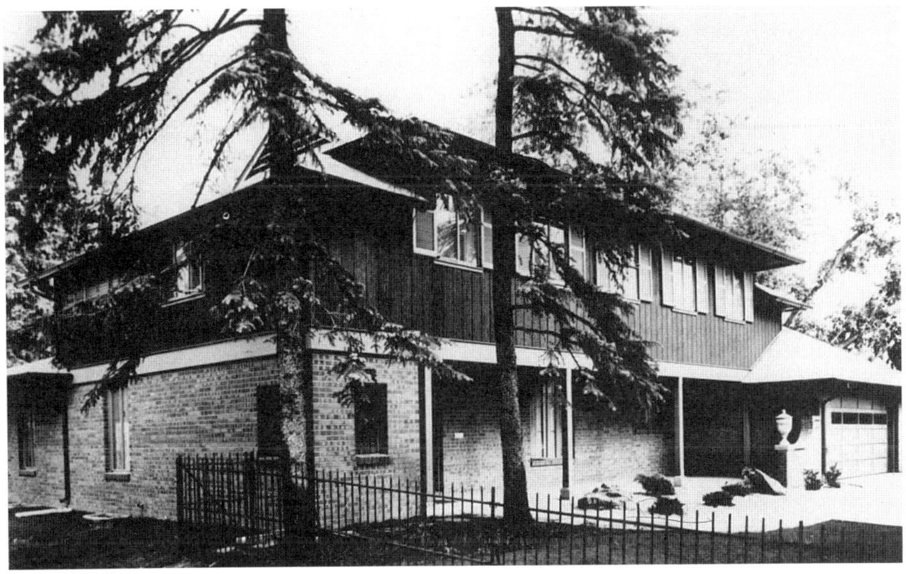

The corner house was built for Nina and John Fleming Kelly. The urn on the pedestal was saved from the Berger mansion. (Courtesy William S. Falkenberg)

served as an advisor to the administration during several budget crises.

At 120 Lafayette is a one-story, cinder-block house with contrasting brick trim and dentils under the hipped roof. A quiet brick walkway leads to the side entrance. White brick quoins decorate the corners. The house, built for Judge Alfred C. Hicks, was bought by Douglas and Aleen Carruthers and was still occupied by Carruther's widow in 1999.

Flamina Elaine "Nina" and John Fleming Kelly lived in the corner house at 100 Lafayette until they sold it to Governor John A. and Anne Love. Nina chose an urn from the old Berger garden to punctuate the garden wall near the front garage. The red brick first floor is topped with a beige textured stucco second floor and hipped roof. The "noise wall" on 1st Avenue matches the beige stucco and is separated by red brick pillars.

At the same time they bought the house, the Kellys built a house at 140 Lafayette for Nina's mother, Princess Elaine Willcox Odescalchi, who had divorced the Hungarian Prince Balthasar Gialma Odescalchi in 1948.

This L-shaped house with a distinctive mansard roof was designed with an extra safety feature. Subsequent owner Mary (Mrs. Giles) Filley said, "The Kellys built a bomb shelter for their mother, themselves, and their children. Giles used it as a wine cellar." Filley, who bought the house in the 1970s, was a pulmonary physiologist at the Webb-Waring Institute for Medical Research associated with the University of Colorado Health Sciences Center in Denver. The deceptively small-appearing house has a spacious living room, a dining room, seven bedrooms, four-and-a-half baths, a greenhouse, and a hot tub.

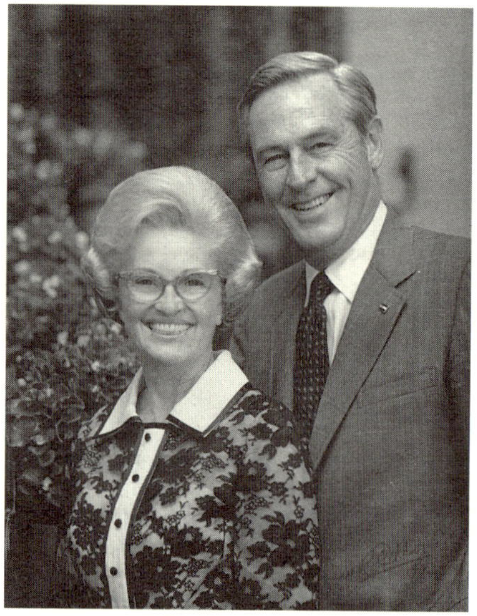

Governor and Mrs. John A. Love bought the house at 100 Lafayette Street from the Kellys. (Courtesy DPL Western History Department)

19
120 HUMBOLDT STREET
Built: 1912
Architect: Jacques Benedict

This Tudor house was described by architect Edward D. White, Jr., as an especially distinctive design of Jules Jacques Benois Benedict's. The cross gables, half timbering, patterned brick, and leaded windows are all good examples of the style. The graceful three-sided, two-story bays on the front and side are topped with stone balustrades under the gables. A brick walk and steps lead to the open side-entrance porch overlooking the garden.

The house was built for Madge and William Harper Huff early in the development of Park Club Place. At that time homes along 1st Avenue luxuriated in wide lots that served as grandstand seats for the weekend polo games at the Denver Country Club. Their open view was limited when a house was built to the south six years later. After Huff died in 1926, his widow continued to live in the house for another three decades.

In 1995 the house was sold to Joyce and Frederick V. Coville, an orthopedic surgeon at Swedish Hospital. "The house is highly livable for an older home. It has not been modernized. The old wood and spirit of the house have been kept up," said Joyce, who is involved with Habitat for Humanity and Central Presbyterian Church.

Striking are the many diamond-shaped, leaded windows throughout the house, even in the postwar rear sunroom addition. Over the entry bay is a circular stairway with the original carved wood banister. The

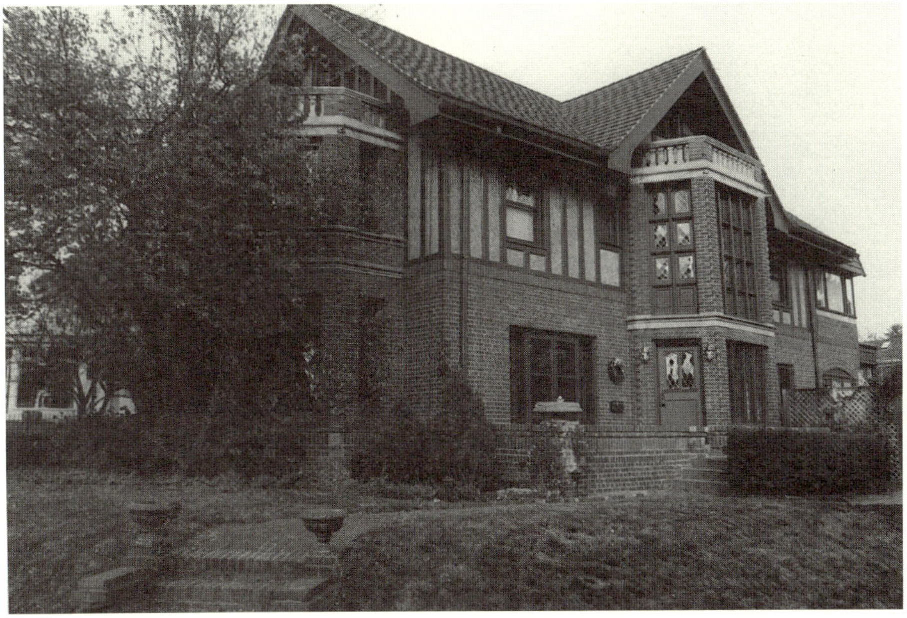

This Tudor revival house at 120 Humboldt Street is an especially distinctive design of Jacques Benedict.

original front driveway has been cut off by a catalpa tree, and a two-car alley garage was built with a lightweight concrete tile roof.

20
140 HUMBOLDT STREET
Built: 1912
Architects: Fisher and Fisher
Remodeling: 1981
Architect: Jonathan Saiber

Another Fisher and Fisher design was the symmetrical Greek Revival house Bethuel Webster built in 1912. The one-story entry portico was supported by round, fluted, free-standing columns with a white balustraded porch above. Keystone lintels marked the first-floor windows while elaborate, full transom lights surrounded the door. The wrought-iron fence is divided by brick pillars.

When the Websters moved away, the Philip K. Alexanders bought the house. They were expecting their third child, Bruce, and they felt that 300 Lafayette was too small. Philip Knox "P.K." Alexander graduated from East High and Dartmouth College. He liked to farm, and at one time he owned nine ranches in Colorado.[14] He also had a woodworking shop where he loved to putter. "Each year Pappy would make doll beds for the Santa Claus Shop," said daughter-in-law Gladys Barkalow (Mrs. Philip, Jr.) Alexander.

After P.K. married Edwin Kassler's daughter, Ruth, he signed on at the First National Bank the year after his father, Hugh J. Alexander, became president. P. K. became senior vice-president and brought two sons, Philip K., Jr., "Pete" and Bruce, into banking before his retirement in 1958. President John Evans said of them, "One of the rare privileges of my banking career has been to be associated so closely with three generations of the Alexander family."

The Alexanders' middle son, Hugh "Brud," married Ellen Shafroth, granddaughter of Governor John F. Shafroth. Unfortunately Brud died of a chronic heart disease a few years after the birth of their daughter, Anne.

Pete, who followed his father to Dartmouth, returned to Denver and married Gladys Barkalow, the daughter of Denise Barkalow. Pete became a vice president of the International Trust Company from 1940 to 1960. "However, Pete was really an outdoor mountain man," his wife said. He had majored in zoology at college and enjoyed working at the Denver Museum of Natural History, now the Denver Museum of Nature

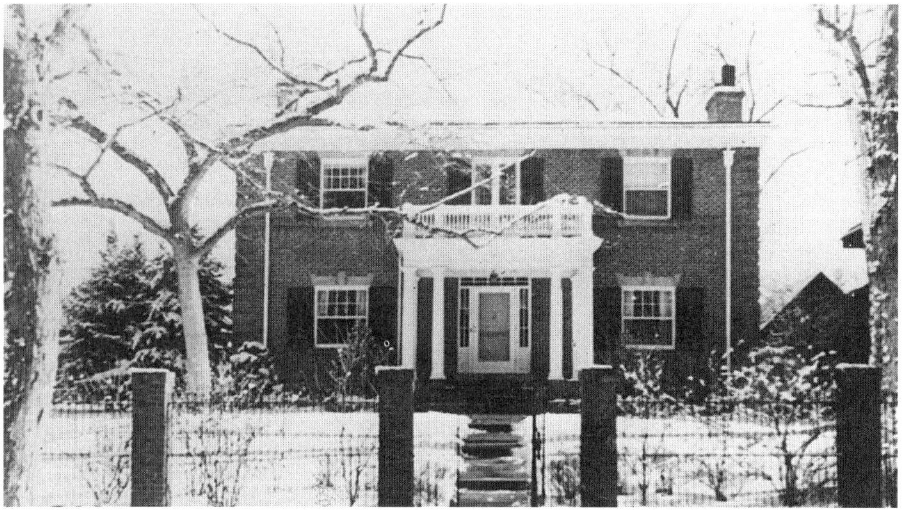

[ABOVE[
This house at 140 Humboldt Street, built in 1912 as a Greek Revival house . . .
(Courtesy Bruce Alexander)

[BELOW]
. . . was gutted and remodeled into a contemporary home in 1981.

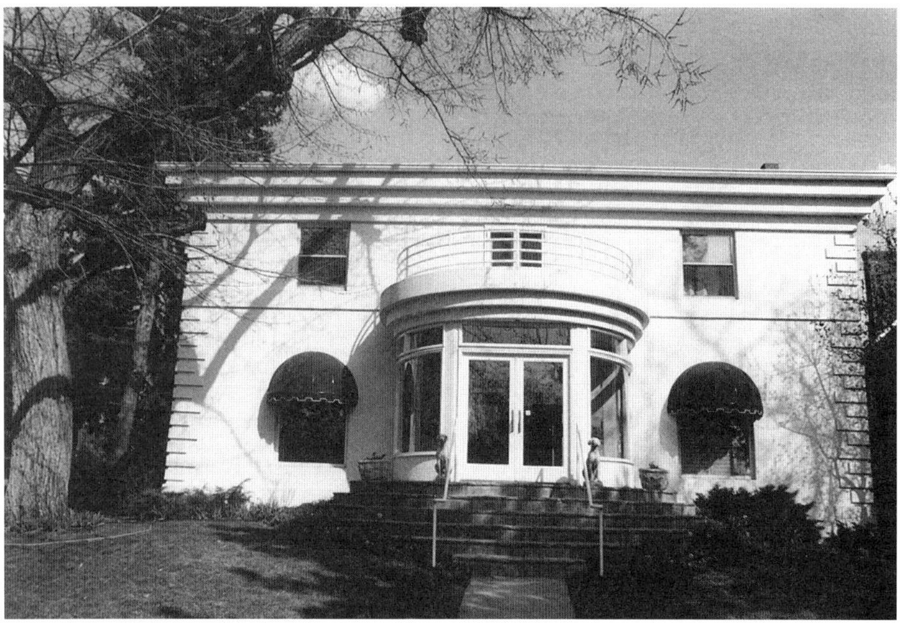

and Science, painting animals and scenes of nature, and researching and writing meticulously documented family histories. Pete retired from banking after 20 years to pursue his interests in natural history, Colorado history, and art.

Bruce married Phyllis "Chick" Safarik, the daughter of a prominent Denver physician, who subsequently followed in her mother-in-law's footsteps by presiding over the Junior League of Denver. She served as executive director of the Institute for International Education for 13 years. After retiring from the bank, Bruce continued the family tradition of service to the community. He took the job of executive director of the Denver Botanic Gardens, then served a term as Denver Manager of Parks and Recreation.

Harley and Lorraine Higbie raised five children at 140 Humboldt during the sixties and seventies.

On July 8, 1981, a building permit was issued to new owners Sanford D. and Toni-Dee Kaiser, who retained architect Jonathan Saiber to "remodel the entire interior" of the house in a post-modern eclectic style. The Greek Revival facade was replaced by a semicircular, glassed-in porch with a molded unadorned cornice. Walls were removed and the rooms were opened up into large spaces with plenty of sunlight. In the glass-enclosed vestibule is a two-floor spiral staircase. The old staircase was replaced by the master bedroom suite, including a tub at the foot of the bed, an exercise room, a library, and a nursery.[15] "They really remodeled a seven-bedroom house into a one-bedroom house," said Lorraine Higbie.

The Kaisers had to move soon after the remodeling, but it was enjoyed by the next owners, the Sidney Shlenkers, who added a pool and dressing rooms in 1987.

Although the Historic District had been formed in 1979, the Landmark Committee of the Country Club Historic Neighborhood had not drawn up design guidelines, so the remodeling plans were not reviewed. Bruce Alexander, who grew up in the house, saw the remodeling at a Dora Moore house tour. "There's a circular stairway in the foyer. At the entrance is an oversized cardboard cutout of the owner, extending his hand in welcome to any visitor," he said. "I couldn't recognize any room in the house. I couldn't even find my own bedroom."

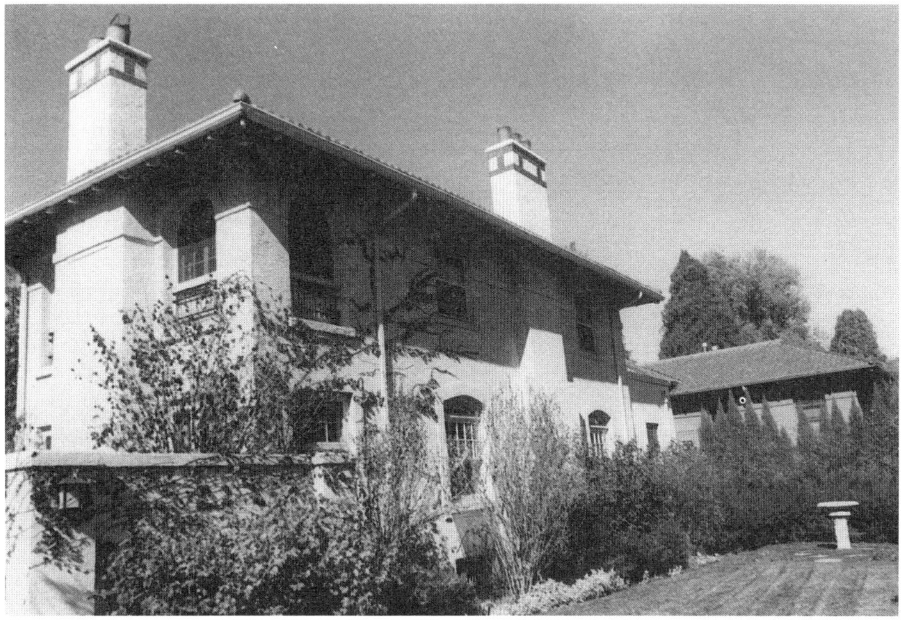

When this house at 135 Humboldt Street was built on 12 lots in 1908, the extensive south garden overlooked the Denver Country Club golf course.

21
135 HUMBOLDT STREET
Built: 1908
Architects: Fisher and Fisher

Several early homes along 1st Avenue, built in the second filing of Park Club Place between 1st and 3rd Avenues, included extensive grounds facing the Denver Country Club.

The southern half of Block 7 of Park Club Place was sold in August 1907 to Lina Bell Kountze Brown, daughter of Mary Estabrook and Charles Brewer Kountze. She and her husband Samuel Ritter Brown, built a Fisher and Fisher-designed two-story, beige stucco, Mediterranean-style house on the eastern 12 lots and moved there with their three-year-old son, Samuel Ritter Brown, Jr. Elaborate gardens extended from the house to dirt-covered 1st Avenue. Because Lina Bell's cousin, George Berger, built on the western half of the block, there was no alley between the houses.

The unadorned front entryway is marked by two urns on the east stucco wall. This opens onto a stone terrace that overlooks the gardens, now walled off from 1st Avenue. Window openings have arched heads above and flat arches below. The two chimneys towering above the low-pitched, red tile roof are trimmed with geometric designs of red brick.

Unlike the rest of the Kountze-Berger clan, Samuel Brown was not a banker. The son of a Denver pioneer, he was a philosopher and author whose book, *When Dreams Come True,* is a novel about old Mexico. As a man of wealth, Brown championed the natural, simple way of life, as contrasted with the wealthy superficial civilization in which he found himself. "He is the example par excellence of the rich man who, seeing the injustices of our economic and social system, has devoted his life to the solution of the underlying workings of a society which raises a few, while it crushes the many," reported the *Daily News* on December 8, 1912.

In 1913, retaining 32,118 square feet of land, Lina Bell sold the western half of the property to her cousin, George Bart Berger, Sr., son of Margaret Kountze and William B. Berger, who had also built a Fisher and Fisher-designed house on 12 lots.

During the early 1920s the Humboldt Street house was occupied by a prominent businessman, Leopold Henry Guldman. One of many German-Jewish immigrants, Guldman left his home at 18, arriving in Denver in the early 1870s. He established the Golden Eagle Dry Goods store at 16th and Larimer, and the large gold-painted eagle carved for the top of the store symbolized his love for his adopted country. A biography of Guldman states: "No more devoted, patriotic or enthusiastic resident ever lived in Denver, or Colorado, than he, because Colorado and Denver had given him his chance, and he appreciated it."[16]

Guldman repaid the community by helping reverse the financial crisis during the Silver Panic of 1893 by using cash to purchase and secure bank certificates of local banks.[17] A solarium was dedicated to him at National Jewish Hospital, where he had served on the board for 32 years as "one of its staunchest friends and supporters."[18]

John G. Lowe; his wife, Edith, and two children, John G., Jr., and Catherine moved into the house in 1930. Lowe built a swimming pool in 1933 for his son who was afflicted with cerebral palsy and added an elevator two years later. He maintained the family business, Lowe Brothers Paint Company, with his brother, accumulating enough wealth to purchase a collection of rare valuable paintings that adorned his Humboldt Street house. Lowe was a trustee of the Denver Art Museum, and the family was socially prominent in the community.

Some years later his wife instituted divorce proceedings, alleging cruelty. The interlocutory decree was granted only months before Lowe's strange disappearance in 1937. Lowe boarded a boat en route to Boston from New York City, but never disembarked. "Police believed Lowe had walked in his sleep and plunged into the ocean, tho [sic] when his body was found he was fully dressed and the key to his stateroom was in the pocket of his coat," reported the first page of the August 28, 1937, *Denver Post.*

Edith continued living in the house with her handicapped son and Catherine's daughter, Frances, whom she raised. Neighbor Meredeth "Merce" Moore (Lea) used to go over to play with Frances. "The house was formally furnished with antiques to complement the collection of rare paintings. . . . They had a butler, a cook, and a chauffeur. That's where I learned to use a finger bowl—at every meal," she said.

Edith Lowe remained in the house until the mid-1980s when she died, leaving the art collection to various museums. Nobody knows more about Humboldt Street than Charles M. "Charley" Moore, who grew up at 301 Humboldt. He remembered these Lowe paintings and commented: "My favorite picture of that house is of Mrs. Lowe, a 90-year-old, four-foot, ten-inch woman, pretty much living there by herself with this large collection of fabulous paintings. When she died she gave them to museums, which were then responsible for this priceless collection so they immediately sent out a contingent of armed guards to protect this windfall. The security system in that house went from one little 90-year-old lady to armed guards patrolling the grounds with guns."

Jeffrey W. and Mary Ross have lived at the house since 1992. "The house had been completely renovated by the couple here before us, Page and Jay Cowles," Jeff said. "They landscaped and terraced, taking advantage of the huge lawn between the house and 1st Avenue. A porch off the dining room replaced the swimming pool, which was buried long ago. It was too much of a liability, anyway." Mary pointed out the windows that had been enlarged or made into doors that brightened the rooms, previously kept subdued to preserve the paintings.

After three years of renovation, the Cowleses were transferred to Minneapolis during a housing recession. Without a wall to buffer the growing traffic noise on 1st Avenue, they had trouble selling the property. Their friends, the Rosses, rented for a year, then bought it. Proud to own one of the earliest houses in the Country Club district, they have preserved and enhanced the charm of this historic home.

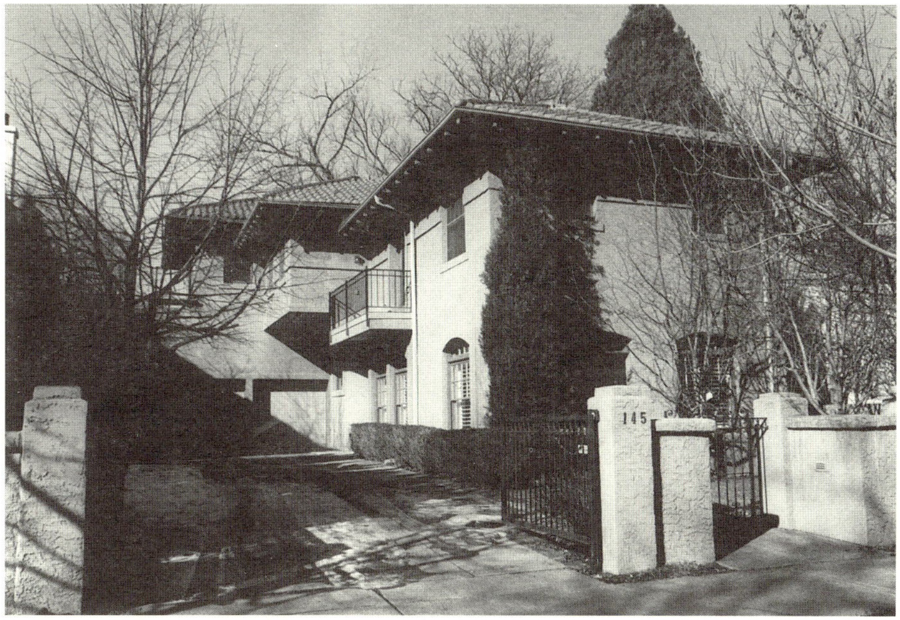

The house at 145 Humboldt was split off from the house to the south, turned 90 degrees, remodeled, and sold as a separate house during the mid-1980s.

22
145 HUMBOLDT STREET
Architect: Fisher and Fisher
Built: 1908
Detached: 1988
Remodeling:
Gordon Lewis Associates

In the mid-1980s, 135 Humboldt became a house divided. Gordon Lewis Associates, Architects and Contractors, bought it, detached the north wing, turned it 90-degrees clockwise, added a family room and terrace, painted it a rust color, and sold it as a separate house, now 145 Humboldt Street.

"It [135 Humboldt] had been a rambling old mansion, really too large for today's lifestyles," Lewis said. "Furthermore, the north wing, which had been added, interrupted the proportions architect William Fisher had intended. The answer was division."[19] The horizontal trim, the eyebrow windows, the belt course, and the red tile roofs confirm the common ancestry of the two houses. The newer house has become a six-level, four-bedroom contemporary home with a large living room opening onto a private patio and garden.

23
160 HUMBOLDT STREET
Built: 1956
Architect: Paul Atchison

The small, two-bedroom, red brick retirement home that Paul Atchison designed for himself and

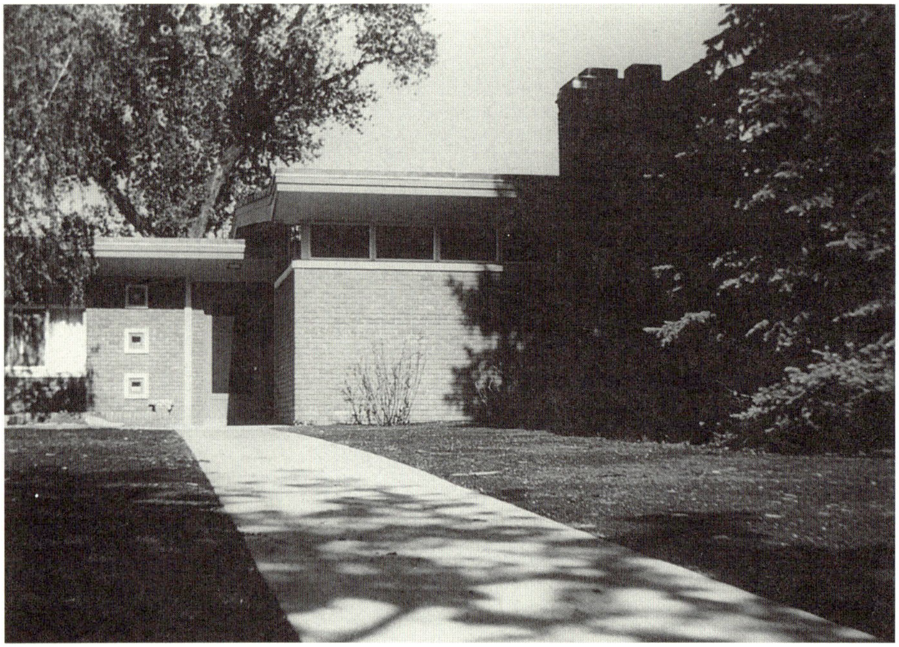

Architect Paul Atchison built a small retirement house for himself at 160 Humboldt Street in 1956. Subsequent owners have added wings and a second floor. (Courtesy Robert Atchison)

his wife, Mary, is now a 6,450-square-foot "pop-top." "The site was a big carriage house with living quarters above, belonging to the 1908 house to the north [180 Humboldt]," said their son, Philip, also an architect. "My father wanted to live in that area. He grew up poor and wanted to live in a neighborhood with rich people."

The house is a modified International style with ribbons of clerestory windows. "I would describe the house as eclectic contemporary," Philip said. "The fact that the roof turns up was because my father had a liking for Japanese buildings. Also, he wanted soft common brick and had to get it from Missouri."

After studying architecture, Paul worked in the offices of architects Jacques Benedict, Temple Buell, Victor Hornbein, John Gaw Meem, and Alan Fisher before opening his own firm in 1937. Among his Denver designs is a charming little house at 340 Lafayette that he designed for his mother-in-law in 1927. He also designed a home at 2015 East 4th Avenue and the famous "Cinderella House" built at 5010 East 6th Avenue in Hilltop in 1935. This house, built to attract residents to the area, was auctioned off at a theater drawing and won by a penniless couple from Brooklyn.

There have been two owners of the Humboldt Street house since then. John "Tim" and Janet Tyler put in a master suite and a therapy pool for Jan in the late eighties.

James and Merrillyn Shroads bought the home in 1990. "We remodeled 90 percent of the house, adding a second floor," Jim said. "We didn't take out the pool, but we covered it with our family room. The pool is still there underneath the television set."

24
180 HUMBOLDT STREET
Built: 1908
Architects: Sterner and Williamson

The lovely, red brick, eclectic Greek Revival house at 180 Humboldt Street seems to be set back in the woods, so lush are the 90-year-old evergreen trees that surround it. However, when Aaron Dennison Lewis built it in 1908,[20] the house was sitting in a wheat field from the former John J. Riethmann farm.

Lewis, who came to Denver in 1880, made a mark in the community by running one of the great dry goods houses of Colorado and the West. "Only goods of the best quality and highest grade have stocked the counters and shelves of A. T. Lewis & Son Dry Goods Company,"[21] a firm he ran with his father, Aaron Thompson Lewis. Later, four of the ten lots were sold to architect Paul Atchison, who tore down the old carriage house to build a retirement house to the south in 1956. (see 160 Humboldt)

In 1954, Robert "Jim" and Janet Widmer and their four children, Deborah, Nancy, Judith, and Robert, Jr., lived in the big house at 180 Humboldt for eight years. Nancy (Widmer Freeman) described the 4,776-square-foot house: "On each floor there was one room the same size—the billiard room, the living room, and upstairs, the master suite. There were three bedrooms and a bath on the third floor that were built for servants. . . . The neighborhood was a great place to grow up because it was safe and there were so many kids. We all got along, and we played Sardines and Hide and Seek all over the neighborhood."

On the west side of the three-story asymmetrical house is a large front entry porch supported by two-story paired round white Ionic columns. This is offset on the north by a wide two-story bay containing multipane, double-hung sash windows with keystone lintels. White pedimented trim surrounds the paneled arched door. On the third floor, the low hipped roof is punctuated by three gabled dormers trimmed with dentils. "We loved the house, but it always needed work," said Janet Widmer. "We had a carpenter practically living with us."

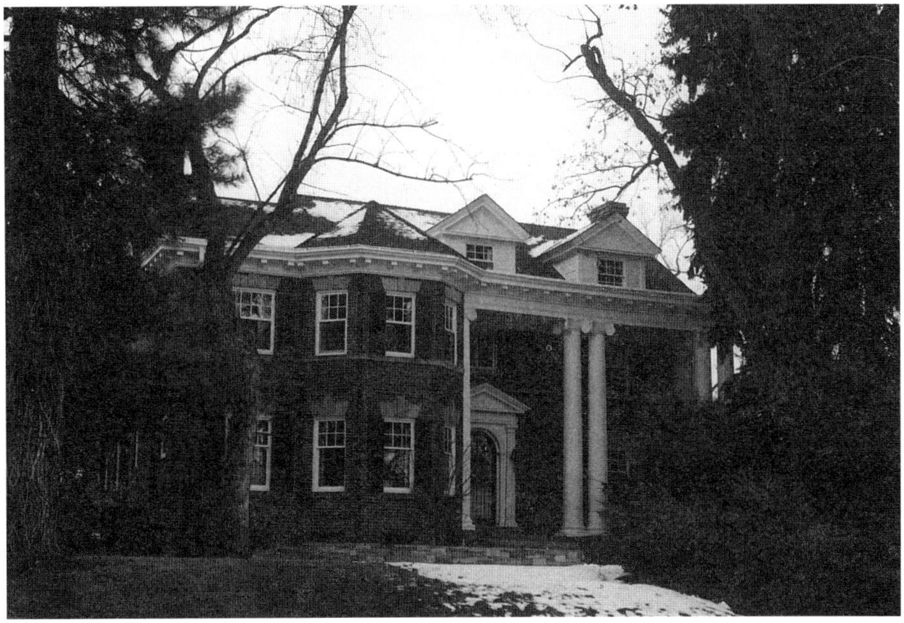

In 1908 this brick house at 180 Humboldt Street was built on 10 lots amidst the wheat fields of the former Riethmann farm.

After the Widmers left Denver, Dr. Thomas H. Coleman and his wife, Lorraine, moved in with their three daughters. The house is surrounded by tall evergreens and bushy junipers. "During the winter of 1998 we found a fox sleeping very comfortably in the sunshine on our south brick terrace," said Lorraine. "Once we even found two mallard ducks in our tiny pond. Back in the bushes Tom found three eggs that they had laid." The lush growth is borne out by Jim Shroads, their neighbor at 160 Humboldt, who calls their property "the Colemans' rainforest."

25
177 HUMBOLDT STREET
Built: 1929
Architect: Henry James Manning

This three-and-a-half-story mansion was built by Austrian immigrant A. C. Kalmus between 1929 and 1931. Kalmus was widely known at the time for his women's apparel shop, A. C. Kalmus Sample Shop, on 15th Street. The house was later occupied by his son-in-law, Martin Bechtold. "Marty told me that his father-in-law went back to New York every month, had his own room at the Waldorf, and bought a lot of fashionable samples which he sold in his stores," said Humboldt Historian Charles M. "Charley" Moore. "It was very popular in Denver because they were the latest styles and people never saw another dress like it."

Although Kalmus lived only three years in the house, his wife lived on there until 1947. "During the war," Moore continued, Marty and Mildred came to live in the house with her mother, bringing their son, Bruce."

Bechtold, a native of Indiana who was educated in Denver Public Schools, was a director of the Florence Crittenton Home for unmarried mothers and active in the United Fund. He also dabbled at managing some of his range properties. In 1949, Mrs. Kalmus had a

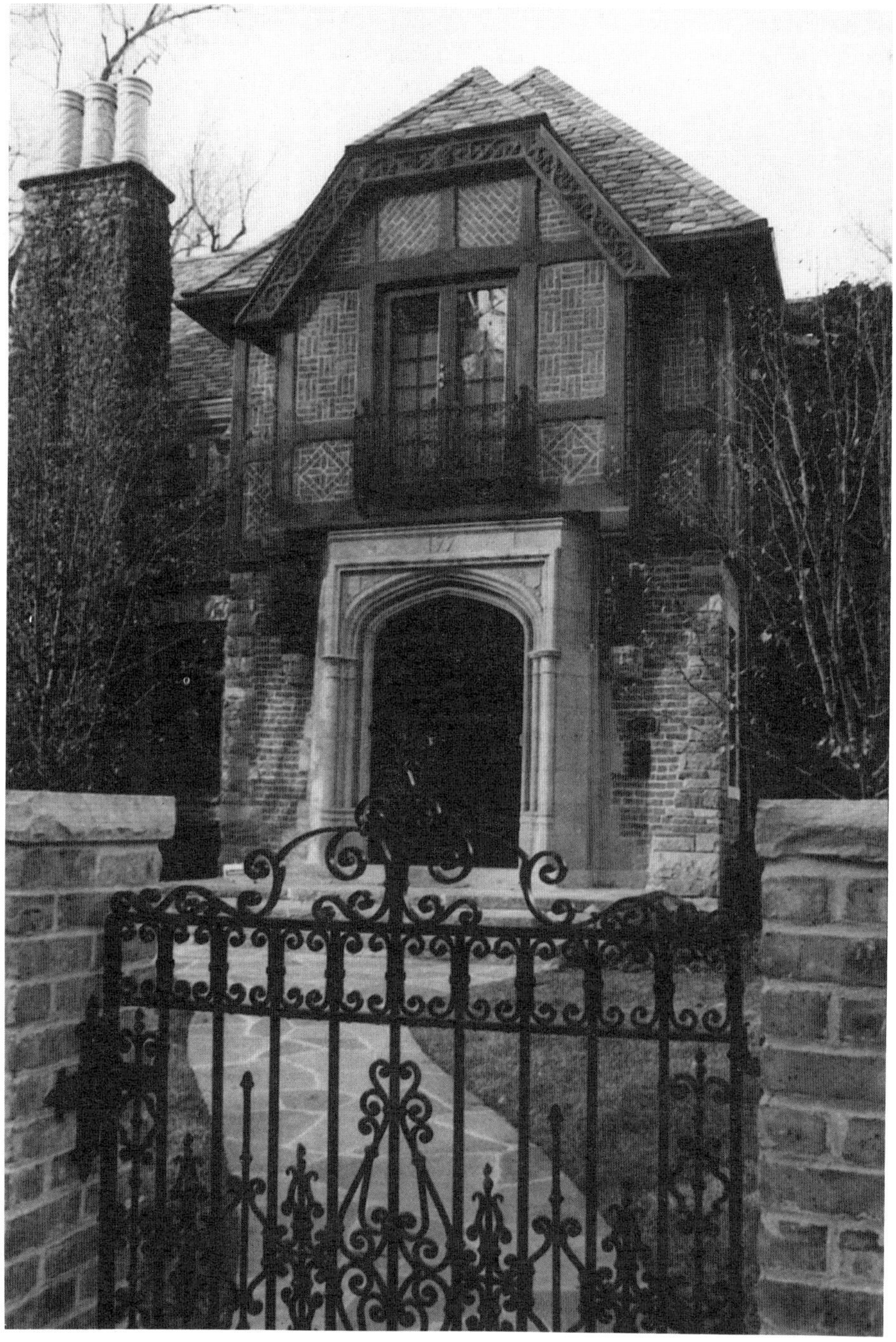

[RIGHT]
The elaborate 300-foot iron fence bordering the property at 177 Humboldt Street was originally built by ironworkers imported from Jamaica in 1929.

fatal stroke near the pond in their backyard. "When Mrs. Kalmus died, her trust fund kicked in and enabled Marty and Mildred to live there pretty independently," Moore said. "However, the house was kept in the trust."

Although their son, Bruce, lived out of town, his daughter, Bitzie, used to visit her grandparents. "It was fun to play with her," said Katherine "Kim" Millett, a neighbor at 320 Humboldt Street. "When I went over in the late fifties, Bitzie and I wanted to play around the pond, but her grandmother said, 'Come watch color television. It will be good for you.' I had never heard of color television then." This pond was the future home of Huey, Dewey, and Lewey, three white pet ducks. Nancy Widmer Freeman, who lived across the street at 180 Humboldt, said, "When Bitzie lived there for a year, Mrs. Bechtold let us play dress-up. She had bought her whole trousseau in Europe."

The Kalmuses had traveled extensively and bought many objets d'art for their homes. "Marty was convinced thieves were going to rob him. He kept loaded guns throughout the house and asked me if I would stay with them to help guard the house," said Moore, who lived at the Bechtolds' house during the year before they died within 48 hours of each other in 1970. After their deaths Moore found out that most of the priceless "objets d'art" had really been replicas.

Kalmus spared no expense when building this modified Tudor-style house. For the elaborate wrought-iron stair railings, front door, trim, and 300-foot-long fence that borders two sides of the 21,900-square-foot lot, he imported Jamaican ironworkers. "They set up a forge right in the front lawn to manufacture the wrought iron on the spot," said Moore.

When the home was built, their daughter Mildred was already married. The 6,300-square-foot house was, therefore, built for a couple. There were only three main bedrooms, each with private baths and sitting rooms. Moore described the house when he lived there: "At the end of a long hallway, down the back stairway, through the kitchen pantry, and up the stairs to a passway over to the garage, there were two bedrooms and a bath for the servants."

During the 1980s, Gail Heitler Klapper lived there with her husband, neurologist Jack Klapper and their children. Gail, an alumna, and later a trustee, of Wellesley College, is a prominent lawyer. She was defeated in a close run for attorney general of Colorado in 1982. During the nineties she was president of the Denver Chamber of Commerce.

The house has elaborate decorative detail. The south truncated gable is half-timbered. Beside it, off the master bedroom, is a stone balcony overlooking the spacious side yard with a deep pond in the southwest corner of the property. Topping the tall chimney are three carved stone chimney pots. The heavy-wood front door is paneled with wrought-iron trim. Decorative brick surrounds the balcony door, while carved wooden bargeboards line the truncated gable above. Leaded glass is set in the bay windows as well as the doors on the master bedroom cabinets. Over the stairway are three large Gothic windows with thick translucent glass. The three-floored attached garage is between the levels of the house with a bedroom above, the furnace below, and below that a pump for the well in a little sub-basement cubbyhole.

When private investor Michael Kennedy and his wife, Kelly, bought it in 1998, they spent a couple of years renovating the house by updating the plumbing and wiring, stripping layers of paint off the rusted 300-foot fence and the circular stair railing and trim. They also pushed up the roof, covered it with slate, and finished the attic rooms. They completely renovated the house, preserving its historic charm. "We're trying to sandblast and strip to restore the house to its original beauty. What we can't restore we're replicating, like some of the molding on the wall," said Kelly Kennedy.

Nancy Widmer said, "I think this is the most beautiful house in the neighborhood. The staircase is so graceful, and the sunroom had those beautiful tiles forming a pond."

26
301 HUMBOLDT STREET
Built: 1908
Architects: Sterner and Williamson

In 1908 realtor Augustus F. Fisher engaged architects Frederick Junius Sterner and George Hebard Williamson to design this $10,000, three-story brick square house at 3rd and Humboldt. Architect Edward D. White, Jr., commented, "It has a Dutch Colonial look." It has a deep wrap porch, later glassed in on the south, a two-story bay window with a roundel on the south, and a carriage house at the back. Decorative brackets support the deep eaves of the medium-pitched, hipped roof. The ornate, flared Mission-shaped dormers are distinctive. Ownership changed every decade or so until architect Thomas Edgar Moore moved there with his wife, Ruth, and seven children after their return from Grand Junction in 1952.

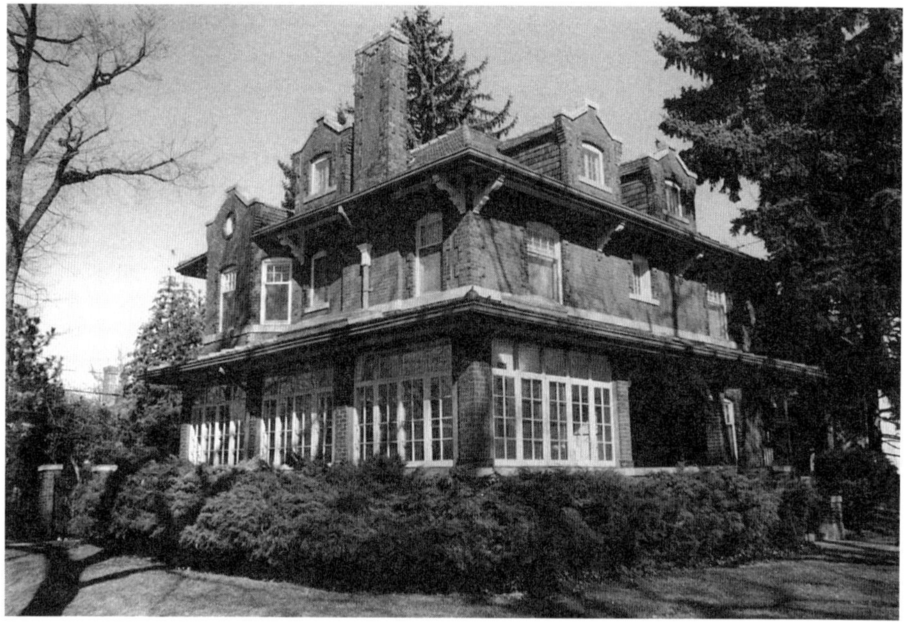

The three-story house at 301 Humboldt Street housed the family of architect Thomas E. Moore.

One of the children, Charles M. "Charley" Moore, is a gregarious raconteur and the recognized authority and historian of Humboldt Street in the Country Club neighborhood: "The house at 301 was pretty full when we were there. We used the side porch for sleeping in summer. There was a coal chute with an outside staircase. When I wanted a room to myself I was given the room in the basement and found the staircase a very handy exit in the middle of the night. Youngest child, Dorsey Moore, said, "There were only four bedrooms on the second floor, so we made the third floor into two bedrooms to house all of us."

Other Moore children are Michael, a past director of Denver Opportunity, who is presently manufacturing AirLift, a backpack to carry oxygen, which is a reproduction of the original Snugli baby carrier. Tom "Tim" was in the international division of Gates Rubber Company, while engineer Christopher "Kit" ran a construction company in Montrose, Colorado. Jinny teaches school in Carbondale. Hugh owns the general store in Gold Hill, Colorado, and novelist Dorsey lives in Denver.

Thomas was the second son of Harold W. Moore, founder of H. W. Moore Equipment Company, a firm that supplied machinery for building roads, dams, and mines. Harold Moore was a cattleman in Brush, Colorado, before coming to Denver.

He lived at 1410 High Street in a large beautiful Colonial home nicknamed "The House of a Thousand Candles" because of its many windows that let light stream into every corner. Author Meredeth Nicholson lived there and had published a mystery book of that name in 1905. Tom was brought up in this house with his older brother, John, later of 369 Humboldt Street, who carried on the equipment company. Their youngest brother, interior designer Richard, lived at 181 Franklin Street.

Tom Moore studied architecture at Yale and was the first to design a precast concrete form for geodesic domes. He designed many Denver residences before his death at 61 in 1970.

Subsequent owners of the Humboldt Street house have "enlarged the house and jazzed it up," Charley said. They incorporated the side porch into the living room and pushed out the back to extend the kitchen. The outside staircase is now enclosed. This is the only staircase to the basement, as the inside stairs are closed up.

The Moores loved to sing and formed a talented and lusty choir. Every Christmas eve they would pack the family in the car and visit friends, caroling on their doorsteps and spreading good cheer.

The talented Moore family chorus caroled friends and neighbors on Christmas eve. (Courtesy Charles M. Moore)

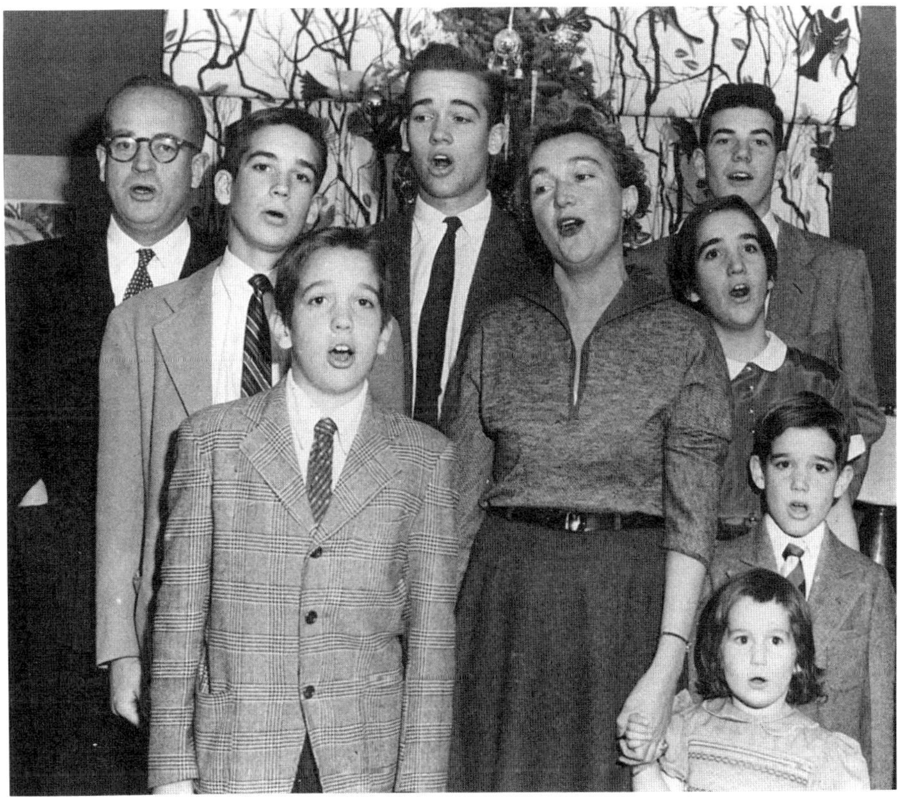

27
300 HUMBOLDT STREET
Built: 1910
Architects: Marean and Norton

Although Robert W. Speer bought his 3rd Avenue and Humboldt Street lot in 1904,[22] he had just started his first two terms as mayor of Denver and didn't get around to building a house until 1911,[23] just before his first two terms ended. As the secretary of the Park Club Place Land Company, Speer had his pick of lots in this subdivision.

As mayor, Speer's priority was to create a "City Beautiful" with green parkways lined with trees and landscaped gardens. For his own house he chose architects Albert J. Marcan and Willis A. Norton, who designed such Speer-initiated projects as the Greek Theater in Civic Center and

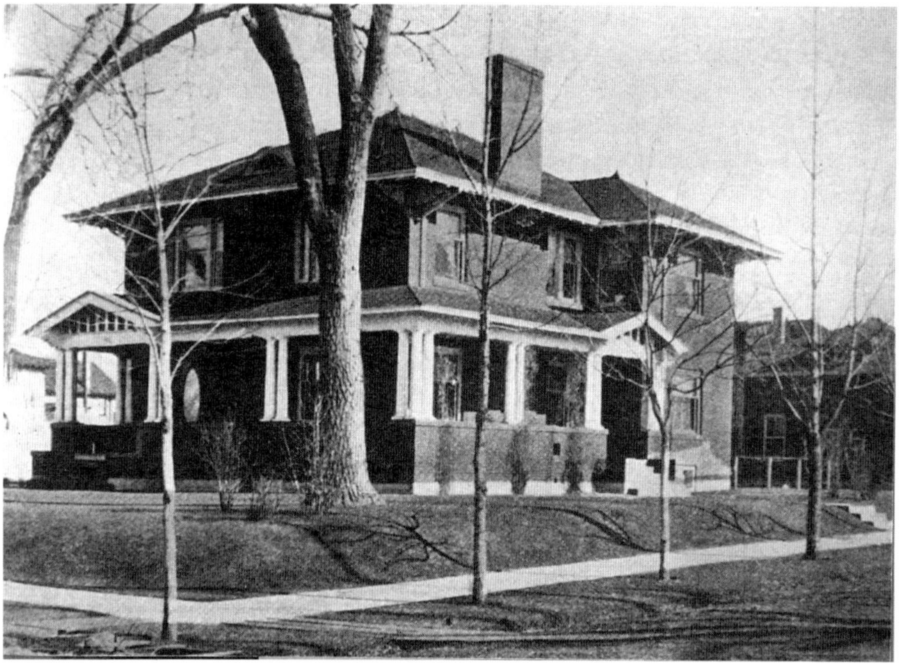

In 1904, Mayor Robert W. Speer, secretary of the Park Club Place Land Company, chose the corner of 3rd Avenue and Humboldt Street for his own home. (Courtesy Denver Planning Office)

the Greek Pavilion in Cheesman Park. For Speer they designed a two-story, brick, square house with a wide wrap porch supported by paired round columns. The west and south pedimented porch entries are half-timbered. The medium-pitched hipped roof is supported by brackets. A two-story carriage house with a door to load the hay lies next to the alley.

Although Park Club Place had been platted evenly, an alteration occurred in the lot sizes. Charles M. Moore, the Humboldt Historian, told the story: "The architects drafted beautiful plans for the house and gardens. Speer was terribly pleased, but there was a discrepancy: the plans were too big for the lot. No problem. As mayor and secretary of the Park Club Place Land Company, the alleys between Humboldt and Franklin were simply moved to the east." Sure enough, the distance from Humboldt to the alley is 163.96 feet and that from the alley to Franklin is 132.5 feet.

In 1882 Speer had married an old Pennsylvania school chum, Kate Thrush, after heroically saving her from drowning in a lake when their rowboat capsized. Speer brought her to Denver where he had already settled with tuberculosis in 1878. After Speer died in office in 1918, his widow continued to live at 300 Humboldt with her sister, Lucie Frederick. Kate continued some of her husband's community projects during her 96 years and died, childless, at 300 Humboldt Street in 1956.

Before her death she gave her prized possession to her neighbor, Ruth (Mrs. Thomas E.) Moore, who lived across the street at 301 Humboldt. "Mrs. Speer never had any children," said Charley Moore. "When our family moved across the street to 301 Humboldt with seven kids, she loved it. She would sit in her upstairs window and watch all of us coming on our bikes. One day we came home from church and Mom said, 'While you're all in your Sunday clothes we're going to go across the street because Mrs. Speer is going to give us a gift.' We all stood in the downstairs hallway because Mom didn't want us all piling in on her, but she wanted her to know that we were there. When Mom went upstairs, Mrs. Speer said, 'Now Ruthie, I've had such pleasure watching your family I want to give you my most precious possession'" It was the plaster model that the artist,

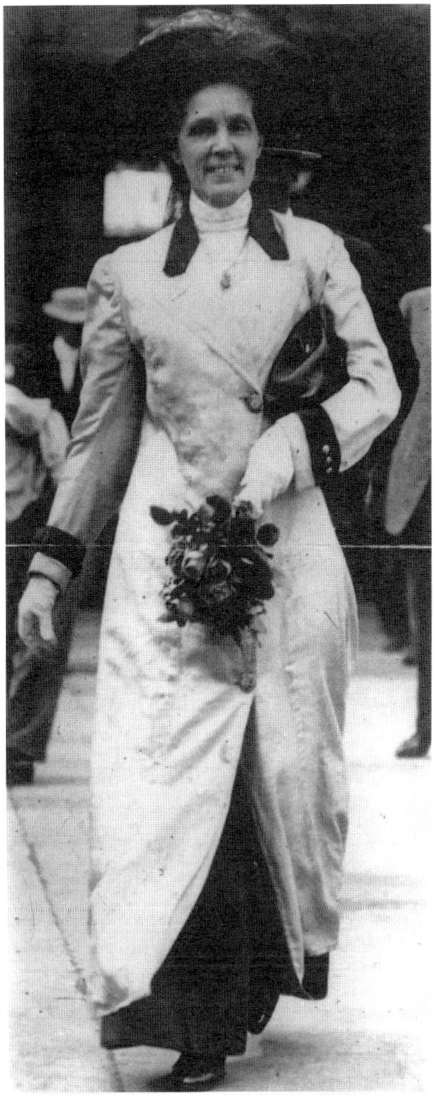

After her husband died, Kate Speer continued living in the house at 300 Humboldt Street. (Courtesy DPL Western History Department)

Mable Landrum Torrey, had used for the famous statue of Wynken, Blynken, and Nod at Washington Park and given to Kate Speer after Speer died. The Moores took the model home, but when they moved out of the house, Charley donated it to the Colorado Historical Society. The society thought the model a fake because the artist's name was erroneously spelled Mab<u>el</u> instead of Mab<u>le</u>. Through the persuasive efforts of W. "Bart" and W. M. B. "Bill" Berger, the society loaned it to the Children's Pavilion of the Denver Public Library where it is displayed for all to enjoy. Now the nonprofit organization Park People arranges to have bronzes made by well-known sculptor Frederik "Rik" Sargent to raise funds for its projects.

"Speer was one of Denver's most individualistic mayors," wrote Charles A. Johnson, author of *Denver's Mayor Speer*. "He never displayed personal flamboyance, but his plans for Denver had a certain majestic quality that will forever distinguish his administration."[24]

After Kate Speer died, Ralph and Patricia Ball lived there from 1958 to 1975. The Balls added a sunroom at the back. Their daughter, Jody, took over the carriage house when she was a teenager. "I used it as a sewing room and plastered the walls with collages of the glamorous covers from *Mademoiselle* and *Seventeen* magazines."

Then David D. and Aspenite Mary Stein Dominick moved in. Dominick, a duck hunter and avid bird-watcher, was president of the Denver Audubon Society. The nephew of U.S. Republican Senator Peter H. Dominick, he headed a major environmental federal agency for the Nixon administration. The Dominicks lived at 300 Humboldt with their three sons during the eighties.

28
320 HUMBOLDT STREET
Built: 1908
Architect: Maurice B. Biscoe

This has been the home of two architects involved with St. John's Episcopal Cathedral. That building, located at the crowded downtown site of 13th Avenue and Clarkson Street, is officially named St. John's Church in the Wilderness.

Architect Maurice B. Biscoe designed this house for his family while representing a firm of Boston architects when they were building the cathedral. Biscoe was associated with the Fisher, Fisher and Biscoe firm while in Denver, but always maintained his Boston affiliations. In about 1924 he returned to Massachusetts where he died in 1953.[25]

Besides the cathedral, Biscoe designed buildings at Colorado College in Colorado Springs, Colorado

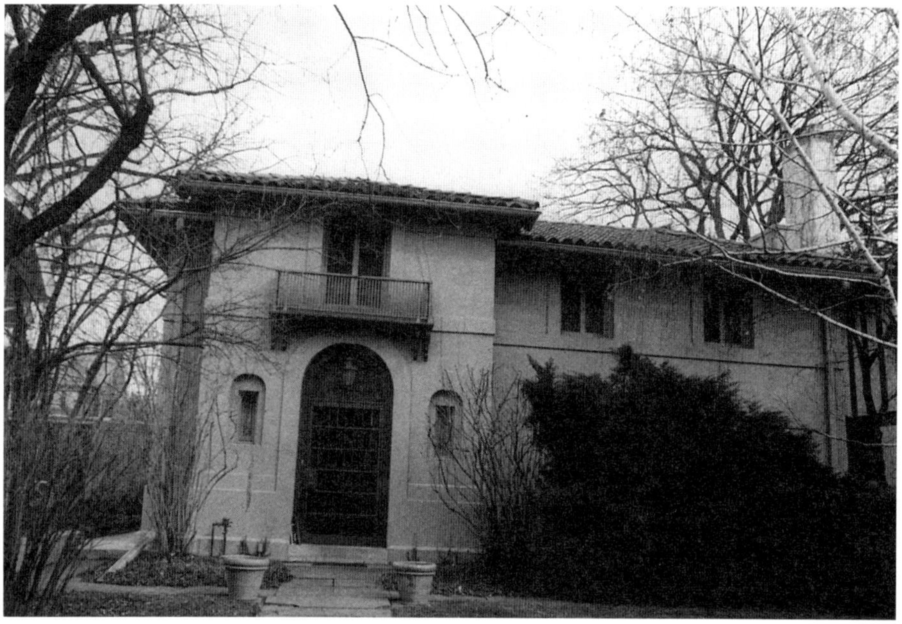

When architect Maurice Biscoe came to Denver to supervise the construction of St. John's Episcopal Cathedral, he built this Spanish house at 320 Humboldt Street for himself. (Courtesy Betsy and George Hoover)

General Hospital at 9th Avenue and Colorado Boulevard, and most of the buildings at Clayton College at Colorado Boulevard and 32nd Avenue (now Martin Luther King Boulevard). He was a founding member and first president of Denver's Cactus Club, often performing in theatrical productions at their outdoor stage, the Cactorium, on Lookout Mountain. He designed homes for several Cactus Club members.

Biscoe designed his own southwestern stucco home in an L-shape that frames a gracious patio off both the living room and dining room. The French doors off the living room led onto a distinctive arcaded porch. The tree-filled front lawn of the Spanish house is enclosed by a low, yellow stucco wall that matches the house. It was originally adorned with a garland of chains that was dismantled during the metal shortage of World War II. The brick garage off the alley was built in 1919. In 1924 a family room and master bedroom suite, designed by William E. and Arthur A. Fisher, were added to the rear of the house by Burdick Simons, who lived there for 28 years.

During the fifties, Dr. William Dickson Millett lived there with his wife, Alice, while raising four children, William, Jr. "Pete;" Katherine "Kim," who is married to Michael Nevin; Elizabeth (Mrs. John H. Cochran), and Margaret "Peggy" (Mrs. Arthur M. Zemach). Millett was the son of rancher and investor Daniel A. Millett and a brother of Helen (Mrs. Karl) Arndt. After graduating from Yale and serving for two years in the Army, he finished medical school and a residency in pathology at the University of Colorado, then practiced at St. Luke's Hospital.

During this time the house at 320 Humboldt Street had a temporary addition. A playhouse between the house and the garage was a stopover for Dr. Millett as he paused on his way to work for a "cup of tea" with his two youngest daughters, Elizabeth and Peggy.

Although the house had four bedrooms and a sleeping porch, the rooms were small, the children grew larger, and the Milletts moved to 180 Franklin Street. They sold 320 Humboldt Street in 1962 to the Calvin W. Kunz, Jr., family. Kunz was a part owner of the Denver Broncos until 1965, then became part owner of a short-lived soccer team, the Dynamos. He also served as president of the Highlander Boys. After his sports career he turned his energies to real estate investment. After a year of ill health he died at 63 in 1983.

In 1979 another architect, George Hoover, bought the house. He and his wife, Betsy, enclosed the patio porch and shut off the back stairway to add a powder room and enlarge both the kitchen and the small bedroom above. Hoover, like his early predecessor, Maurice Biscoe, was working on plans for St. John's Cathedral. Hoover, chairman of the Department of Architecture in the University of Colorado and a partner of the firm of AR7 Hoover Desmond Architects, served in 1998 as chairman of a committee to draft a master plan to remodel the beautiful historic cathedral at 13th and Clarkson.

29
330 HUMBOLDT STREET
Built: 1910
Architects: Sterner and Williamson

At 330 Humboldt, directly south of Lester Bridaham's house at 350 Humboldt Street, lawyer George Alan Smith built a small $2,000 brown brick Bungalow in 1910 designed by the firm of Sterner and Williamson.[26,27] The house has a low-pitched gabled roof, wide overhanging eaves, and a full-length front porch supported by square columns on a low brick wall. The two gabled dormers that interrupt the roofline, like the north wall of the house, have white wood trim that looks like timbering.

After the Smiths had lived there for six years, Lester B. Bridaham's widow, Alice, moved into the house with their only child, 18-year-old Lester, Jr. In 1920, Lester left to study at Cornell and the Massachusetts Institute of Technology, but after working briefly as a chemical engineer, he "was corrupted by art," as he said in a taped interview.[28] He attended night school at the Art Students' League in New York. "I consider my life was all wasted before I discovered art," he said. His artistic talents were supported by the Work Progress Administration Art Project during the Depression. "The WPA Art Project gave dignity and purpose to my life," he said.

After Lester had left for college, Alice married her neighbor from 301 Humboldt, Charles S. Haughwort, vice-president of the American National Bank. After Alice died, Charles continued to live at 330 Humboldt until his death five years later. Charles left his entire estate to his stepson, Lester Bridaham, Jr.

Lester Bridaham's widow, and later his son, lived in this house at 330 Humboldt Street.

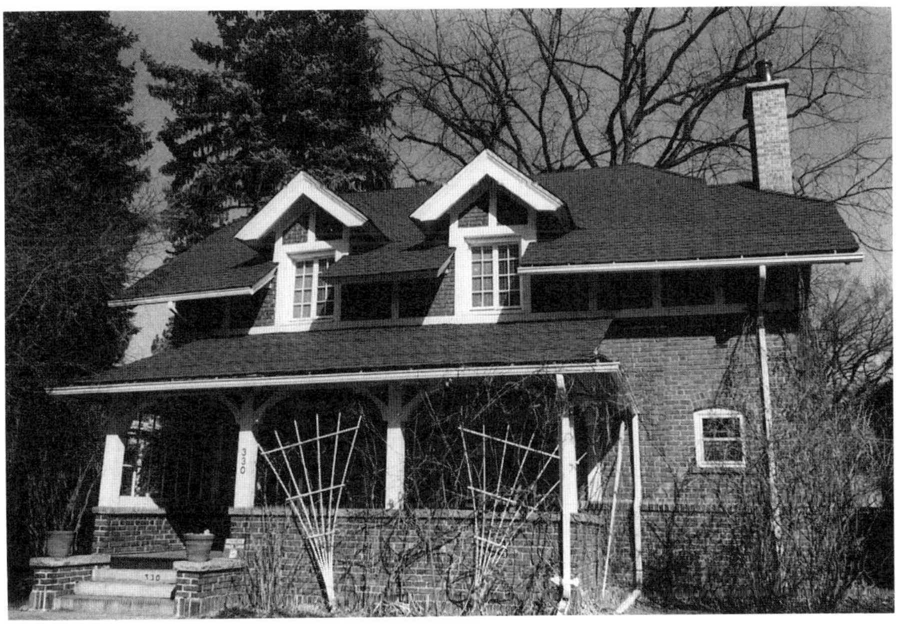

Bridaham returned to the house with his wife, Dorothy, and daughter, Vivian, and lived there for the next two decades. He taught painting in the public schools, but was most proud of the fact that five of his prints were accepted by the Victoria and Albert Museum in London as part of their permanent collection. Lester Bridaham, Jr. retired in 1987 and moved to his daughter's home in Bozeman, Montana, where he died in 1992.

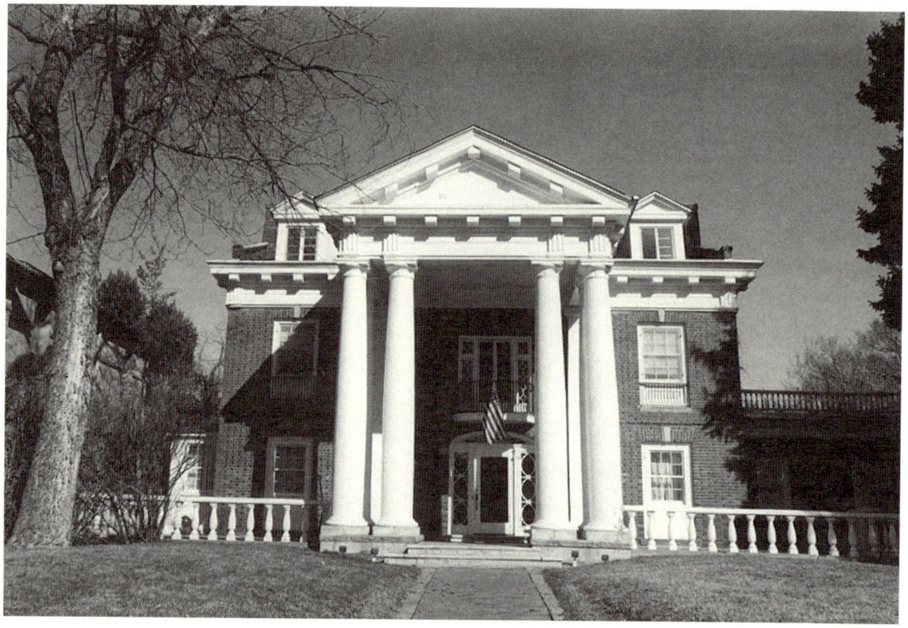

This grandiose Greek Revival house at 350 Humboldt is one of the earliest inPark Club Place. Interestingly, the doorway between the columns is slightly off center.

30
350 HUMBOLDT STREET
Built: 1905
Architects: Sterner and Williamson

At 350 Humboldt Street, Lester B. Bridaham, Sr., took out one of the first building permits in Park Club Place on March 1, 1904, for a three-story, red brick Greek Revival house. Architects Sterner and Williamson designed an entrance portico with a triangular pediment and four dramatic, two-story, white Doric columns. The starkly symmetrical house is approached by a long, straight brick walkway, but interestingly, the front door and window above are slightly to the right of center. Two steps lead to a wide, open balustraded front porch, which is echoed on the balcony above the addition to the south. The house is set back on the lot to leave a spacious front lawn. The surrounding wrought-iron fence, separated by brick piers, lends grandeur to the property.

"During the forties, that front lawn was a great place to play Kick the Can with Tom Simons and Joan and Patsy Prey (Tanner)," said Gerald Moore, who grew up at 369 Humboldt Street.

Born in Pennsylvania in 1872, Bridaham came to Denver in 1896. With his experience working in a pharmacy since the age of 16, he formed a partnership with druggist Frank J. Quereau, who lived at 379 Marion Street. It soon became "the largest wholesale and jobbing drug house between the Missouri River and the Pacific coast," said Thomas Ferril in *Sketches of Colorado*.

Community-minded, Bridaham became a director of both the Associated Charities Society and the Chamber of Commerce. He was well known as a philanthropist and was a popular and entertaining social figure, serving as vice-president of the Denver Country Club at one time.

"There are not many people who would not exchange places with Lester B. Bridaham. . . . He has grown to a position which is "out of sight," as the saying goes, and—well, he's a "corker" and he plays such a game of golf! Oh, he's just about right, Bridaham is," wrote B. F. White in his 1904 *Representative Men of the West in Caricature*.

In 1912, Bridaham's brilliant success was curtailed by business losses. He sold his stock in the drug company, his home at 350 Humboldt, and his automobile. His occasional melancholy episodes ended abruptly at 7 A.M. on October 9 when he went to a friend's office building at 16th and California to make a dramatic six-story somersaulting leap to the courtyard below. Claude Boettcher said, "this unfortunate end is regrettable for he was one of the most likable men in the business and social circles," reported the October 19, 1912, *Denver Republican*.

The house was then occupied by James Quigg Newton, a prominent dealer in municipal and corporate securities. Newton was the first chairman of the Denver Housing Authority, established in 1938. He was also the father of J. Quigg Newton, Jr., mayor of Denver from 1948 to 1955, who spent his first four years in this house.

A brick sunroom was added in 1917. By 1920, Frank C. Cullen, president of the Automobile Sales Corporation, was living there with his wife Gertrude; his brother Neal K.; and his niece, Marion Warfield.[29]

Neal married Olga Lakusta, daughter of the elegant, wealthy Russian lawyer Nicholas Lakusta and his wife, Clara. The Lakustas occupied the house for the next four decades. In 1960, Mrs. Lakusta inherited a large estate worth $1.6 million from her sister, Mrs. Louis J. Sauer, who had visited them often during her last few years. The Sauers were original landowners of a lot in Park Lane Square.

During the 1990s, contractor Charles Jordy moved into 350 Humboldt and renovated the house, despite unfortunate episodes of repeated vandalism during the process. In October 1998 he informed the neighbors by letter that he had "oil poured on my back terrace furniture, obscene remarks carved into my car, and damage to the vehicles in my yard." The vandals were never apprehended.

31
335 HUMBOLDT STREET
Built: 1937
Designer: Writer Brothers, Inc.

A much respected and formidable woman lived at 335 Humboldt Street during the fifties and sixties. The granddaughter of Senator and Mrs. Nathaniel P. Hill and William Bart Berger, Charlotte (Mrs. Alexander) Barbour showed a special fondness for both plants and animals. "Her love of Nature . . . was deep and compassionate," wrote Childe Herald. "Those mountains, the flowers, the animals, the birds, were intimate companions."[30] She donated generously to both the Denver Botanic Gardens and the Dumb Friends League.

Her father, Charles Bart Berger, died before she was born, and much of her childhood was spent in the mountains with her grandmother (Margaret Kountze Berger) at the Berger estate in Estabrook, near Bailey, Colorado.

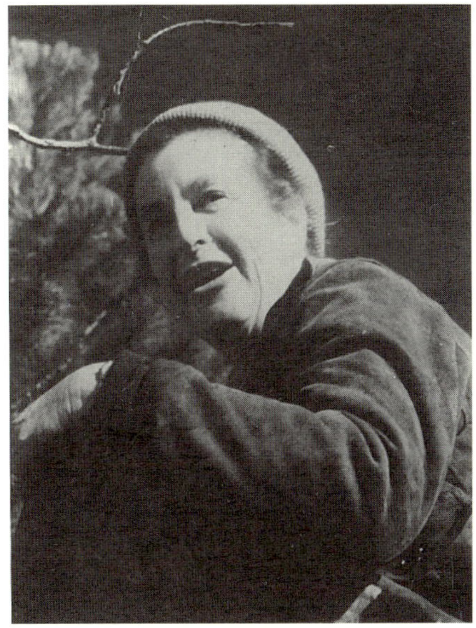

Gardening was a passion of the formidable Charlotte Berger (Mrs. Alexander) Barbour, who lived at 335 Humboldt Street. (Courtesy Denver Botanic Gardens)

Her love of animals was a priority. Once, when Robert A. and "Marge" Priester went out of town, they asked Charlotte Barbour to keep their dog for them. Barbara (Mrs. Field) Benton told the story: "A dog who stayed at Mrs. Barbour's gets ground beef to eat. While they were away the Priesters' son would go over to play with his dog and be informed, 'He's getting ready for lunch,' or 'He's gone to bed.'" The frustrated boy would have to retreat in disappointment.

When pediatrician James E. Russell, Jr., and his wife, who owned the house to the north, 345 Humboldt, retired to Arizona, they rented their house. One day Charlotte knocked on the tenants' door. Their dog had spent all day yapping in anguish because he was shut into a small doghouse between the two houses. Charlotte objected strenuously to their treatment of the dog and was sternly told to mind her own business. She did. She called the Russells, found she could purchase the house, then demolished it and planted a vegetable garden on the site.[31] When she died, Charlotte Barbour left $1 million to the Dumb Friends League.

The first occupants of the house had been Dr. and Mrs. Duval Prey. Their daughter, Patsy (Mrs. Ira) Tanner, said, "The neighborhood was fun. I used to play with the (Robert) Stearns girls [at 319 Lafayette] and swim at the Lowes' swimming pool [at 135 Humboldt]. That was our country club."

Dennis and Betty Lynn Jackson bought the home in 1972. Having rented 401 Humboldt from journalist Robert and playwright Mary Coyle Chase, they had their eye on this house. Betty Lynn heard about it while helping start the Junior Board of the Dumb Friends League with benefactor Charlotte Barbour. "We used to raise money with fashion shows sponsored by Montaldos. Their models would parade the ramp, each with a well-groomed, stylishly dressed dog from the Dumb Friends League," she said.

Dennis Jackson, a lawyer with Holland and Hart, a mountain climber of the 100 highest peaks in Colorado, and an avid gardener, was delighted with the two lots to the north and planted 11 fruit trees there before they moved in. "We had a bumper crop in 1998," Betty Lynn said. Now he has corn, okra, artichokes, three types of red raspberries, yellow raspberries, and blackberries."

The symmetrical, two-story, red brick house was originally built with a two-car attached garage and three-quarter basement by the Writer Brothers in 1936 for a cost of $15,000. On either side of the arched entryway are two large bay multipane windows.

The Jacksons water-blasted the white paint off the brick walls and added a short serpentine wall in front of the garden. The entrance is defined by a short, curved brick wall near the sidewalk with a planted pedestal urn. Two large urns flank the entrance.

32
369 HUMBOLDT STREET
Built: 1922
Architect:
Merrill Hoyt

"I've lived in this house for 70 years," said Dorothy Moore Pate in the year 2000. She moved to 369 Humboldt Street when she married John Crary Moore, who managed his father's H. W. Moore Equipment Company until his death in 1968. John Moore and his two brothers, Thomas of 301 Humboldt and Richard of 181 Franklin, were raised in the "House of 100 Candles" at 1410 High Street. The John Moores' two sons, Gerald W. and John, Jr., spent their childhood playing on the wide lawns of Humboldt Street.

The well-proportioned, two story, red brick Georgian Revival house, designed by Merrill Hoyt, was built for Edwin S. Kassler, Jr., son of prominent real estate investor Edwin S. Kassler of 300 Lafayette Street. The cornice of the medium-pitched, hipped roof displays a row of dentils. The symmetrical house has quoins of patterned brick, and

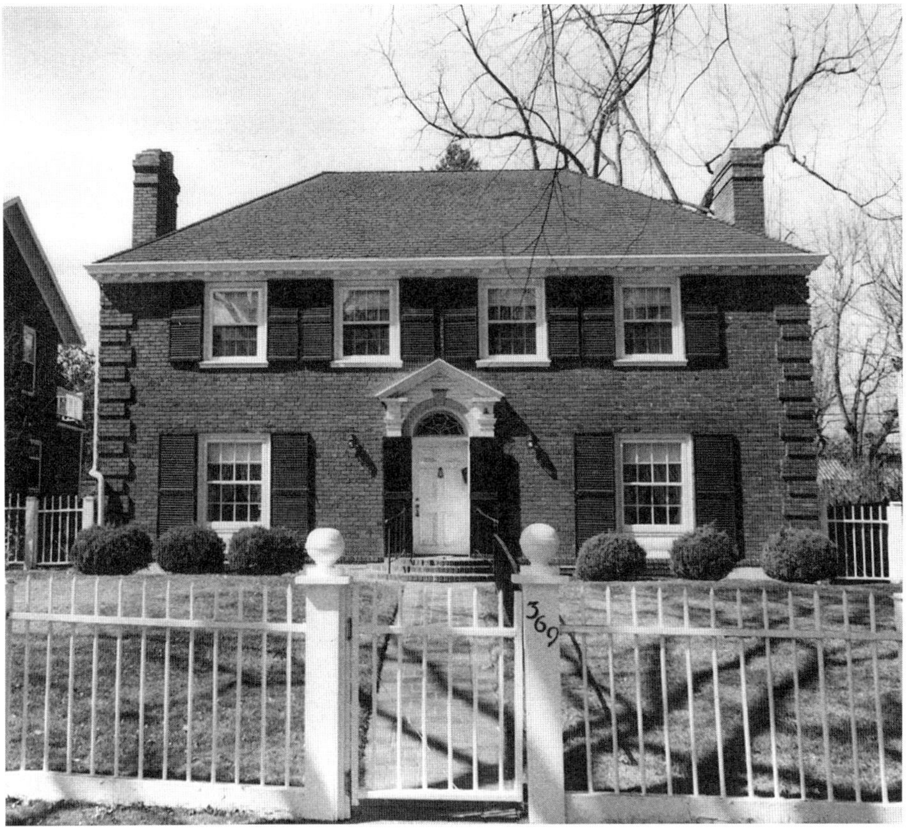

Dorothy Moore Pate has lived in this lovely Georgian Revival house at 369 Humboldt Street for over 70 years.

an arched leaded fanlight decorates the pedimented door surround.

In 1924, Kassler founded the farm mortgage banking business of Kassler and Company, later Kassler Mortgage Company. After he moved, while building a house at the newly developed Polo Club, he sold the house to the Moores. Dorothy Moore Pate said, "After several years Ed would meet me on the street and say, 'Want to sell the house back to me?'" When her physician, Dr. Frank McGlone, made house calls, he called it "one of the prettiest houses in Denver, inside and out."

Some time after Moore's early death, his widow married Richard E. Pate, Jr., owner of the Davis and Shaw furniture store. Pate moved into this house from his own lovely Georgian Revival house at 490 Race.

33
370 HUMBOLDT STREET
Built: 1907
Architects: Fisher and Fisher

This house was the headquarters of a bantam cock-fighting business in the early part of the century. Pioneer Colorado attorney Bethuel Webster engaged architects William and Arthur Fisher to build the house, and he lived there with his family until 1911 when he built the house at 140 Humboldt Street. His namesake son, called Beth, and Beth's friend, Bruce Tidwell of 315 Humboldt, jointly owned an Irish Gray bantam fighting cock. "They would ride their bicycles from 3rd and Humboldt to 2123 Downing to put on some handsome cock fights," reported the *Rocky Mountain Herald* on August 16, 1952. "Beth, looking for knockouts rather than kills, had humanely rigged up tiny boxing gloves to fit the spurs of the cocks." Beth later moved to New York City and became president of the New York Bar Association.

His father, Bethuel, had arrived from Pennsylvania in 1876 "at the age of five or six" with his father, Grove, a descendant of John Webster, fifth colonial governor of

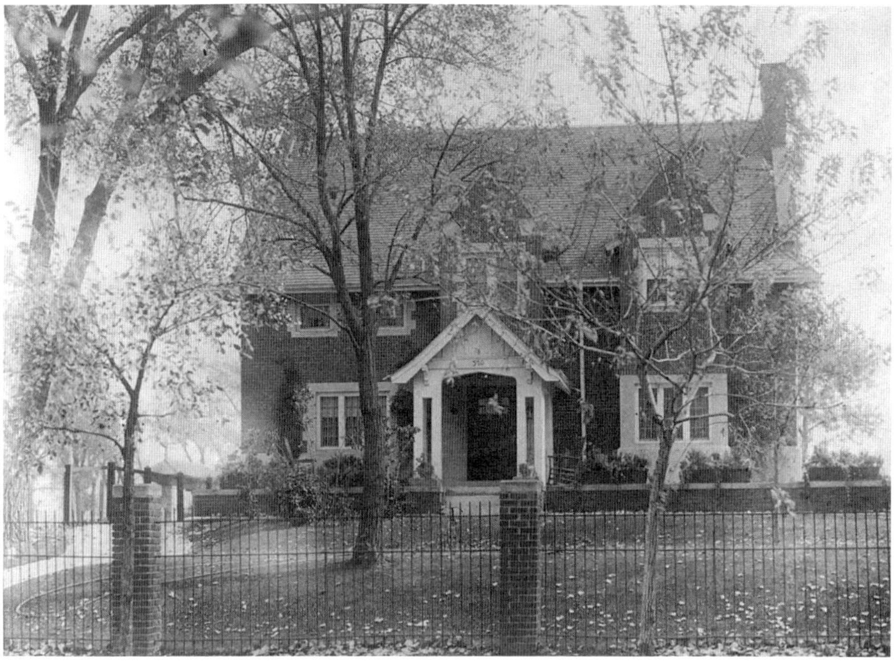

[ABOVE]: *For five decades the John Kennedy, Jr., family lived in this Fisher-designed 1907 house at 370 Humboldt Street. (Courtesy Jane Kennedy Garnsey O'Donnell)*
[BELOW]: *Like many houses early in the century, the Kennedys raised chickens in their backyard. (Courtesy Jane Kennedy Garnsey O'Donnell)*

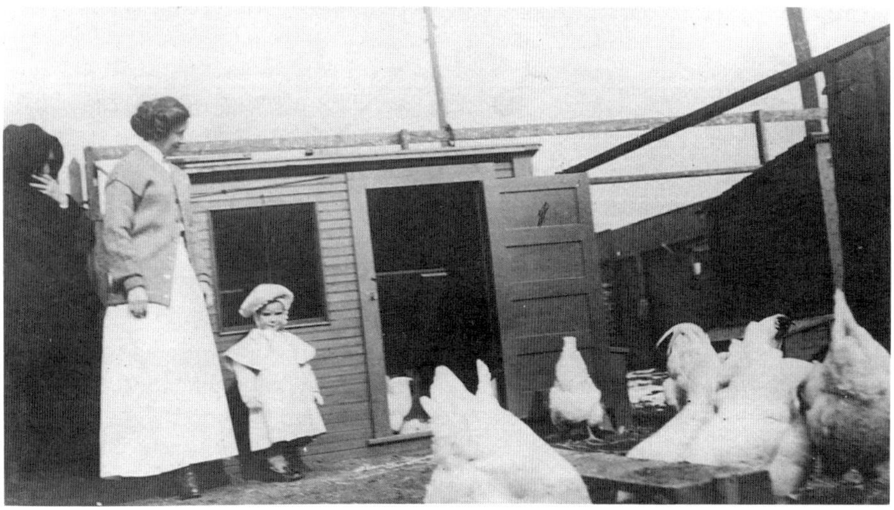

Connecticut. Bethuel, Sr., "attended Denver High School and graduated in the first law class at the University of Colorado at Boulder in 1893."[32]

Because he arrived in 1876 before statehood, he was known as a "Son of Colorado."

Fisher designed a two-story brick house with a steeply-pitched side gable. Two gabled dormers with side walls break the front roofline, each with two double-hung sash windows. The pedimented entry porch is supported by paired square columns. On either side of the entrance are strips of three multi-pane sash windows.

In 1912, John M. Kennedy, Jr., moved there with his wife and three children. Like most families of that era, the Kennedys built a chicken house in back. Apparently Kennedy dreaded going outdoors in the freezing cold at 5 A.M. to let the chickens out, so he rigged a pulley system from the door of the chicken coop to his daughter Jane's bathroom. "With a simple tug he could let the chickens out all over the yard, then go back to bed," said Jane Kennedy Garnsey O'Donnell. Eventually the chicken house was made into an art studio for Jane, who had majored in art at Vassar College. Later she lived in the house with her husband, Walter Garnsey, and their children until the 1960s. Garnsey was from Greeley, but after an eastern education at

Phillips Exeter Academy and Yale University, he moved to Denver and became president of the Stokes Canning Company.

Onetime chairman of major funds for the Republican Party and ambassador to Lesotho, Africa, Keith Brown; his wife, Carol; and their four children lived there during the late fifties and sixties.

While Pam and Lucien Wulsin, chairman of Baldwin United, lived there from 1975 to 1987, they painted the house, landscaped, and put a breakfast room on the back.

In 1998 the Bryan Tontons remodeled the house with a large addition on the back and a garage off the alley where the Kennedys had raised their chickens. The side driveway and curb cut were filled in and grassed for a large front lawn, as recommended by the Landmark Committee's *Design Guidelines*.

34
375 HUMBOLDT STREET
Built: 1922
Architects:
Merrill and Burnham Hoyt

This beige stucco Italian Colonial Revival house is a design of the Hoyt brothers early in their partnership, established in 1919. Rounded arches frame the windows and the simple entrance door. A terra-cotta medallion is mounted above. The east bedroom opens onto a wrought-iron balcony. The house was built for Weir Orford Merryweather, secretary-treasurer of the Salt Creek Oil Company. For four years this was the home of his daughter, Anne (Mrs. Edward B. Close, Jr.).

For almost 40 years the house was occupied by Olga and Virgil L. "Deke" Board, an electrical engineer, who helped form the Public Service Company of Colorado and served as the general superintendent. He was a loyal member of the Church of the Ascension at 6th Avenue and Gilpin Street.

When Alison and Bruce Stocks bought the house, they built an addition using the original 1929 plans drawn by Burnham Hoyt. The Landmark Committee approved this addition, and a sunroom, a kitchen, an upstairs bedroom and bath were added in 1995. "I think they did a particularly nice job with the addition," said close neighbor to the south Dorothy (Mrs. Richard) Pate.

A large, rare copper beech tree shades the front of the house. "We were told it was flown in from Kew Gardens in London. There are only three of them in Denver, I believe," said Alison. "People come here to measure it and study it."

The house at 375 Humboldt Street was designed by the Hoyts soon after Burnham joined the firm of his brother, Merrill. The copper beech tree is rare.

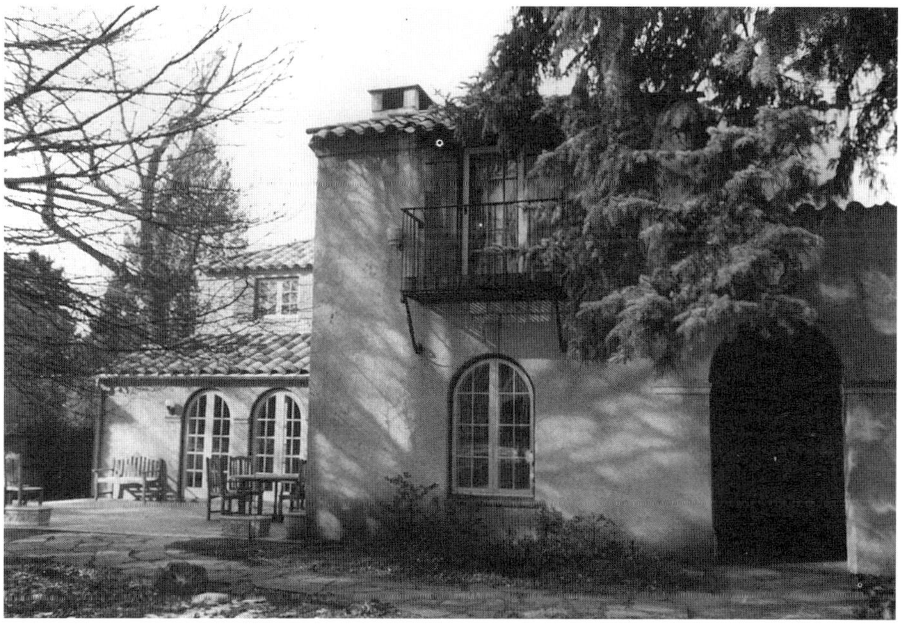

TOUR 2: COUNTRY CLUB PLACE

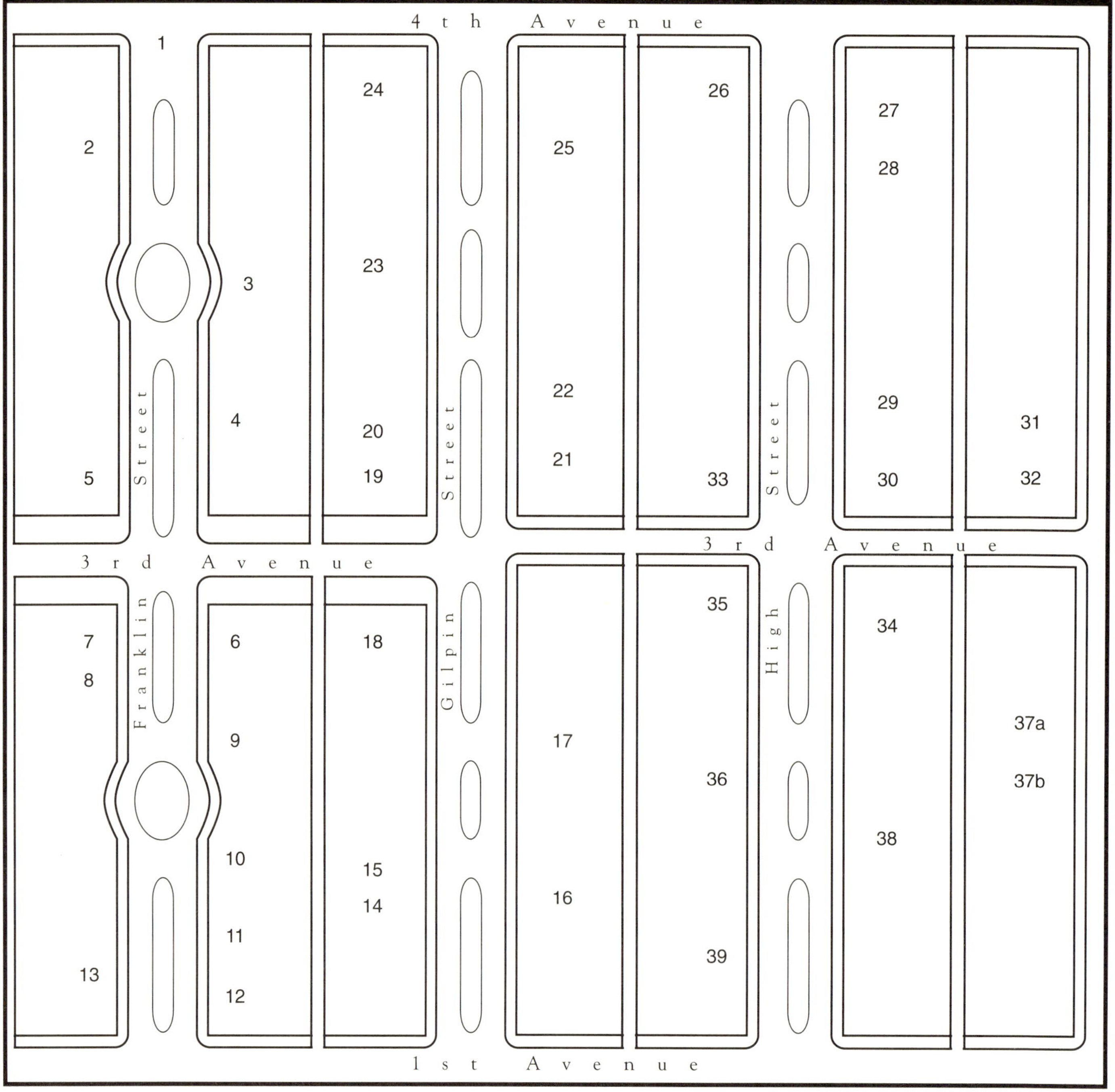

TOUR #2

1 Gates and tree
2 381 Franklin Street*
3 350 Franklin Street
4 314 Franklin Street*
5 305 Franklin Street*
6 180 Franklin Street*
7 181 Franklin Street*
8 171 Franklin Street*
9 160 Franklin Street*
10 120 Franklin Street*
11 110 Franklin Street*
12 100 Franklin Street*
13 103 and 109 Franklin Street*
14 111 Gilpin Street*
15 141 Gilpin Street*
16 128 Gilpin Street*
17 170 Gilpin Street*
18 1640 East 3rd Avenue*
19 1625East 3rd Avenue*
20 323 Gilpin Street*
21 300 Gilpin Street*
22 330 Gilpin Street*
23 355 Gilpin Street*
24 385 Gilpin Street*
25 380 GilpinStreet*
26 399 High Street*
27 380 High Street*
28 360 High Street*
29 320 High Street*
30 300 High Street*
31 310 High Street
32 200 High Street†
33 301 High Street*
34 190 High Street*
35 195 High Street*
36 149 High Street*
37 170 and 180 High Street†
38 140 High Street*
39 101 High Street*

* Buildings which contributed to the character of the neighborhood, resulting in listing as a Historic District in the National Register of Historic Places in 1979.

† Modern buildings compatible with the character of the District.

[Opposite Page]
The tour of Country Club Place begins at the Spanish gate at 4th Avenue and Franklin Street and includes Gilpin and High Streets.

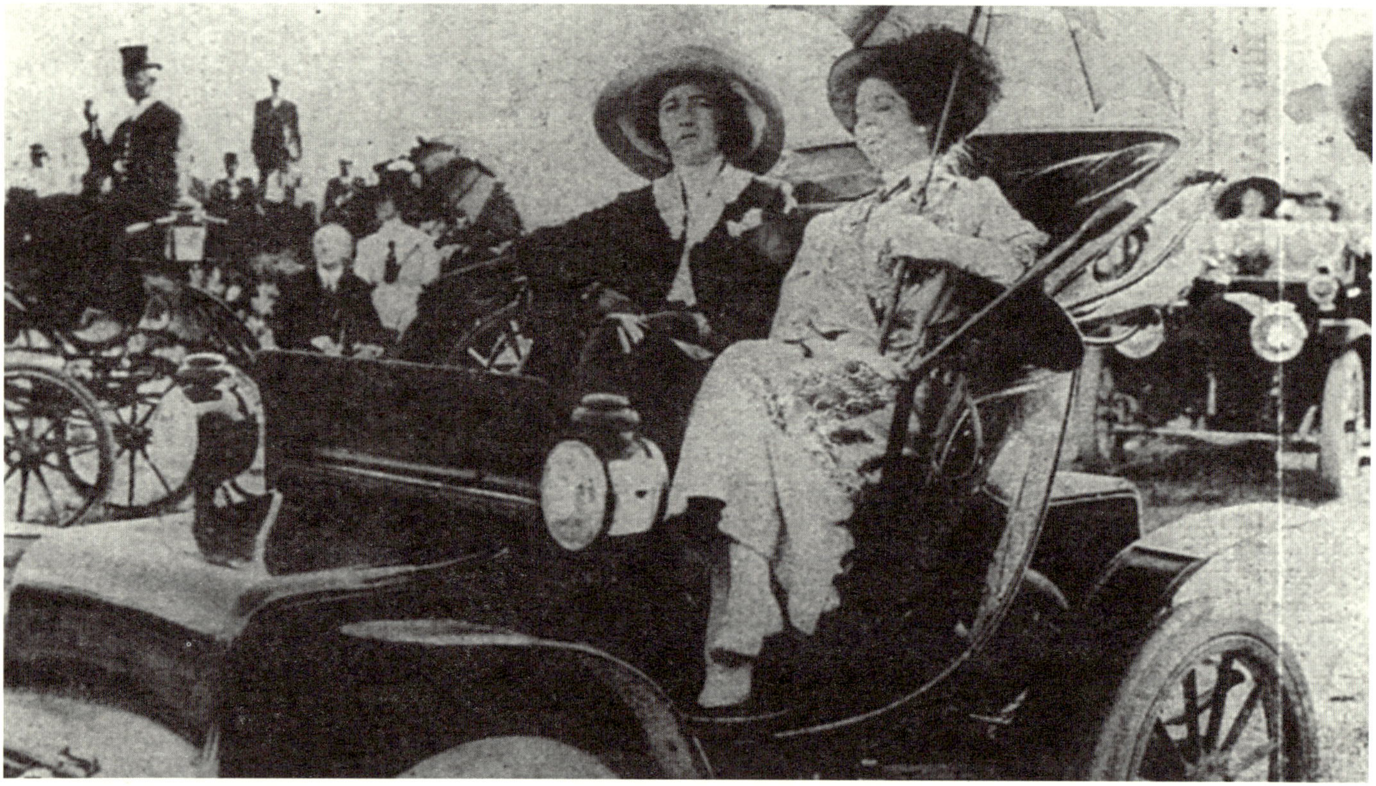

Members were driven to the Denver Country Club in carriages, with and without horses. Mrs. Raymond Sargeant arrived from 181 Franklin Street. (Courtesy DPL Western History Department)

~ Tour 2 ~

1
ENTRANCE GATES
Built: 1903
Architect: William Ellsworth Fisher

When the Fourth Avenue Realty Company bought 240 acres of John Jacob Riethmann's wheat farm in August 1902, they planned to build the Denver Country Club, but reserve 40 acres for residential development. Before putting residential lots on the market, the realtors retained architect William Ellsworth Fisher to plat the area into three wide streets rather than the four streets included in the neighboring western subdivision, Park Club Place. Each street would have a parkway down the center, and each would have a distinctive entrance gate on 4th Avenue. The most elaborate of these gates was built on Franklin Street, the original entryway from 4th Avenue through the residential area to the Denver Country Club. The entrance was changed to Gilpin Street in 1957.

The proposed plans for these gates were described in the August 6, 1903, *Denver Times*: "From the top of each gate the structure comes to a gradual incline, until a four-foot brick wall is reached, which extends all around the addition. The gateways have drinking fountains, upon each side of which is a niche containing statuary. The gates, when constructed, will be the fanciest things of the kind in the country." These proposed plans were not implemented, nor are they included in the collection of Fisher papers in the Denver Public Library Western History Department.

The signature Franklin Street gate spans the whole street. A 10-by-24-foot wooden platform with a sloping, tiled hipped roof with exposed rafters covers the entrance. Supporting this are two large, square, paneled stone columns that connect on either side to Mission-style arches over each of the sidewalks. Often called the "Spanish Gates," these form an appropriate setting for the many Mediterranean-

The entrance parkway along Franklin Street to the Denver Country Club was marked with Mediterranean entrance gates designed by William Ellsworth Fisher.

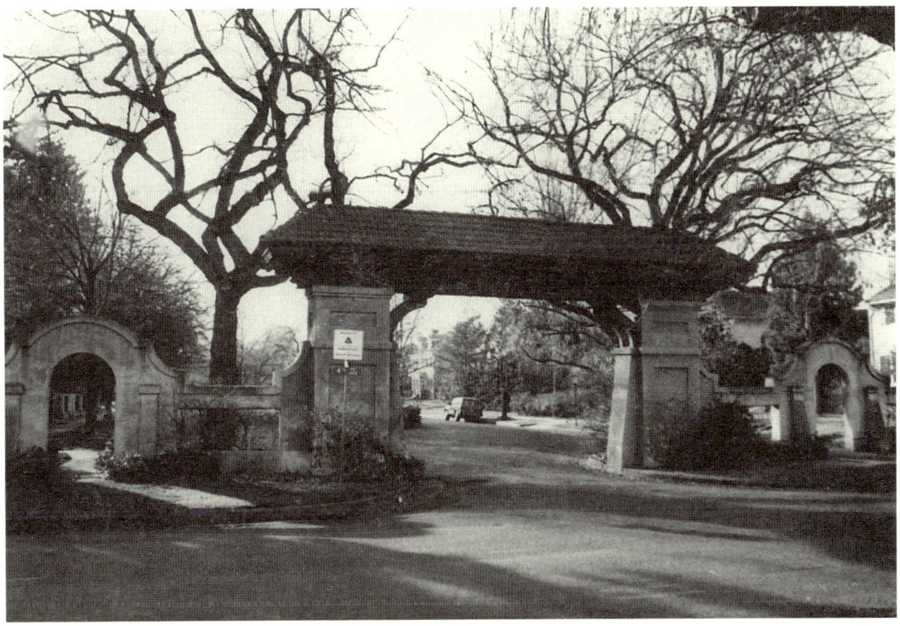

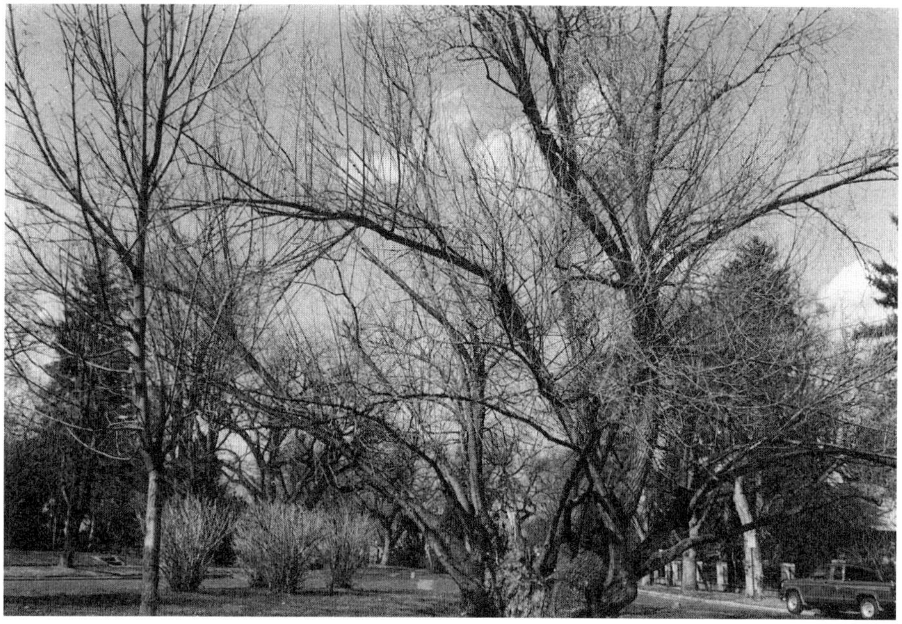

A linden tree on Franklin Street Parkway, has entertained generations of neighborhood children. The neighbors protested when the City wanted to remove the sickly tree, so gangrenous limbs are chopped off periodically.

style houses designed by the Fishers as well as other prominent architects. The similar gates at Gilpin and High Streets do not cover the whole street but stand as pillars on each side, connecting with the sidewalk arches. The original four-foot wall along 4th Avenue connecting these gates has been broken up and replaced with other materials by individual home owners.

Within the Franklin Street median is a historic old linden tree. During the 1970s the City wanted to destroy it because it became gangrenous. However, the neighbors made such a protest that it is still there, with more limbs amputated each year.

"The kids would meet and picnic there. It was so big and full that children could play and hide in it," Bobby Benton said. "That tree is a real landmark." "It's one of the few trees around we could climb," said Elizabeth Millett (Cochran), who grew up in the neighborhood during the sixties.

2
381 FRANKLIN STREET
Built: 1922
Architect: unknown

The $18,000 house built for Guilford and Vera Jones[1] is a two-story, Mediterranean-style structure with arched windows and doorways both outside and inside the house. The windows, trimmed with wrought-iron balconets, have fanlights in the arches that are echoed in the single garage door.

Living there briefly during the early thirties was George Hamlin Shaw, a candidate for the U.S. Senate in 1930. Shaw had moved west at the tender age of 13 because of allergies and worked on a ranch in Oregon. After earning his way through the University of Colorado undergraduate and law schools, he formed the firm of Lee, Shaw and McCreery. He married and had three children, Mary (Mrs. John Evans), Richard H., and Dora "Dody" (Mrs. Peter Neidecker), who was born in the house.

For almost four decades an honorary officer of the Most Excellent Order of the British Empire resided in this house. Judge Eliot Watrous was a prominent Denver International lawyer and former French consul when he received this award from Queen Elizabeth. Watrous, a Yale Law School graduate, had practiced international law in Paris from

1926 to 1939.[2] Later he was president of the Denver branch of the English Speaking Union for eight years. He also received the rank of commander of the French Legion of Honor from the government of France.

In 1963, Field and Barbara "Bobby" Benton bought the house. "I had been to an estate sale after Judge Watrous died and fell in love with the house," Benton said. Benton served as a municipal judge from 1959 to 1962. He then returned to his law firm of Holland and Hart. In 1982 he was appointed judge of the Probate Court, a post he held until his retirement in 1995.

The Bentons landscaped their five lots with a patio and garden to the south, designed by landscape architects Elaine (Mrs. William Cable) Jackson and Gladys (Mrs. Richard) Kirk. They then closed off a little sunroom next to the patio. At the back of the house they paved the wide driveway between the alley and garage.

The two-car garage has one entrance on the east and one on the west for a very practical reason. From the east a narrow driveway runs north of the house to what looks like a one-car garage. Inside, there is another space with a garage door on the west leading to the alley. "During Prohibition, bootleggers would come up the little dirt alley in the dead of night and park in that garage to sell their wares," Benton said. Dody Neidecker confirmed this: "When my father was running for office, there was usually some form of liquor in the house," she said.

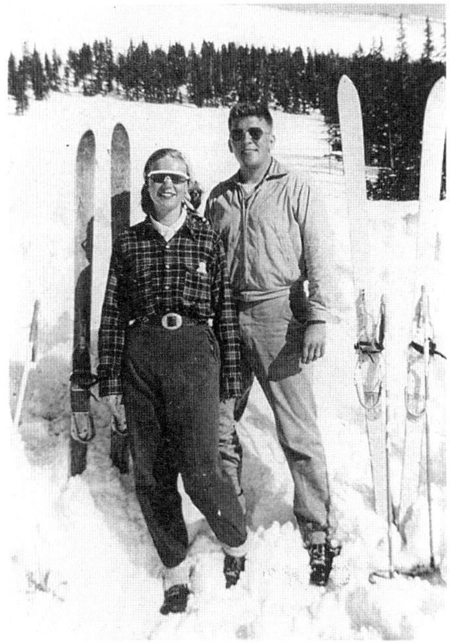

When Field and Bobby Benton bought the house at 381 Franklin in 1963, they were spending their weekends flying down the slopes on wooden skis. (Courtesy the Field Bentons)

This Mediterranean-style house at 381 Franklin Street actually has a two-car garage. There is another entrance off the alley.

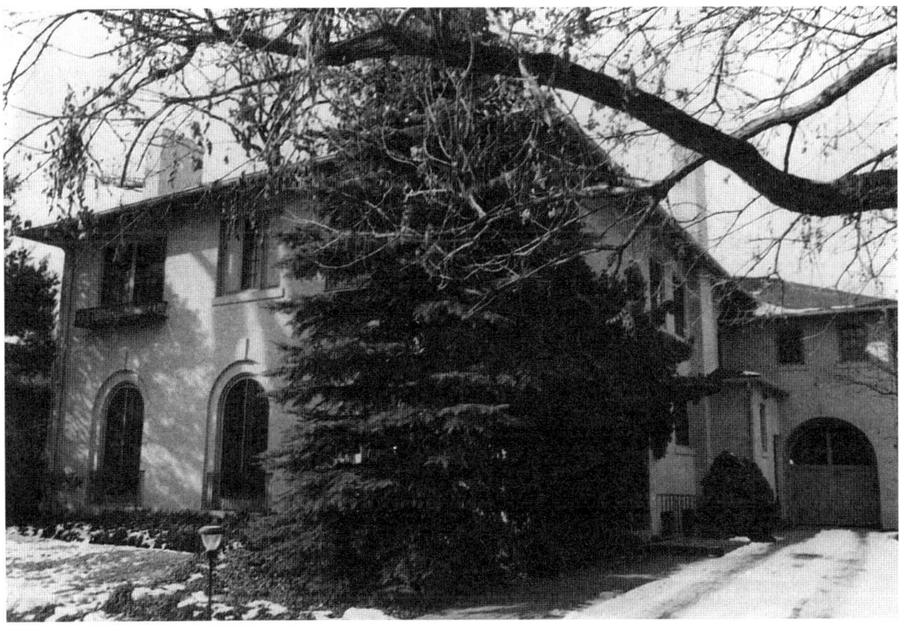

Franklin Street, being the original entryway to the Denver Country Club, has the most elaborate gate marking the 4th Avenue end of the spacious landscaped median. "We love this location," said Bobby Benton. "Turning through these gates is just like coming into a park."

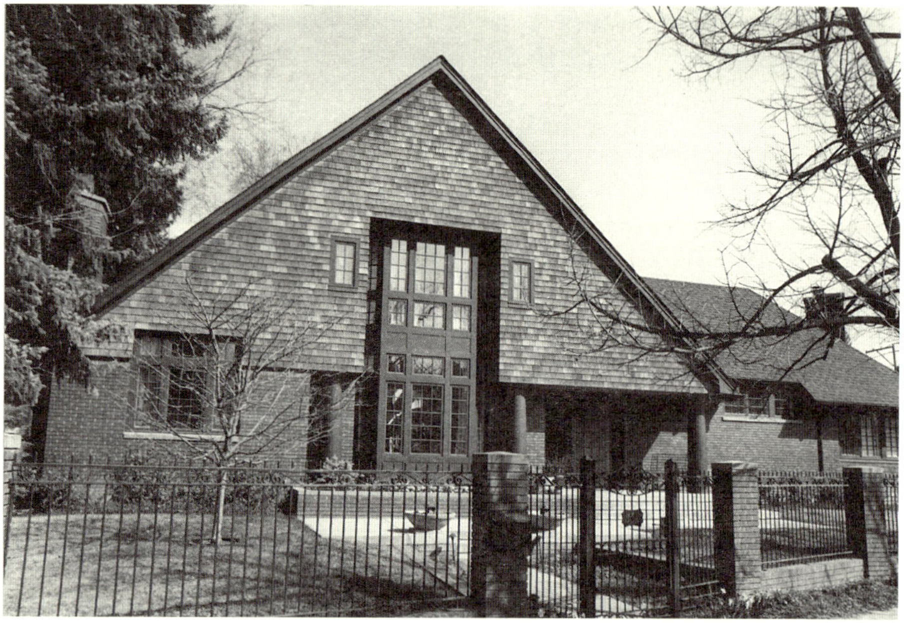

In 1995, this Shingle-style house, designed by David Tryba, replaced a one-story California Bungalow at 350 Franklin Street.

3
350 FRANKLIN STREET
Built:1917, architect unknown
Rebuilt: 1995
Architect: David Tryba

In 1917 a one-story California Bungalow with an open summer house and pergola was built at 350 Franklin Street by Milton Guldman. Guldman, who emigrated from Germany, was the vice-president of his brother Leopold's highly successful Golden Eagle Dry Goods Store. Leopold lived at the huge estate at 135 Humboldt.

In the 1930s the Edwin F. Cowperthwaites took possession when their son, Arthur T., married Blanche "Bammy" Taussig. The newlyweds moved into her family home at 305 Gilpin (later 1625 East 3rd Avenue). Shortly afterwards another son, George, married Blanche's sister, Josephine.

During the fifties and sixties the president of Gardner-Denver, civic leader Ben Essig lived at 350 Franklin with his wife, Ethlyn. Among his community activities, he served as president of the Denver Zoological Foundation, of the Manufacturers' Association of Colorado, and for three terms as the president of the Chamber of Commerce.[3] Essig died in 1972 at the age of 80.

During the 1990s the property was purchased by Barbara and David B. Sheldon, who tore down the house and rebuilt in 1995. The architect of this new chalet-like, 5,190-square-foot house was David Tryba. He planned the two-story multipane glass entry to be recessed into the dominant front shingled gable, which is flanked by two small windows on the second floor. To the south a porch is supported by two round columns. A see-through, wrought-iron gate protects the property. "He didn't want to duplicate another style in the Country Club district," said Barbara Sheldon, former board member of Historic Denver, Inc., and current board member of Colorado Preservation, Inc. "We had a certain plan of rooms that we wanted, and the house just formed. Tearing down the old white stucco house was not comfortable for me," she admitted. "We lost a lot of the original character of the house, but we consulted with many people and couldn't adjust the architecture to fit our floor plans."

Tryba admitted that the building is controversial. "I enjoy working in historic districts," he said. "There were some other Shingle-style houses down the block and we were trying to blend them with, but add some life to, the neighborhood."

"When we built, the architect talked with the Country Club Historic Neighborhood, Inc. [CCHN] Landmark Committee about our plans," said Barbara Sheldon. "We were out of the loop as we did not talk with them directly. We love the house, and I always wanted to live in this district. It has a feeling of space and trees, like out in the country where I was brought up, and it is still in the heart of the city."

A number of residents and architects have commented that the new house doesn't fit in with the neighborhood. Robert L. and Virginia Dean, across the street at 355 Franklin, were sad to see the little house go. "We used to watch our friends, the Essigs, having breakfast in the big front window every day, being served by a maid in white-aproned uniform—a bygone era," said Ginny nostalgically.

Mona Ferrugia was chairman of the CCHN Landmark Committee at that time. "I like the originality and think it adds variety and charm to the area," she said. "It's an example of what we would like to see in the neighborhood—good quality of contemporary design rather than replicas of the old traditional styles."

4
314 FRANKLIN STREET
Built: 1911
Architect: Glen W. Huntington

The gabled Tudor residence at 314 Franklin is a truly "Bosworth" house. The building permit issued to Helen R. Bosworth at 324 Franklin in 1911[4] was on land that was later incorporated into 314 Franklin Street, a house later occupied by the family of Helen S. and Robert G. Bosworth for five decades. The two families were not related to each other.

The first Helen Bosworth, at 324 Franklin, was married to Edwin M. Bosworth, president of Union Realty and Investment Company which traded stocks and bonds. When they left the little one-and-a-half-story house with the single-car brick garage in 1921, the owners of 314 Franklin snapped up the land and demolished the house to expand their own house to the north.

The first building permit for 314 Franklin had been issued in 1913 to Darius A. Barton,[5] secretary and treasurer of Home Savings and Trust Company. He built the Glen Wood

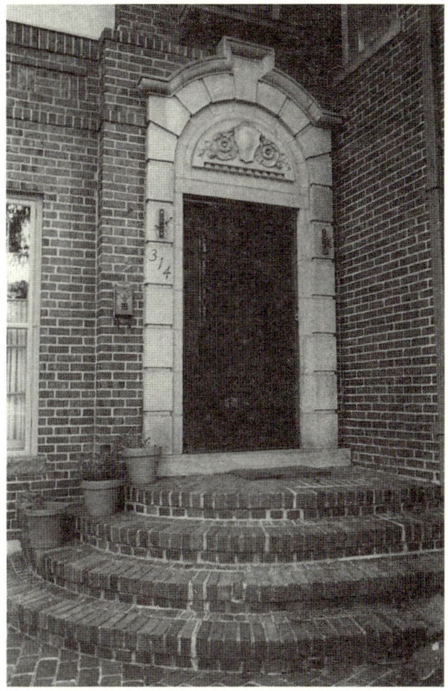

The Tudor Revival house at 314 Franklin Street was owned by two unrelated families named Bosworth.

Huntington-designed, $10,000, two-story, red brick house. The arched door surround of carved stone displays a floral design at the center. At the front of the house the balcony over the sunroom is protected by a low, solid-brick wall. Under the truncated front gable are two third-floor sash windows.

After a couple of years, Barton sold the house to Cassius A. Fisher, an eminent scientist and mining engineer. As a founder of the firm Fisher and Lowrie, he was internationally

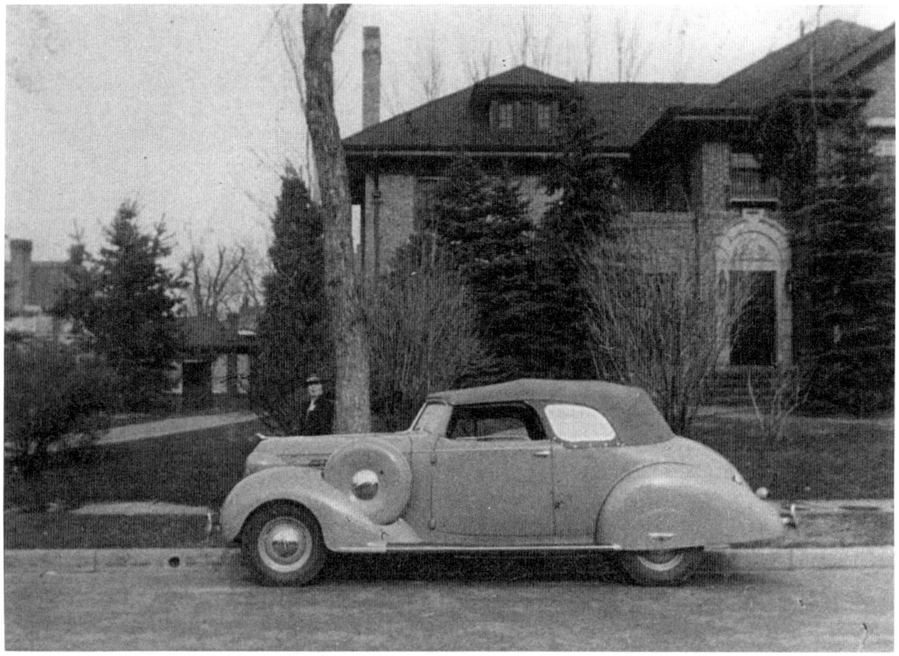

Robert G. Bosworth; his wife, Helen; and their three children lived at 314 Franklin Street in 1937. (Courtesy Barbara Bosworth Pilling)

known for his work in writings on mining and geology. For several years he worked for the U.S. government as assistant chief of the fuel section of the Geological Survey and was in charge of the U.S. Navy fuel expedition to Alaska in 1912. His social connections included the Denver Club as well as the Royal Society of London.

It was Fisher who incorporated the land at 324 Franklin Street into his own house. "When Fisher owned the house, he bought the little house to the north, tore it down, except for the garage, and expanded 314 with a beautiful library and gardens to the north, but he kept the garage," said subsequent owner Dr. Robert G. Bosworth, Jr. When the house was sold in 1998, the little brick garage was still there, perched next to the alley beside the larger two-car garage and dog run.

A few years after Cassius Fisher died of a heart attack in 1930, the house was bought by lawyer Robert G. and Helen S. Bosworth. Here they raised their children: Helene, Barbara, and Robert, Jr. The senior Bosworth was graduated from East High School, Princeton, and Harvard Law School before entering the firm of Pershing, Bosworth, Dick and Dawson. He belonged to both the Law Club and Bar Association, and was elected to the state Senate in 1939 where he was majority leader. He is remembered for his humor and wit. Known as "a very sharp man with a verse,"[6] his salient poems about fellow legislators are bound in a leather-covered book presented to him by his colleagues during his six-year term.

His histrionic talents were well used. The University Club's *Twelfth Night* production relied on Bosworth for much of the script. During the Cactus Club theatrical performances in the twenties, Bosworth was frequently on the rustic stage at the Cactorium in the woods of Lookout Mountain.

After his death in 1954 the house was occupied briefly before it was purchased by his son, Dr. Robert G. Bosworth, Jr., a physician in internal medicine who graduated from the University of Columbia College of Physicians and Surgeons. He, and his wife, Alice, lived there for another 30 years, bringing up their children Sally, Patricia, and Robert, III, along the spacious Franklin Street parkway before moving to 2115 East 4th Avenue. Dr. Bosworth followed in his father's footsteps presiding at the University Club

Twelfth Night performance from the musicians' loft of the College Room, garbed in the traditional crown and robes of the Mighty King.

During the eighties and nineties, Frank A. Kuegler, economist for the Colorado National Bank, lived at 314 Franklin with his wife, the former Monty Campbell, and their family.

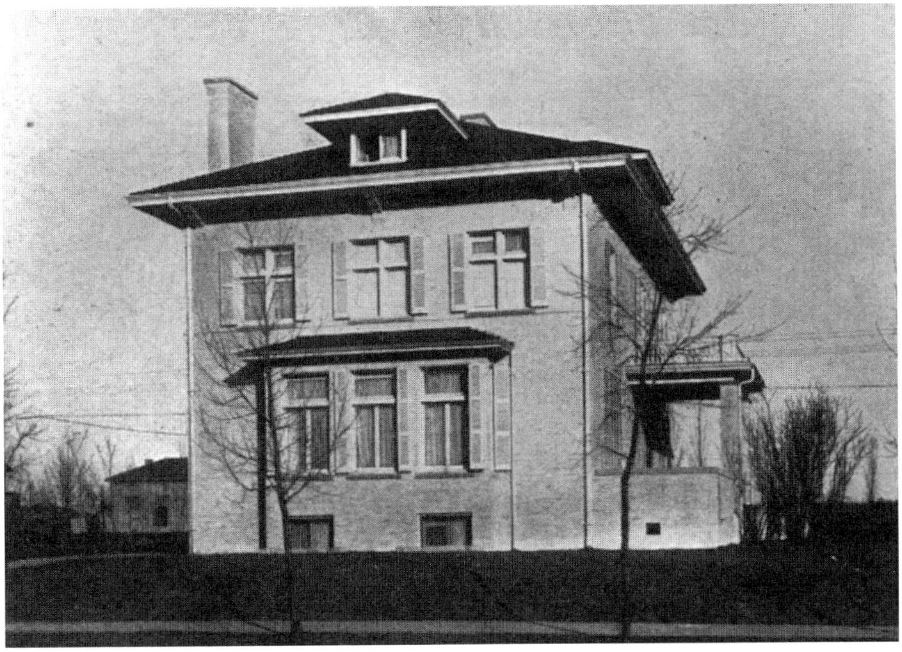

A large western wing has been added to this 1907 house at 305 Franklin Street. (From Denver Municipal Facts, courtesy DPL Western History Department)

5
305 FRANKLIN STREET
Built: 1909
Architect: unknown

A member of the Berger banking family lived in this house from 1951 to 1971. Merriam Bart Berger was the son of George Bart and Carrie Merriam Berger of 124 Lafayette Street. From this old Berger homestead on Lafayette, Merriam attended Corona School, Broadway Latin School, and East High School. The 1918 flu epidemic forced him to drop out of college. However, he followed the family tradition by joining the Colorado National Bank as a messenger boy in 1920 and rising to president in 1958.

Berger moved to 305 Franklin with his second wife, Elizabeth, daughter of Colorado Governor Alva B. Adams. Their son, W. Bart Berger, was raised there: "It was great growing up with that parkway in front. In those days 3rd and Franklin was a fairly lazy little intersection. Once, when a friend and I set off a pile of gunpowder with a lighted cigarette, the 20-foot-high flame hardly fazed the neighbors. It was high drama!. But the streets were so empty no one was hurt."

The big, brick, $7,000 Denver Square house was originally built for president of the Englewood Lumber and Coal Company William H. Endner. Under the wide, overhanging eaves was a decorative frieze. The sash windows are flush with the outside wall. A two-story addition to the west has its own double-door entrance, and above it double doors open from the master bedroom onto a balcony. The third-floor, hipped dormer is centered on the front facade.

6
180 FRANKLIN STREET
Built: 1907
Architect: Glen W. Huntington

Edward T. Wilson, president of Continental Oil Company, installed his own gas tank and pump beside the chauffeur's quarters in the garage

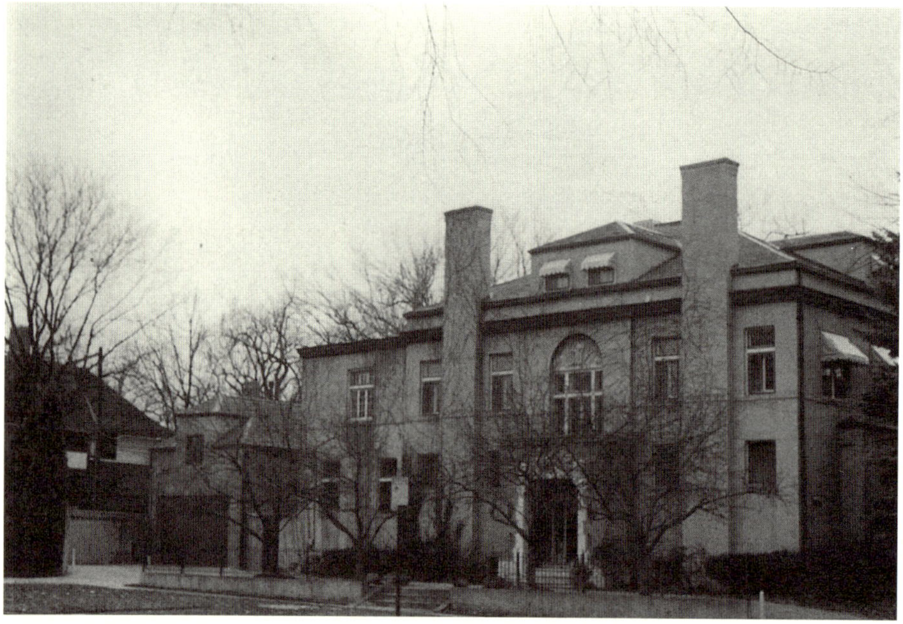

First owner of this 1907 house at 180 Franklin Street was Edward T. Wilson, first president of Continental Oil Company. The house was completely renovated between 1998 and 2000.

of his house at the corner of 3rd and Franklin. In 1907, when he moved into the newly built Italianate brick house, designed and partially built by Glen Wood Huntington, gas stations and mechanics were rare to nonexistent. For Wilson a motorcar was a necessity.

The family of seven, plus servants, occupied the 10 bedrooms, four-and-a-half baths, spacious living room, and pool room in the basement, complete with an indestructible old pool table and tall viewing chairs. "John Mitchell [his next-door neighbor] and I practically destroyed it, the way we attacked it," said Robert Bruce "Robbie" Wilson.

During construction the first occupant of the house appeared. Youngest son Robbie said, "One day the police discovered an escaped murderer living in the foundation. He thought the empty, unfinished basement was an ideal place to hide out from the cops."

In 1919 the Wilsons extended the library south with a small porch added to the west beyond French doors. Over the library addition a bedroom opened up onto a balcony next to a tall elm tree—an effective midnight escape route for adventurous teenagers.

During the twenties, Fisher and Fisher transformed the living room into an English drawing room. First they bricked up two small openings on either side of the fireplace facing north. The papered ceiling was replaced with a Wilderhope plaster ceiling and cornice. The fireplace mantel was faced with Antwerp Black Marble, and fine oak, linenfold panelling was installed on the walls.[7]

After Edward Wilson died, their son, Robert Wilson and his wife, Valentine, who had been living there, sold to the William D. Milletts in 1962. The elegant Tudor living room was a major attraction for meetings, musicals, and receptions. In 1964, when the Milletts took their four children on a grand tour of Europe, six-year-old Peggy, while visiting the sixteenth century great room in the royal palace of Henry VIII at Hampton Court, England, remarked, "This room looks just like our house." It was time to go home.

The Milletts added a patio to the south and revelled in the spaciousness of their new home, full of hidden nooks and crannies. "'Dan Fisher' [an imaginary character] lived in an extensive alcove under the eaves, reached through the back

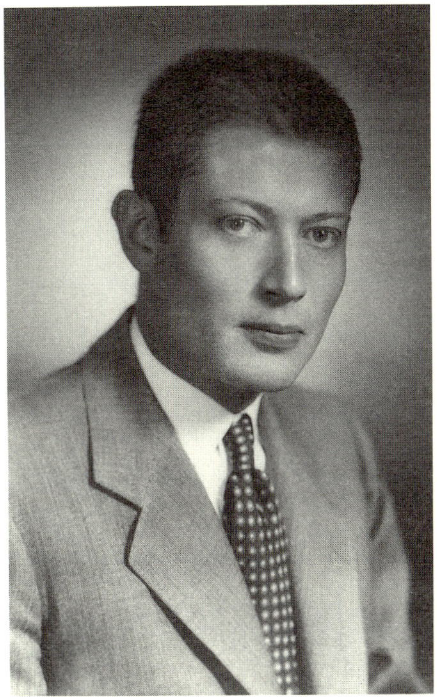

The William D. Milletts owned the house at 180 Franklin Street from 1962 until 1974. Millett was the chief pathologist at St. Luke's Hospital. (Courtesy Alice Millett Bakemeier)

door of a closet in one of the maids' rooms. "We were invited to tea parties there," added Elizabeth Millett (Cochran). Neighbor Jody Ball (Albrecht) remembers Kim's (Katherine's) "Leprechaun's Cave," a large closet off a third floor bedroom, lavishly furnished with an old mattress and a lamp for reading. "The door was only high enough for a leprechaun," said Peggy (Margaret Millett Zemach). In the basement, William "Pete" Millett, Jr., became something of a pool expert while Elizabeth entertained a healthy representation of her many friends around this irresistible attraction.

Dr. Millett, a pathologist at St. Luke's Hospital, was a devout churchman at St. John's Cathedral; a president of Protestant Episcopal Church Homes, Inc.; and a founder and president of the board of Spalding House, now Spalding Rehabilitation Hospital. When he died at the age of 49 in 1970 he was chief pathologist and president-elect of the medical staff at St. Luke's Hospital.

When artist Ramon Kelley bought the house in 1976, he immediately remodeled the chauffeur's quarters over the garage into an art studio, cutting a large window in the north wall. Two years previously, he had become the only Denverite voted to membership in the prestigious American Watercolor Society. Born in poverty in Cheyenne, Kelley had no formal art training until the 1950s after he finished a stint in the Navy. Since then, he has won several awards and has exhibited at the Canyon Road Gallery in Santa Fe, The Gallery in Palm Springs, and Gallery West in Denver.[8]

The house, bought in 1998 by the preservation-minded Warren and Denise Cohen, underwent extensive renovation. The magnificent oak-paneled, Fisher designed living room has been left intact, "but to let in more light, the original windows flanking the fireplace were opened and fitted with authentic lead glass by a specialist in Littleton," said Denise Cohen. The gas tank was removed and the garage remodeled and attached to the house. Walls were removed on the second floor to make a master suite. The basement is remodeled to include a dance floor with pool table, an exercise room, and a wine-tasting room off the wine cellar. "We want to have little dinner parties down there," Denise said. The house was completely rewired and replumbed.

7
181 FRANKLIN STREET
Built: 1907
Architect: unknown

A few years after stockbroker Raymond E. Sargeant arrived in Denver in 1903, he built one of the first houses in Country Club Place. His three children grew up amid wheat fields and vacant lots just one block from the Denver Country Club where Sargeant could easily duck over for a game of golf.

Born in Cleveland, Ohio, Sargeant went to Colorado Springs before coming to Denver to form the brokerage firm of Sargeant, (W. Oscar) Malo and Company, one of the first Denver members of the

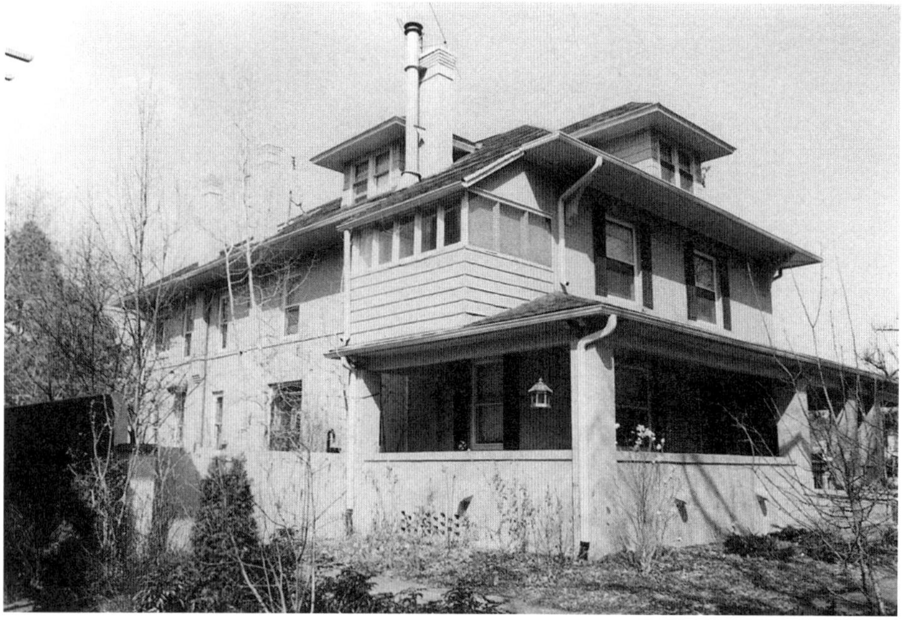

This large Foursquare house at 181 Franklin Street was built in 1907 by the Raymond Sargeants.

New York Stock Exchange. He and Malo managed one of the largest real estate transactions of the time, the purchase of the $2 million Equitable Building.

Charles M. "Charley" Moore told the story that "early each morning, Sargeant would read the paper and rock on his front porch, watching the trolley roll up 4th Avenue. He could see all the way to the end of the line at Clayton Street, and when it started back down 4th he would amble down Franklin Street to catch a ride downtown." Sargeant lived at 181 Franklin until failing health at the age of 73 led him to end it all in his study. His wife, Beatrice, lived there for another two years.

"We used to always go down to that house for a huge formal Sunday dinner. To my grandmother's dismay, my father used to snap the paper doily away from under the finger bowl without spilling a drop," said granddaughter City Councilwoman Polly Sargeant Flobeck. Flobeck's father, manager of Harris, Upham Company. Raymond, Jr., and his wife, Frances (Pyeatt), lived in the Country Club district at 2124 East 4th Avenue where they raised three children.

In 1957 the house was bought by Zina Minette "Zinny" (Spore) and her husband, Richard Merideth Moore, brother of Thomas Edgar and John Crary Moore at 301 and 369 Humboldt Street, respectively. Moore, a partner of George Bethune, opened a design and contemporary Swedish furniture store at 2412 East 3rd Avenue. The building, designed by Moore's brother, architect Tom Moore, "helped set the standard for unique retail stores in the early Cherry Creek North area," reported the *Denver Post* on July 30, 1998.

The house at 181 Franklin is a large Foursquare with seven bedrooms. The front of the wrap porch extends to make a porte cochere over the driveway leading to the garage. The driveway has since been removed and planted to make a fenced garden. The Moores' daughter, Meredeth "Merce" (Lea), described the classic long upstairs hallway with bedrooms off either side: "Ours was far enough away from Mother and Dad that we could talk across the hall," she said. "There was only one bath for all of us."

In 1967 the Moores moved their three children to Aspen where Richard bought the old railroad station for an interior design store, adding a small branch shop at the Hotel Jerome. The Moores returned to Denver in 1988 after he retired.

The owner of the house during the eighties was Craig Barnes, a congressional candidate and chairman of Common Cause.

8
171 FRANKLIN STREET
Built: 1906
Architect: Edwin H. Moorman

Another early house was built at 171 Franklin Street. Although a building permit was taken out by Emma S. Miller on November 26, 1906, the house may have been constructed earlier. The owner since 1987, Lorna Grindlay Moore, said, "The front porch was caving in on us. When we rebuilt it, we found some old yellow 1905 newspapers tucked in the cracks."

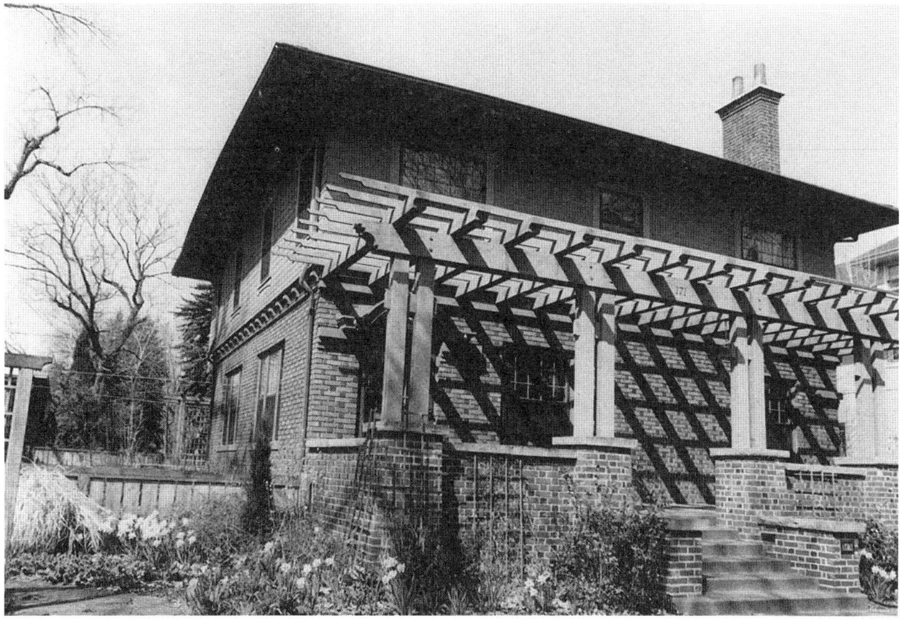

The walls of this 1906 Crafstman-like house at 171 Franklin Street are of Flemish-bond brickwork design.

The house, considered "neo-Craftsman," by architect Edward D. White, Jr., retains such elements of the Craftsman style as a wide full-length front porch supported by paired square columns on the low brick wall. Carved porch beams cast decorative shadows on the floor and walls, which are of Flemish-bond brickwork design (alternating headers and stretchers in each brick course, horizontally and vertically). The low-pitched, side-gabled roof has wide overhangs and exposed rafters.

The first occupants of this house were Claude and Honore Sachs, who first appear in the city directory in 1907. Sachs was owner and publisher of *The Mining Investor*, one of four such periodicals covering the all-important mining industry. In 1911 the Sachs built the house to the south, 165 Franklin Street.[9]

By 1910, Charles L. Wellington, general traffic manager of the Colorado and Southern Railroad, moved in with his wife, Martha. Born in East Cambridge, Massachusetts, Wellington gained much experience in railroading, in both Detroit and Chicago, before coming to Denver. He was well situated in Country Club Place to enjoy his hobbies of billiards and golf at the Denver Country Club.

The next owners were realtor-investor Alfred H. Parker; his wife, Edith; and their daughter, Ruth, a friend of Ruth Hollister (Mrs. Dudley Smith) who lived at 103 Franklin.[10] In 1927 they sold it to Frank and Katherine Hoart. Frank was a long time manager of the Brown Palace Hotel. The Hoarts sold a year later to lawyer Erl Ellis.

Florist Arthur Bush and his wife, Almeda, made this their home for three and a half decades. Bush worked for Daniels and Fisher before starting his own floral business at

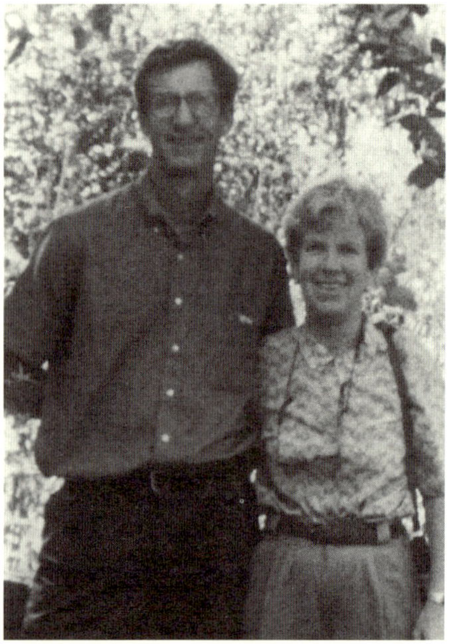

Lorna and William Moore took great care to restore Craftsman elements of the house at 171 Franklin Street when they purchased it in 1987. (Courtesy the William Moores)

6th Avenue and Marion Street. Almeda chaired the Denver Symphony Guild and was active in the Denver Lyric Opera Guild. A devout Christian Scientist, this dignified and gracious woman lived to the age of 90.

In 1987, when Lorna and William Moore bought this Bungalow, Lorna found it, "shall we say, underwhelming." The house was run-down and the shingles were painted white. They called architect Philip Greenberg, who saw the Craftsman elements in the house. "We began remodelling in April 1988, stripping the oak woodwork, sandblasting the fireplace, and adding a new kitchen with Craftsmen-styled cabinets." They also built a two-story addition with a communal living space, a spacious upstairs study, and a guest room.

In a paper presented to the Denver Fortnightly Club, Lorna explains that "the Craftsman movement was an effort to preserve natural materials and simplicity at the beginning of the twentieth century when the machines of the Industrial Revolution were threatening to take over human acts."

9
160 FRANKLIN STREET
Built: 1906
Architect: unknown

Another early house on Franklin Street was built in 1906 by Edwin L. Scholtz, president of the Scholtz Drug Company. Of his chain of four drug stores, the one at the corner of 16th and Curtis, just opposite the Tabor Opera House, was especially well known. This historic corner, bought in 1860 for $700, was originally the site of a rustic, one-story Baptist church. Intended as the basement of a much more sumptuous

An art studio was added to this two-story Bungalow at 160 Franklin Street by long-time resident and artist, Gertrude Freeman.

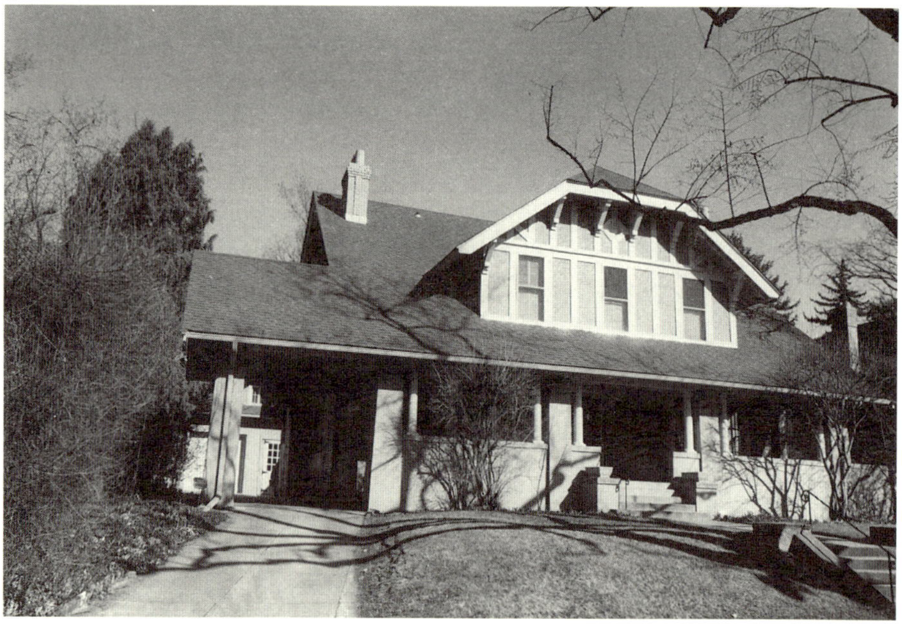

structure, this cabin, called the "Baptist Dugout," was built in 1867.[11]

This, the largest of seven Scholtz drugstores, was where Denver's business elite met at the "large white marble soda fountain, serviced by white-jacketed colored boys."[12] Lime, cherry, and orange phosphates were squirted out of fountain spigots for the downtowners perched on leather-cushioned, revolving stools at the counter. Cigars, pipes, perfumes, and Cashmere Bouquet soap were popular items. Natural sponges hung like bunches of bananas, and Sen Sen, sassafras, and pennyroyal were sold in abundance.[13]

The prominent Scholtz was the first president of the proud Sons of Colorado, an organization started in Colorado's thirtieth year of statehood, 1906. Its purpose was to sponsor a monthly publication to "deal with conquests of the brave men who blazed the trail in the strenuous days when crossing the plains meant peril to life."[14] While chairing the first-anniversary celebration of this august group, Scholtz ended his flowery speech, "Who is it that will say that the good citizens of our state shall not set apart . . . the first day of August of each year . . . to honor the occasion that gave to Colorado the birthright of statehood?"

Scholtz retired from business in 1920, and the house was bought by Roch and Celeste Savageau, who lived there with their two children,

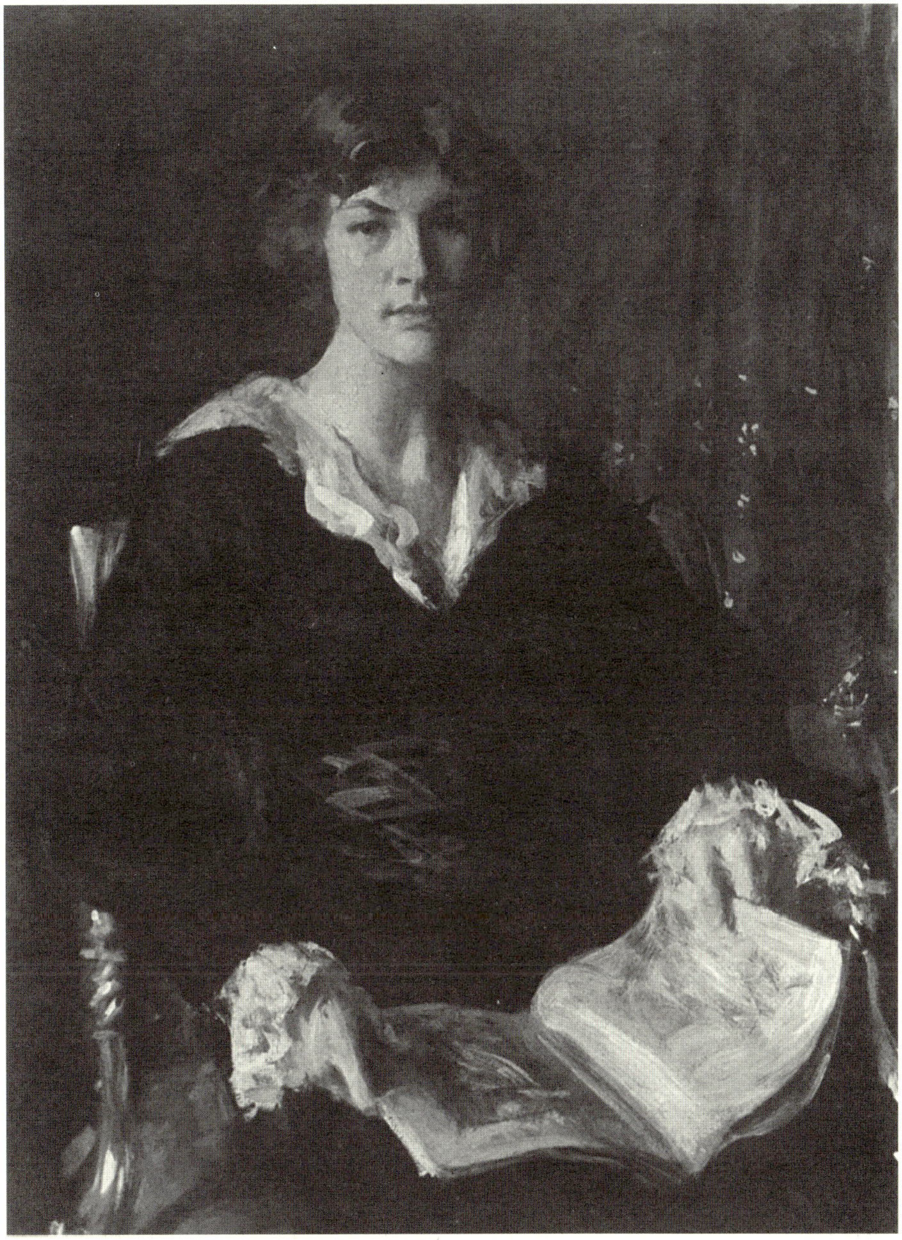

Gertrude Savageau Freeman studied painting with William Merritt Chase, who painted this portrait of her while she was studying with him. It is one of three Chase paintings owned by the Denver Art Museum. (Courtesy Joe Freeman)

Raymond and Gertrude. After Celeste died it was occupied first by their son, Raymond, and then their daughter Gertrude with her husband, real estate developer William Bradley Freeman, from 1958 until Gertrude's death in 1992.

Gertrude was an accomplished painter and good friend of artist Elizabeth Spalding, daughter of Episcopal Bishop John Franklin Spalding. "Often Elizabeth would stop by her house, run in the front door and call out, 'Off we go, Gertrude, into the foothills,' and Gertrude would gather up her easel and paints for a jaunt to the countryside," recalled Elizabeth (Mrs. Emerson) Ellett.

One of the Denver Art Museum's paintings by William Merritt Chase is of Gertrude, done while she was studying with him on Long Island during the summer of 1915. It was featured on the cover of the May/June 1992 issue of the Denver Art Museum magazine *On and Off the Wall*[15] after Gertrude donated the painting following her death. "My parents were most reluctant, when asked by Chase, to grant permission to paint their daughter," Gertrude told neighbor Kim Millett. Roch Savageau would not buy the painting as he thought the decolletage was too deep and made her look too mature. Later, Gertrude bought it from Chase's widow. "The painting is one of three Chases owned by the Denver Art Museum. At one time it hung on the sixth floor," said her grandson, Joe Freeman.

The large, two-story Bungalow with a wide front porch supported by large square columns extends north to form a porte cochere. A large truncated gable with timbering dominates the front facade. The wide eaves are supported by triangular braces. Gertrude Freeman made the back of the house into an art studio. She welcomed her next door neighbors, the William D. Millett children, to her studio, where she painted individual portraits of each of the three older ones.

"She told me that once, while her husband was terminally ill, they made a grand world tour, she always carrying her sketch pad and easel. In her dining room she hung a series of about 30 of these paintings," said frequent visitor Kim Millett. "She loved drawing people and was fascinated with the way African women would drape their colorful clothes." Joe Freeman remembers these pictures: "Now the paintings have been distributed, some to me, some to my brother, others from her estate." Sidney (Mrs. Caleb, Jr.) Gates bought six of these, and they hang in the staircase of their home at 100 Franklin Street.

10
120 FRANKLIN STREET
Built: 1909
Architect: William Ellsworth Fisher

For almost all of his 97 years, mining engineer Everett Humphreys Parker lived in this white, painted brick house built by his father, engineer Richard A. Parker, for $8,000 in 1909.[16,17] The house was designed by his friend and neighbor to the south, William Ellsworth Fisher, and the two houses originally faced the garden between them. Large bay windows facing the front and south sides of the house have balconies above with elaborate wooden balustrades. The wide, low-pitched, hipped roof has paired brackets at the corners.

When Everett Parker took over the house for his own family in 1947, he moved the entry from the south to the north side, replacing the servants' entrance and removing the old pantry with the potato and flour bins. He retained architect Burnham Hoyt to design a study, a powder room, and an attached garage with two new bedrooms. The living-room fireplace is set with Grobe tiles that Mrs. Richard Parker ordered from Boston.[18]

Everett Parker taught topography during World War I and was a lifelong member of the Cactus Club. He was active in the Children's Aid

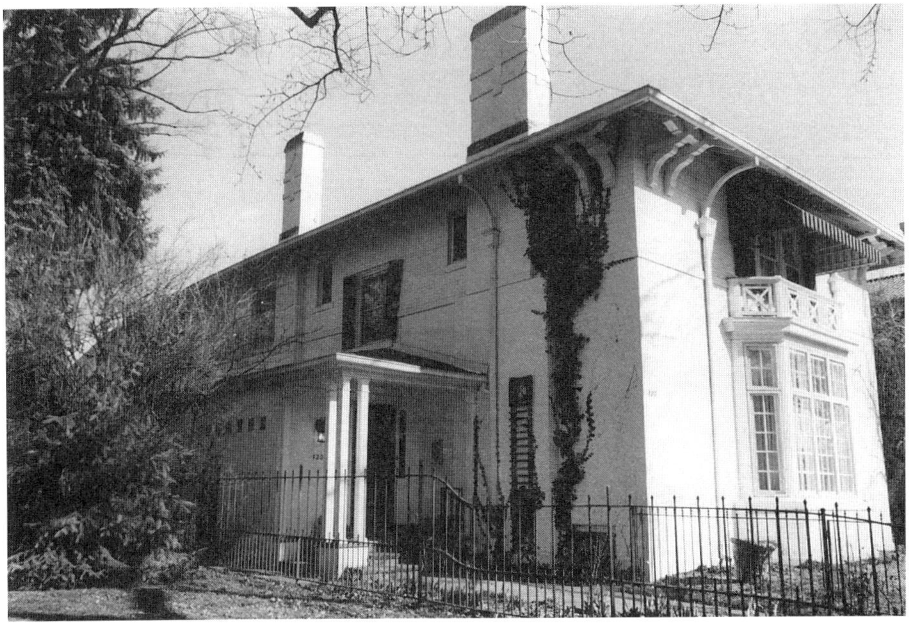

[ABOVE]
Originally this Fisher-designed house at 120 Franklin Street faced south.

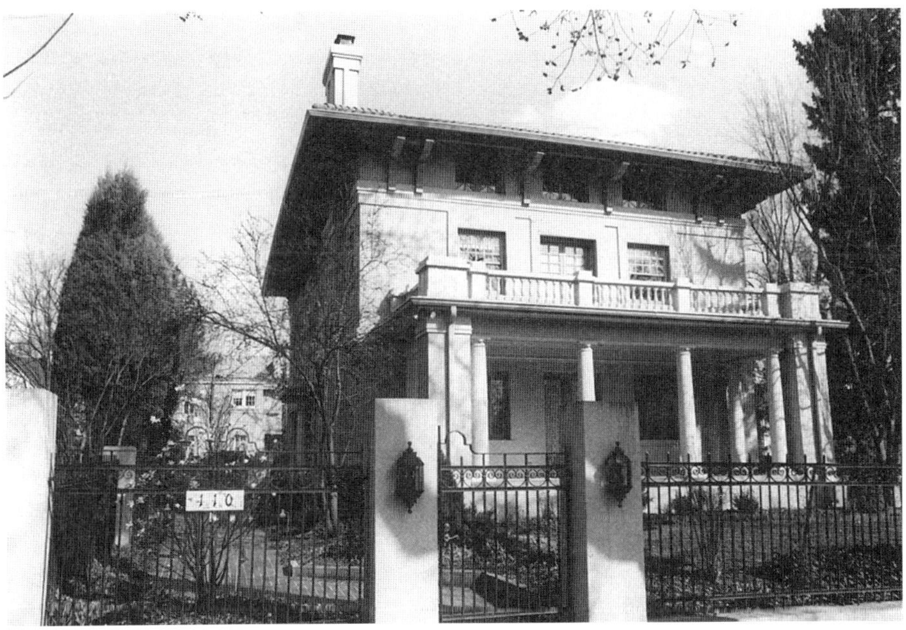

Society, Colorado Family and Children Services, and the Young Adults Club of the Church of the Ascension.[19] He, and his wife, Clare, were staunch supporters of their alma maters, Dartmouth and Smith Colleges, respectively.

After Parker's death in 1991, the house was bought by Margaret Morrissey, daughter of the George R. Cannons.

11
110 FRANKLIN STREET
Built: 1911
Architect: William Ellsworth Fisher

This house was built by William Ellsworth Fisher for himself. Fisher was chosen by the Fourth Avenue Realty Company to design the subdivision Country Club Place, which he laid out with wide landscaped medians on each of the three streets and elaborate Spanish gates at each 4th Avenue entrance.

At 110 Franklin Street, Fisher built a three-story, stucco Italianate home for himself; his wife Clair; his daughter, Katherine; and his son, Alan. (Although Fisher's father was named Allen, and the spelling

[LEFT[
William Fisher built this Italianate house for himself at 110 Franklin Street near the original entrance to the Denver Country Club.

"Allen" appears on the 1910 census report, this son, also a prominent architect, was known as Alan Berney Fisher.) Completed in 1911, the house has a low-pitched tile roof with wide overhangs, much like the gates he designed for the Spanish entrance gates. The large Italian garden to the north of his home included a fountain and lily pond. The north-side entrance portico is supported by Doric columns with a small, stone, balustraded balcony above. Within the house, fumed oak is used for both the paneling in the living room and the staircase trim. The ceiling of the library is of decorative plaster.

Fisher arrived in Denver from Ontario, Canada, in 1885. After some drafting experience, he opened his own architectural office in 1892. His remodeling and residential designs brought him increasing popularity. By 1905 he had so many commissions to design private dwellings, as well as the layout of Country Club Place, that his brother, Arthur Addison Fisher, came to Denver to join the firm. Besides such commissions as the Denver City Tramway Building, the Colorado National Bank, the International Trust Company, Neusteter's Department Store, and the Davis and Shaw furniture company building, the firm of Fisher and Fisher designed 18 houses within the two western subdivisions of the Country Club district between 1906 and 1924.

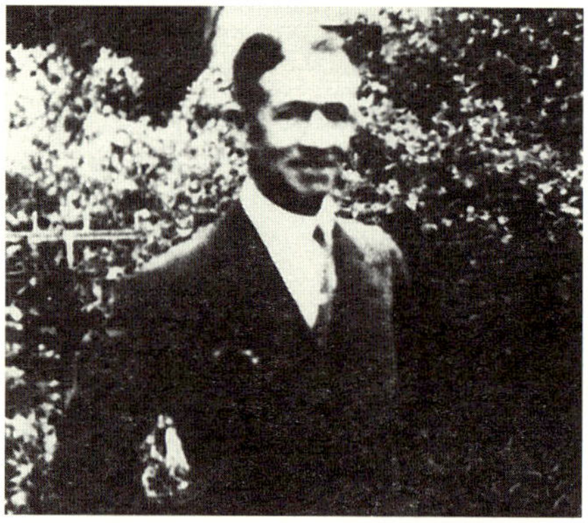

Architect William Fisher in his garden. (Courtesy DPL Western History Department)

William Fisher also built homes in Cherry Hills Village and the Polo Grounds. Later he specialized in hospitals. During the Depression, commissions were few but the firm was retained for several large residences, including that of Senator Lawrence C. Phipps in Bel Caro. After William Fisher's unfortunate suicide in 1937, his son, Alan, joined his uncle, Arthur Fisher, and the firm continued to flourish. Alan was especially remembered for his interest in historic preservation and for his work on the Denver Landmark Commission.

Marjorie "Marnie" and Lawrence A. Jump moved into the house in 1965. As a Dartmouth graduate and 10th Mountain Division member at Camp Hale during World War II, Jump's interest in skiing led him to help launch Arapaho Ski Basin. In 1982 he was inducted into the Colorado Ski Hall of Fame. He died at the age of 75 in 1989.

12
100 FRANKLIN STREET
Built: 1906
Architect: William Ellsworth Fisher

Arthur B. West arrived in Denver from Illinois in the late 1890s to live with his uncle, James E. Rhodes, while attending law school. After joining the firm of Potter, West and Potter, he built a two-story house at 100 Franklin Street,[20] designed by his neighbor to the north, architect William E. Fisher. In 1915 the Franklin Street house was bought by Merritt W. Gano, Jr., who subsequently built a home at 101 High Street. The house was purchased in 1935 by Frank Penn "Bud" Spratlen. He was owner and president of Ready Mix Concrete Company, an innovative business of mixing concrete while it travelled in a truck. Spratlen had organized the company with his father-in-law, Lloyd Brannan, in 1936. Spratlen enjoyed the sports of the day, fly-fishing and duck hunting, and belonged to the Wigwam Fishing Club and the Mile High Duck Club.

After two decades, Spratlen left 100 Franklin, just before his wife died. Caleb F. Jr., and Sidney Brock Gates bought it in 1960, just after 1st Avenue was widened and the Denver Country Club gates were moved from Franklin to Gilpin Street. Gates' father, Caleb, Sr., was a chancellor of the University of

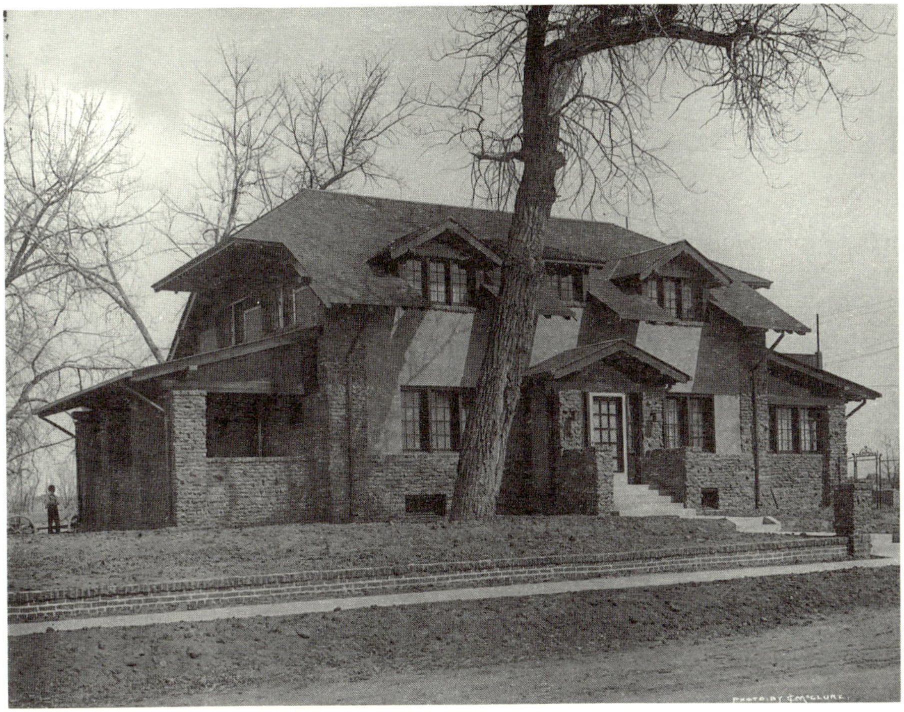

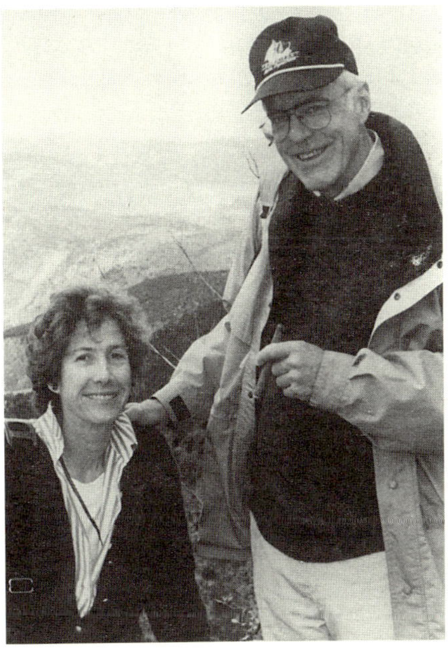

[ABOVE]
This 1906 house of rusticated brick at 100 Franklin Street is shown from gravel-covered 1st Avenue. (Courtesy DPL Western History Department)

{LEFT]
Caleb and Sidney (Brock) Gates purchased the house at 100 Franklin Street in 1960, three years after 1st Avenue was widened. (Courtesy Sidney and Caleb Gates)

Denver and lived at 1640 East 3rd Avenue during his son's childhood. Gates is a senior partner of Denver Investments Advisors, LLC.

This Fisher-designed, rusticated brick house has the typical Craftsman-style, low-pitched hipped roof with exposed rafters and wide overhangs. The full-width front porch is supported by square rough-brick columns that reach to the ground. A side driveway separates this home from that of architect William Ellsworth Fisher at 110 Franklin.

A wall to cut down traffic noise was built after 1st Avenue was widened to accommodate the influx of traffic into the Cherry Creek Shopping Center.

13
103 FRANKLIN STREET
Built: 1906
Architect: William Ellsworth Fisher

The first house to adjoin the original Denver Country Club entrance was General Uriah Shutt Hollister's two-story, symmetrical, beige brick house at 103 Franklin Street.[21] Architect William Ellsworth Fisher, who later built a house for himself across the street, designed this rectangular home with a low-pitched, red tile roof with wide bracketed eaves.

Born in New York in 1838, Hollister was a farmer, schoolteacher,

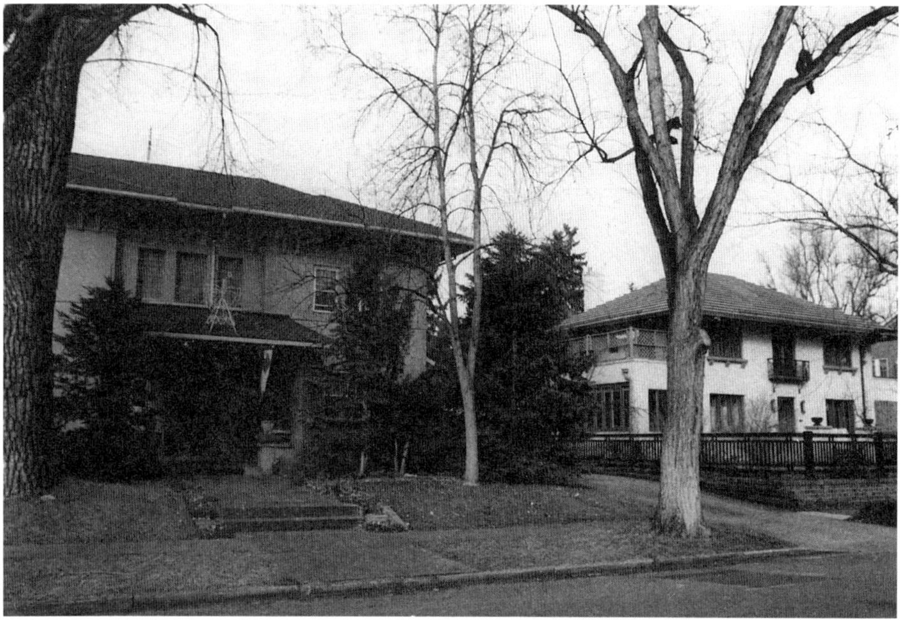

The houses at 103 and 109 Franklin Street were built by brothers Uriah and James Hollister at the original entrance to the Denver Country Club.

soldier, and merchant in his early life. During the Civil War he captained the 13th Wisconsin Infantry, but as his granddaughter, Ruth Hollister (Mrs. Dudley T. Smith) said "Although he was called 'General' he never attained that rank." He became vice-president of the Continental Oil Company, working with his neighbor, CONOCO president Edward Wilson of 180 Franklin Street.

Three months earlier, on July 21, 1906, a building permit was obtained for his son, James M. Hollister,[22] for a 39-by-28-foot brick residence next door at 109 Franklin.

In 1902, Hollister had made an unprecedented trip to Japan. He wrote, "Japan has over 40 million people and, as the country is developed, will have room for 40 million more." He talked about the government-owned farms, and how lucky American farmers were in comparison. He brought back from his tour a fine collection of cloisonne and Japanese pottery.

His wide experience with the West and Native Americans led to his 1903 publication of *The Navajo and His Blanket*, a widely acclaimed book about their lifestyle and the intricacies and subtle colors of Navajo rugs. His love of the Southwest was transmitted to his great grandson, Dudley T. Smith, Jr., who managed the museum shops at the Denver Museum of Natural History and Colorado Historical Society before opening his own store, West Southwest, on Fillmore Street in Cherry Creek North.

A book review in the *Times*[23] states: "The Navajo squaw is said to live in social independence as compared with women of adjacent tribes. The Navajos have many songs, but the Navajo woman is songless, her art being spinning and weaving, to which she devotes her life, silently, almost sadly."

His granddaughter, Ruth Smith, lived with him as a little girl during her teens. "Everett Parker [120 Franklin] was the big boy in the neighborhood, and I loved to play with the Scholtz children [at 160 Franklin] because they had drugstores all over town and we could get free sodas."

In 1911, when President William Howard Taft was breakfasting at the Denver Country Club as a guest of the Colorado Yale Club, the unescorted government car stopped at the entrance, which was right in front of their house. "Will [William Ellsworth] Fisher's daughter, Kath, ran across the street to present him with some flowers. Although I had pangs of regret that the gift wasn't made by me, I realized that she was two years older than I, so it was appropriate for her to do the honors. Of course, there was no security then for the president," Ruth said.

Charles J. "Slide" Kelly, legal counsel for the Public Service Company, lived there during the 1950s. Born in Newfoundland, he came to Colorado with tuberculosis and graduated from the University of Colorado Law School in 1925. His children, John Fleming Kelly (who lived at 100 Lafayette) and Mrs. Thomas P. Owen (who lived at 2025 East 4th Avenue), gave him eight grandchildren. Ralph W. Ball of 300 Humboldt was a student and golfing friend of Slide's: "He was a self-made man and an unquestionable success professionally and personally. . . . with a cherubic smile that lit up a room and a favorite Irish ballad called 'Bridget McHugh,'"[24] Ball wrote of him.

Dr. Giles Filley, a pulmonary specialist at Webb-Waring Institute, lived there during the sixties. "The house was built like a fortress and was in wonderful shape when we bought it from the [Charles] Kellys," said his wife, Mary. "In the cellar was a big playroom and a john with a tub. The sink was on the third floor. The third floor also had three huge bedrooms and a walk-in safe to store all the silver when you went off in the summer. The children had a lot of fun with the safe." There were four boys, the youngest being nine months old when they moved in.

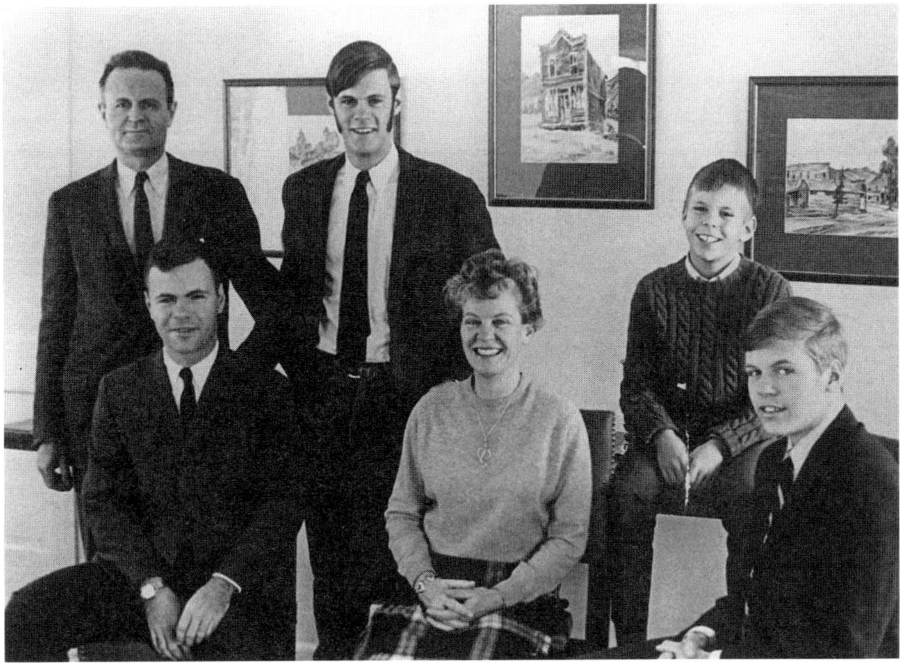

Living at 103 Franklin Street during the sixties were Mary and Giles Filley and their four sons: Dwight; Giles, Jr., "Josh;" Jonathan, and Christopher. (Courtesy the Filley family)

Giles built the wall on 1st Avenue, getting up early every morning before work. "One morning when he was out laying bricks a man stopped his car and said, 'Say, young man, I need some tucking done for my brick. I could use your help.' 'Sorry, I'm all booked up,'" replied the pulmonary physiologist before he biked off to work at the Webb-Waring Institute at 8th Avenue and Colorado Boulevard.

The Filleys sold in 1973 and spent a year in their house in Aspen before moving to 140 Lafayette Street. The present owner is Patricia L. McFee.

14
111 GILPIN STREET
Built: 1913
Architects: Marean and Norton

A parade of influential politicians and businessmen made 111 Gilpin Street their home. It was built in 1913 as a wedding gift to International Trust officer Horace Herbert Brooks and his wife, Jeannette De Sollar, from her parents. The prospective Mrs. Brooks, who insisted that the marriage take place in her own home, spent 18 months designing and furnishing the house

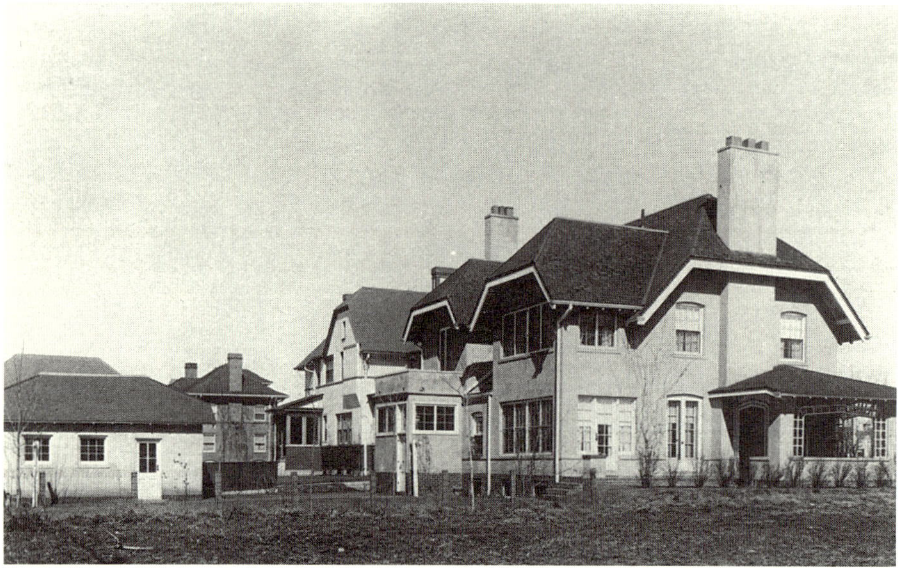

[ABOVE]
When the house at 111 Gilpin Street was built in 1913, the lawn extended to graveled 1st Avenue. In 1999 a large house was built on this property. (Courtesy Anthony Leuthold)

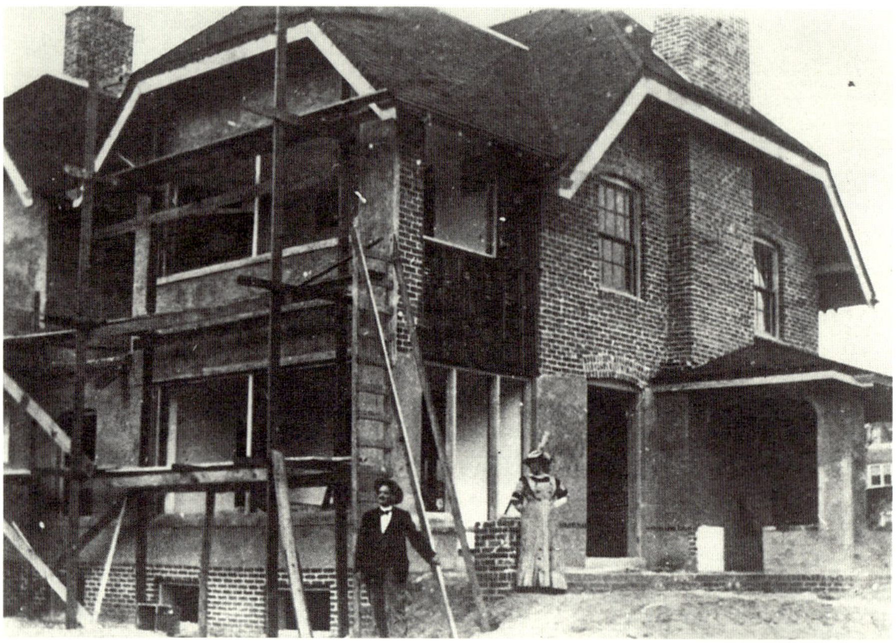

with the help of architects Willis Marean and Albert Norton. The formal ceremony took place in front of the Brittany fireplace of hammered copper. The stairway was built for the future installation of a pipe organ. The house, described as "one of the most artistic in the city," by the *Denver Post*,[25] overlooked the Country Club from the side porch, now enclosed and topped with a second-story extension of the master bedroom. Truncated hipped roofs covering each wing are trimmed with dentils. Architect Edward D. White, Jr., commented that the house has an English roof with sloped gables, like the British thatched roofs. The flat arch covering the simple entrance is repeated over the windows above. Bilateral protruding wings have strips of three windows on each floor.

The next owners were Mary Brooke and James B. Grant, son of Colorado's third governor, and their two children, James B. "Jimmy" Grant, III, and Mary (Mrs. Adolph Coors, III). Grant was in a law partnership with William V. Hodges of 320 High Street and then with Mason Lewis of 575 Circle Drive. Both he and his wife were pillars of

[LEFT]
The prospective Mrs. Horace Brooks, who insisted on a wedding at her own home, spent 18 months designing and furnishing 111 Gilpin Street. (Courtesy Anthony Leuthold)

the Church of the Ascension at 600 Gilpin Street. During the 1930s, Jimmy lived across the street from Philip Gates at 140 Gilpin. "My first playmate was Jimmy Grant," wrote Gates. "He was across the street, and since we weren't allowed to cross it we invented a game. Jimmy's dad brought back empty shotgun shells from his duck hunting. We filled them with water and winged them at each other."[26]

During the sixties, C. R. Kendrick, president and founder of Kendrick-Bellamy Stationery Company moved in with his wife and two children. Kendrick, who had come to Colorado in 1872, lived on a cattle ranch near the future Green Gables Country Club before starting his business career in Denver.

During the early seventies, Tim and Wren Wirth lived in the house for a couple of years, then moved to Jefferson County so that Tim could run for Congress as a resident of District 2. First elected to Congress in 1974, Wirth was an influential Democrat who championed campaign finance reform, reproductive choice for women, deregulation of savings-and-loan companies, and saving the environment. After four successful terms, Wirth served a term in the Senate. He was gearing up for a second term when he suddenly announced he would not run because of the exploding financial costs of campaigning and his frustration with the legislative process. He refunded the contributions to his campaign and was then appointed undersecretary of state for Global Affairs, a post President Bill Clinton created for him. In 1998 he took the job of turning media mogul Ted Turner's promised $1 billion gift to the United Nations into programs to help women, children, and the environment.

The present owners are Merrilyn and Anthony Leuthold, who came to Denver in 1969. Leuthold is president of Leuthold Commercial Properties and is active in Country Club Historic Neighborhood, Inc.

15
141 GILPIN STREET
Built: 1912
Architects: Sterner and Williamson

In 1912 a building permit was issued to a Country Club district pioneer, druggist Frank Quereau,[27] while he was living at 379 Marion Street. Quereau, with his partner, Lester Bridaham of 350 Humboldt, started the largest wholesale drug company west of the Missouri River. After he died in 1918, his widow stayed on with her sister, Mary E. Webb,[28] until the forties when the house was sold to pediatric dentist

This house at 141 Gilpin Street was designed by Sterner and Williamson for Frank Quereau in 1912.

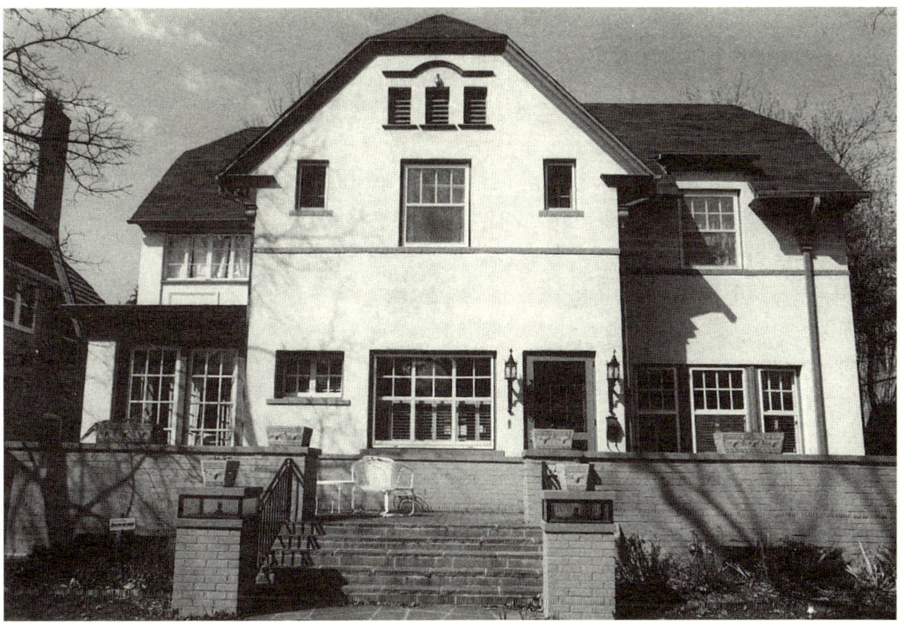

Dr. William P. Humphreys.

Lawyer Howard W. Rea and his wife, Betty, lived there with their three children, Drayton, Kim, and Alison, during the sixties before moving to 200 High Street.

The house was sold to Gladys and Richard A. Kirk, president of the United Bank of Denver. Kirk served on the boards of the Denver Chamber of Commerce and the Boettcher Foundation and as president of Downtown Denver, Inc., and the Botanic Gardens. At the black-tie dinner in 1984 where he was named "Man of the Year" by the American Lung Association, John C. Mitchell, II, told of his successful meeting with Kirk in New York to persuade him to come to Denver to work for the Denver National Bank.[29]

In 1996, carpet and drapery store owner Michael L. Handler took over the asymmetrical house, which is approached by a curving brick walkway leading to a wide, open front porch that is glassed in on the south. The front and side gables are truncated. A four-foot brick wall leading off the front steps now surrounds the house.

16
128 GILPIN STREET
Built: 1909
Architect: Arthur Addison Fisher

Before Arthur A. Fisher came to Denver in 1906 to practice with his brother, architect William Ellsworth Fisher, he was widely travelled. He had attended the Beaux-Arts Institute of Design in New York and had made several trips to Europe to study in France, Italy, Spain, and Greece. His experience earned him recognition as an outstanding architect in classic and northern Italian design,[1] and he brought with him to Denver the Mediterranean influence so prevalent in the 18 Fisher houses in

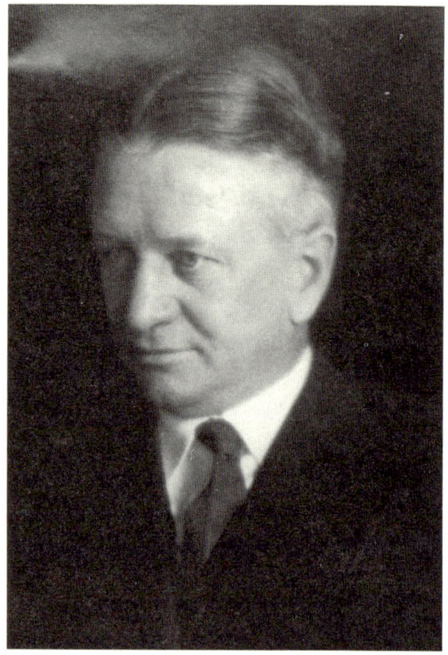

In 1906, Arthur Addison Fisher came to Denver to join his brother, William Ellsworth Fisher, in the prestigious firm of Fisher and Fisher. (Courtesy DPL Western History Department)

Despite his Mediterranean travels, Arthur Fisher designed this English-style cottage at 128 Gilpin Street for himself in 1909.

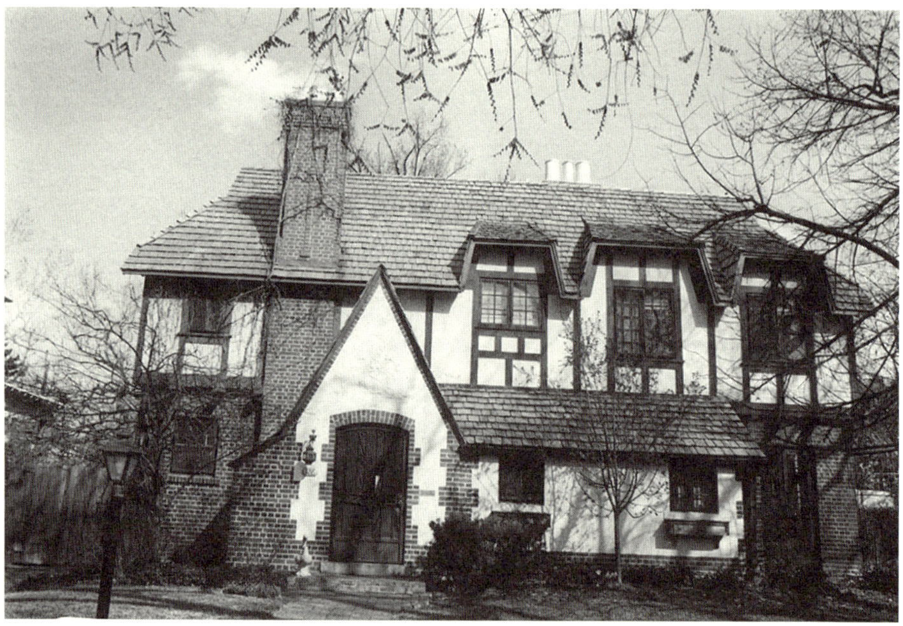

the Country Club district. Arthur Fisher designed the Church of the Ascension at 6th and Gilpin where he was a vestryman and loyal member. After his brother died, Fisher joined his nephew, Alan Fisher, in practice until he retired in 1959.

"The influence and encouragement of Arthur A. Fisher cannot be overlooked. He has been instrumental in developing the use of painting and sculpture in public and semi-public buildings by designing his buildings to carry sculptural adornment or mural painting," reported the *Denver Post*.[30] Some examples are South High School, Midland Bank building, and the Denver Polo Club. "These are the same principles that shed such glory upon Greece, Rome, and the Renaissance cities."[31]

In 1909, Fisher designed this two-story brick and stucco house for himself[32] With all his Mediterranean background it is surprising that he built this English-style cottage with intersecting gables and half timbering on the second floor. An off-center gable covers the enclosed portico at the front entry. Fisher designed a one-story addition to the house in 1923.[33] The house is described in the Denver Public Library's publication, *Lookout*, as "English half-timber house with a fascinating blue door."

The house was built when the district was very young. Fisher's wife, Florence, ran a nursery school. Blanche Taussig (Cowperthwaite-Davis) of 1625 East 3rd Avenue said, "I remember going to kindergarten at the Arthur Fishers' on Gilpin Street. My teacher was named Hypatia Hooper."

17
170 GILPIN STREET
Built: 1913
Architect: Walter E. Rice

This gabled stucco house was occupied for over 20 years by William Ellery Sweet, Jr., the son of Colorado's governor from 1923 to 1925. Sweet, an investment banker, is also remembered for his community activities. He served as president of the Denver Symphony Society and was active in the Metropolitan Council for Community Services, Southwest Denver Community Center, and the Iliff School of Theology. He also carried on the tradition of his father, who spearheaded the YMCA of the Rockies camp in Estes Park.

His well-dressed wife, Georgia, was one of Denver's leading socialites. In 1957 she bought the specialty dress shop Kathryn Kemp, Inc. to manage along with her many civic activities. She chaired the

The Spanish Colonial house at 170 Gilpin Street was occupied by Georgia and William E. Sweet, Jr., the son of the governor from 1923 to 1925.

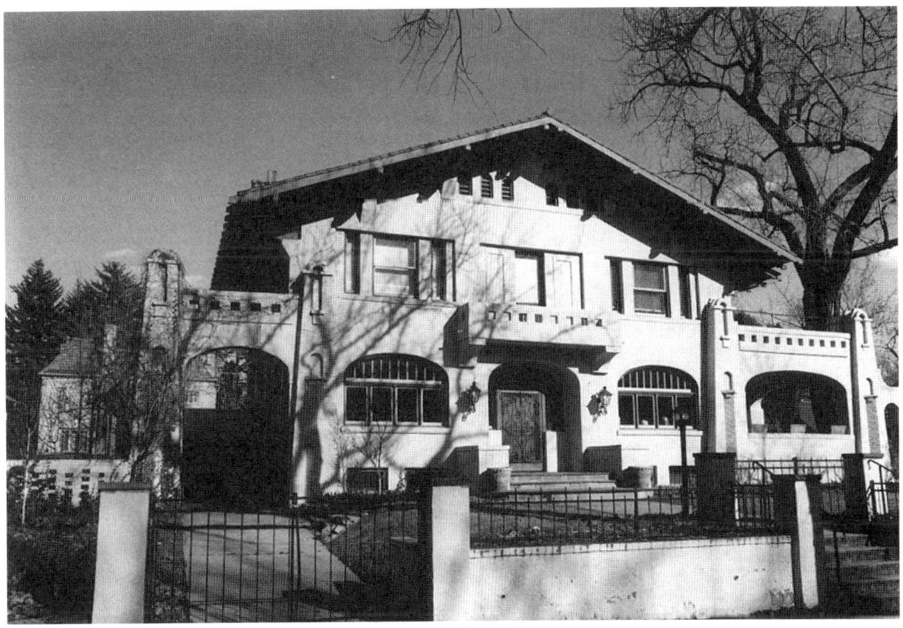

Symphony Guild and served on the boards of the Visiting Nurse, Red Cross, Good Will Industries, and Community Chest. "If you just organize things a little you can get your housework done by 10:30 or 11. Then you can do other things," she told a *Rocky Mountain News* reporter in 1955.[34]

The house was built by Dr. Frank L. Birney, grandfather of Marjorie (Mrs. William Geddes) Temple. Birney, who had studied medicine at Rush Medical School in his native Illinois, came to Denver in 1888 and practiced with his father. After his father moved to California Birney turned to real estate. In the neighborhood he also built the house at 375 Gilpin in 1919.[35]

This house was designed by architect-engineer Walter E. Rice, who arrived in Denver in 1888. Rice then travelled extensively in South America and Guatemala, which inspired him to specialize in Spanish Colonial designs.[36] These are demonstrated here in the stucco construction, balcony, and red tile roof. The porte cochere is balanced by a two-story open porch to the south. Both are decorated with tall, painted brick pilasters at the corners. Wide rounded arches cover both side extensions as well as the entry and the side windows. A balcony above the entry and a wrought-iron fence are Spanish touches.

18
1640 EAST 3RD AVENUE
Built: 1916
Architect: Maurice Biscoe

This house, designed by Maurice Biscoe, was the childhood home of John Clark Mitchell, II; his brother, Quentin; and their sisters, Clara, Elizabeth "Betty," and Catherine.

Their father, Clark Goodell Mitchell, and his sister, Clara (Mrs. Henry C. Van Schaack), had come to Denver from Leadville about 1901, when their father, John Clark Mitchell, transferred from the Carbonate Bank there to become vice-president of the Denver National Bank.

Clark Mitchell, who had graduated from Yale and Columbia in mining engineering, went back to the mountains to supervise a mine in Cripple Creek for six years. However, as the Kiwanis magazine, the *Denver Kiwanian* wrote, "After learning how gold was made, he decided there were easier methods [to find it] and naturally gravitated into Bonds and Investments. . . . He could not escape his destiny of Banker, however, being one by heredity, disposition, and physically."[37]

Maurice Biscoe designed the house at 1640 East 3rd Avenue, at one time owned by the University of Denver as a chancellor's home.

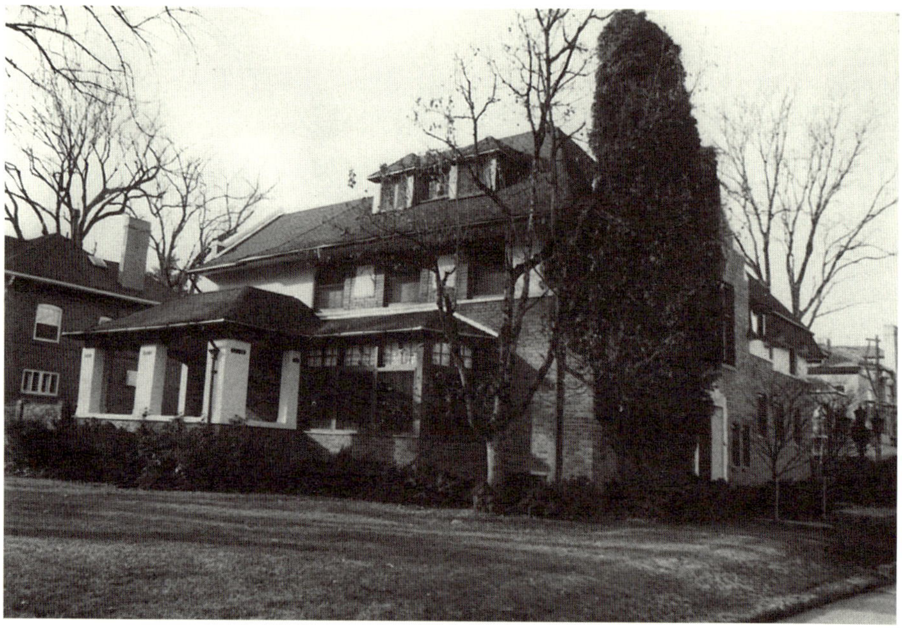

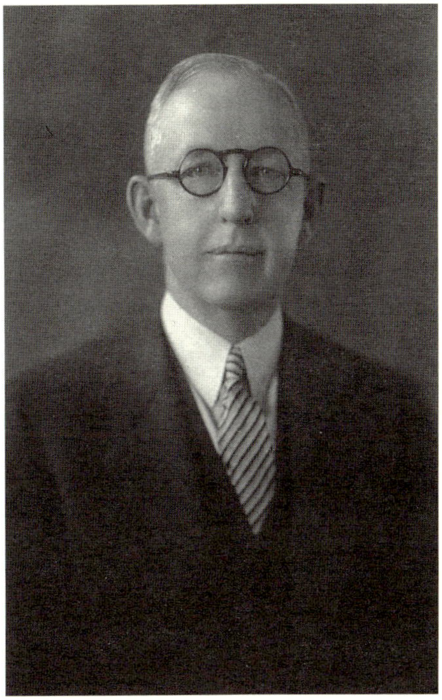

At 1640 East 3rd Avenue Clark Goodell and Ida Mitchell brought up their family of John Clark, II; Quentin; Betty; and Catherine. (Courtesy DPL Western History Department)

Several years after Clark Mitchell married Ida Quentin, the two moved in 1918 into a brick residence on 3rd Avenue built two years before by Dr. and Mrs. Arthur McGugan. McGugan had served in the First World War as a physician. The Mitchells then changed the attic into bedrooms[38] for their growing family. Mitchell was a leader in the Boy Scouts of America, the Community Chest, banking circles, plus an avid golfer. His premature death occurred in 1931 at the zenith of his career while his children were still teenagers.

The neighborhood was sparsely built during the twenties. John played with their next-door neighbor, Robert Bruce "Robbie" Wilson. "There was a vacant lot just north of Parkers [at 140 Franklin] where we built caves," John Mitchell said. "There was a network of covered intricate tunnels," Wilson added. "They were so long we took a hose down to communicate and would yell in one end and listen in the other."

Tennis at the Denver Country Club was a popular family pastime. A special Mitchell Cup tennis tournament is held at the club each year in memory of Quentin and his wife, Eugenie, who were tragically killed in an automobile accident in 1969. Set up by some of his numerous friends, a practice session held on Friday night is followed by a cocktail party hosted by the previous year's winners. On Saturday are all-day matches with 12 to 16 teams participating. The handicap event mixes 2.5 with 4.0 players so that everybody has a good game and a good time, which is the purpose of the memorial.

John, who married Nancy Kountze, daughter of banker Harold Kountze, followed family tradition, both as a vice-president of the merged Denver U.S. National Bank and as a dedicated community leader. In 1962, after serving on boards of the Denver Symphony Society, American Cancer Society, Downtown Denver Improvement Association, Denver Country Day School, Denver Art Museum, and Botanic Gardens, John became executive director of the Boettcher Foundation. The community room at the Botanic Gardens is named in his honor.

Soon after Clark Mitchell's death, the house was sold to the University of Denver as a chancellor's home. Caleb F. Gates, and his family lived there for several years while he was chancellor between 1941 and 1947. His son, Caleb, Jr., spoke of driving across the country from Princeton to Denver with his father when he accepted the position as assistant chancellor. "While we drove out, Dad was notified that the current chancellor had died. Would he take the job of chancellor?" He would. A few years later the house at 360 High was donated by Lawrence C. Phipps for the same purpose, so the university sold the Gilpin Street house.

When Robert Shaeffer Gast, Jr., moved from Pueblo to this house in Denver in 1960, he brought a legacy of prominent Colorado law practice with him. Gast first practiced law in Pueblo with his father, who had graduated from Yale University in 1902. After the senior Gast died, he had joined Senator Alva B. Adams in the firm of Adams and Gast in Pueblo. When he came to Denver, he joined the firm of Kelly, Stansfield and O'Donnell. Gast had served in the Colorado House of Representatives from 1946 to 1948 as a Republican from Pueblo. Ann and Bob Gast joined the Denver Country Club, where their children, Pamela, Corrine, and Richard, III, could swim and skate just a block away.

During the seventies the house was occupied by Carrick A. Hill, owner-manager of the Denver Dry Goods Company.

The first story and walkway of this house are built of red brick. The second story is of beige stucco, echoed in the pillars on the side porch and stone door surround, which has a floral design on the arched pediment. The cross gables are edged with beige trim. The third-floor addition has a hipped roof.

19
1625 EAST 3RD AVENUE
Built: 1909
Architects: Fisher and Fisher

20
323 GILPIN STREET
Built: 1912
Architects: Aaron Gove, Jr., and Thomas Walsh

Perhaps the most loyal and stable person in the Country Club district is Blanche "Bammy" Hallack Taussig Cowperthwaite-Davis. She, her grandparents, and her parents have lived at 3rd and Gilpin since 1909.

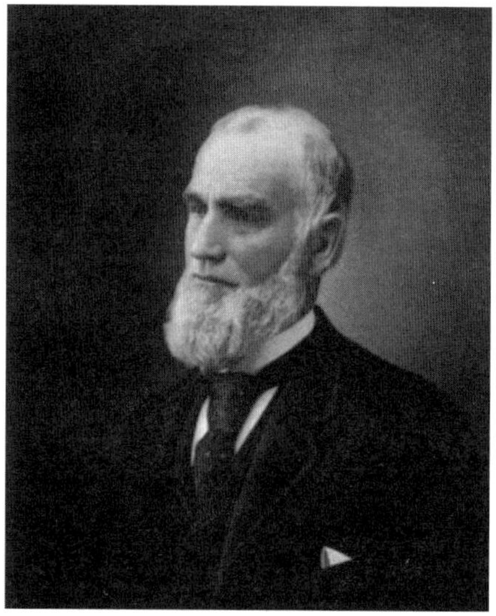

Charles S. Hallack crossed the plains in 1867 and founded the Hallack and Howard Lumber Company. (Courtesy DPL Western History Department)

Her New Yorker grandfather, Charles S. Hallack, "crossed the plains from Kansas with his wagon and his wife, Rachel, in May 1867."[39] With his brother, Erastus S., he started what became the Hallack and Howard Lumber Company, a large flourishing business in rapidly developing Denver. Hallack, who was recognized as one of the foremost businessmen of the city, was especially fond of trees and grass. His elegant home at 17th and Sherman was the first urban residence to have a lawn. "He served for a time as one of the Park Commissioners of Denver, and it was during his administration that the lake at City Park was built."[40] Hallack had numerous real estate holdings, many of which have been retained by his descendants.

In 1919, 13 years after Hallack died, his widow, Rachel, and daughter-in-law gave the city a block of land at 20th Avenue and Irving Street to be used as a park.[41] Hallack Park has rolling hills and is popular for football practice, its bike path, sledding, the playground, and the picnic site. This land is several blocks from the present Coors Field, built in 1995 on a piece of land that had been held by the family for 110 years.[42]

Charles Hallack's daughter, Gertrude, married cardiologist Arnold Steven Taussig. They built the first house on Gilpin Street in 1909, designed by Arthur Fisher, on the corner of 3rd Avenue at 305 Gilpin Street, later 1625 East 3rd Avenue. This beautiful Tudor house is timbered throughout the second story. The entrance was moved to the south during the mid-thirties and covered with a shed-roof portico. Beside it is a two-story, five-sided bay similar to the sunroom on the east, which replaced a sunporch. A wide bay upper window gives a view to the south from the apartment over the garage. The north garden became a home for two ducks. "I won them at the [Harley] Higbie's

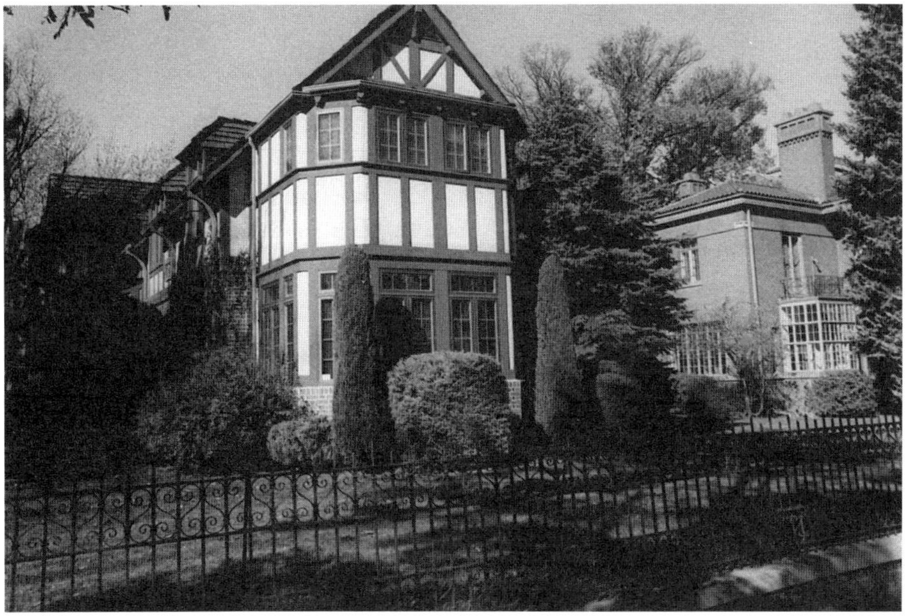

The houses at the corner of 3rd and Gilpin have remained a Cowperthwaite family compound since they were built in 1910 and 1913.

Easter party and brought them home in a perambulator," said daughter Jill (Mrs. Charles) Jones.

After Charles Hallack died, his widow, Rachel, built a house next to their daughter's at 323 Gilpin in 1910 and lived there until her death in 1921. Of lighter red brick, this latter house has a full length front porch supported by square wooden columns. On either side of the two-story projected entry are balconies with iron balustrades. Over the entry is a strip of five narrow windows. To the south a two-story addition holds the sunroom and bedroom with a small balcony.

Arnold and Gertrude Taussig then moved over to 323 Gilpin with their two daughters, Blanche and Josephine. Arnold's brother, Claude, and his wife, Margaret, moved into the corner house at 305 Gilpin. Margaret Taussig was an accomplished woman, receiving a doctorate degree from the University of Denver in 1919.[43]

When Blanche married Arthur T. Cowperthwaite, they moved into 305 Gilpin with the Claude Taussigs, adding a brick house-keeping unit over the garage for themselves and an addition to the north in 1930. Soon, however, they wanted to start a family. "Art and I finally took over the house and remodeled it, hitching the garage to the house," said Blanche. They added a sunporch on Gilpin Street, a front door on 3rd, and changed the address to 1625 3rd Avenue. Claude and Margaret Taussig moved to 351 Lafayette. Meanwhile, Art Cowperthwaite's parents, the Edwin Cowperthwaites, moved to 350 Franklin Street, half a block away. Josephine Taussig married Art Cowperthwaite's brother, George, and lives at her mother's house at 323 Gilpin.

Blanche spent her life as an active businesswoman and community leader while raising five children: Charles Hallack, a lawyer-realtor; the late Arnold Stephen, who headed the realty firm of Cowperthwaite; realtor James; Jill Hallack (Jones); and architect Arthur T., Jr.

As a child, Blanche said dolls and dress-up weren't her thing. "When I was a little girl I only liked boys," she said. "I went into the real estate business in 1953 because I wanted something worthwhile to do." She was a realtor with Blue and Blue Realty Company and active both locally and nationally in the American Association of University Women. In November 1954, she was elected to the state House of Representatives. In December she delivered her fourth child, Jill, before taking office in January one month later.

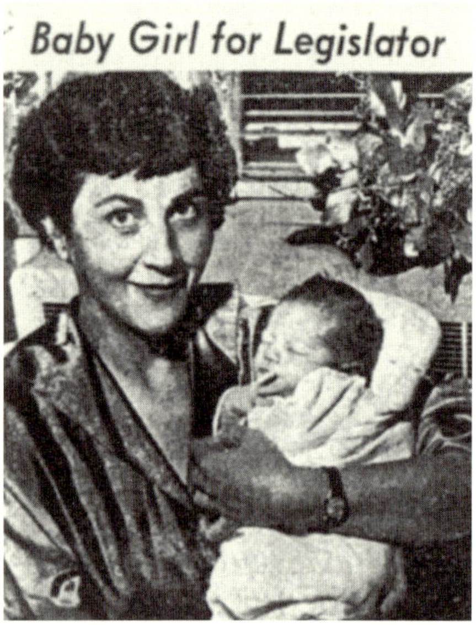

Blanch Hallack Taussig Cowperthwaite-Davis, called "the epitome of the modern woman," was elected to the state house of representatives in 1954, a month before the birth of her daughter.

Because of her interest in the education of women she was appointed chair of the Colorado Commission on the Status of Women in 1970. To demonstrate the prevalence of discrimination against women she shocked the Denver male community by holding a meeting at the Denver Club, "traditional bastion of men and most certainly a stubborn discrimination against women!" noted the *Cervi's Rocky Mountain Journal.*[44] As a result of all her diverse accomplishments, Blanche was called "the epitome of modern women" by Pat Hanna.[45]

Despite her worldliness she has lived her whole life in these two houses in Country Club Place. In 1995, however, her loyalties expanded all the way across Franklin Street when she fell in love with and married architect Rodney S. Davis, who had lived half a block away at 315 Franklin Street for 23 years. "You know, it's a funny thing. I really didn't know Rod very well while he lived there," she said.

21
300 GILPIN STREET
Built: 1910
Architect: Henry James Manning

Vermonter Frederick R. Ross arrived in Denver in 1888, eventually becoming a much-respected citizen and pioneer realtor, specializing in the Country Club area. It was written of him in 1911, "More important than big deals is the striking development of Country Club Place into one of the most beautiful and restricted residential sections of the city. The addition opened six years ago and now contains a number of Denver's most magnificent homes. The streets are 105 feet wide. Parkways are planned connecting Cheesman and Washington Parks that go through here. An artistic wall a quarter of a mile long extends along the 4th Avenue side. The minimum cost of a residence has been established at $6,000. Last summer half a dozen between $12,000-25,000 were built." Buying were Mrs. Charles Halleck, General U. S. Hollister, Erl B. Ellis, Irving Snyder, E. L. Scholtz, W. E. Fisher, and James S. Wright."[46]

During his diggings in the area, Ross had the rare experience of discovering a tooth from a giant mammoth. He donated this lower right molar, M/2 or M/3, of a Pleistocene *Mammuthus columbi* to the Denver Museum of Natural History in 1932.[47]

Ross retained Henry James Manning to design a two-story, light grey stucco, Mission-style house with arched windows beside the door and a flat arched canopy over the front portico. The arch is repeated in a stucco gateway over the side driveway and sunroom windows. Wrought-iron balcony rails trim the upper-story windows.

Ross's elegant home in the heart of the Country Club area was, apparently, a target for thieves. Twice his silverware was stolen. In 1918, one Rudolph Fininaid was arrested when caught digging a "safe" in his own backyard, attempting to dispose of silverware stolen from Ross's home. When police caught up with him, his explanation, "that the rabbits had dug up the stuff in the rear yard of my home," was not convincing.[48] Again in 1930, three men were accused of robbing Ross' home of a "large quantity of

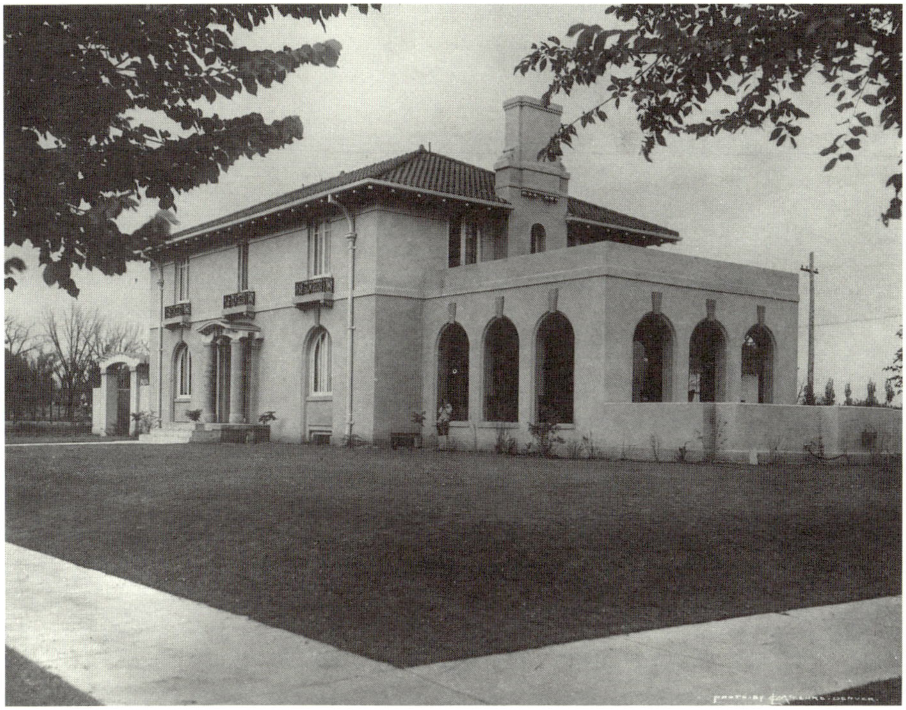

The stucco house at 300 Gilpin Street was designed by Henry James Manning in 1910, one of the early houses in Country Club Place. (Courtesy DPL Western History Department)

silverware, clothing, and household furnishings."[49]

Much respected as president of the Frederick R. Ross Investment Company, the Denver Water Board, and the Denver Real Estate Exchange, Ross is best remembered as president of the Library Commission. During his term the main and several branch libraries were built, two of which are named after him. His portrait, sponsored by City Council and painted by Jack Pohr of Colorado Springs, hangs in the Ross Cherry Creek branch.

Ross died in 1938, and the house was sold to socialite Mrs. David Twigg Chalmers, widow of David, who lived there with her children, Dorrit and David, until they left home.

The house has always been a showpiece. In 1989, when Cile and Ronald Williams bought the house, they used old pictures to guide the repair of the arch over the driveway. "We replaced virtually every window in the house and the windows in the breezeway porch according to historic photographs," Ron said. Sometimes they notice groups of people looking over their house. "Especially in the spring when the tulips are out, tour buses stop and unload so people can take pictures of the house," Cile said. It is obviously a major Denver attraction.

Frederick R. Ross, who helped develop Country Club Place, is remembered as an outstanding president of the Denver Library Commission. (Courtesy DPL Western History Department)

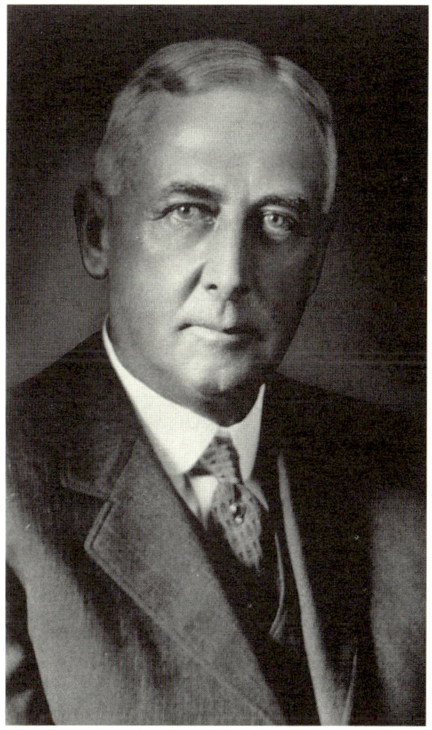

22
330 GILPIN STREET
Built: 1912
Architect: Jacques Benedict

A Benedict-designed house was built in 1912 for Irving T. Snyder, vice-president of Vindicator Consolidated Gold Mining Company. In three years it was sold to lawyer Clayton C. Dorsey, called by a federal judge "far and away the most brilliant lawyer to appear on my bench"[50] and a "man of Supreme Court caliber."[51] Son of Stephen W. Dorsey, a U.S. senator from Arkansas, Dorsey formed the prominent law firm of (Gerald) Hughes and Dorsey in 1911, specializing in corporate law. The political clout of this firm was weighty, with Dorsey a Republican and Hughes a Democrat. When Dorsey died, his practice was taken over by his son, Montgomery Dorsey.

This three-story, English-style gabled house, with a Tudor arch in the door surround, was one of Benedict's early designs. The leaded windows in the dining room and the hand-rubbed woodwork are outstanding. Dorsey's granddaughter, Anne Merryweather (Mrs. Edward) Close remembered "lots of old wood in the downstairs. It was a big, comfortable house. I call it a 'bastard chalet,'" she said. Her stepfather, Montgomery Dorsey, lived nearby at 177 Race Street, where Anne grew up.

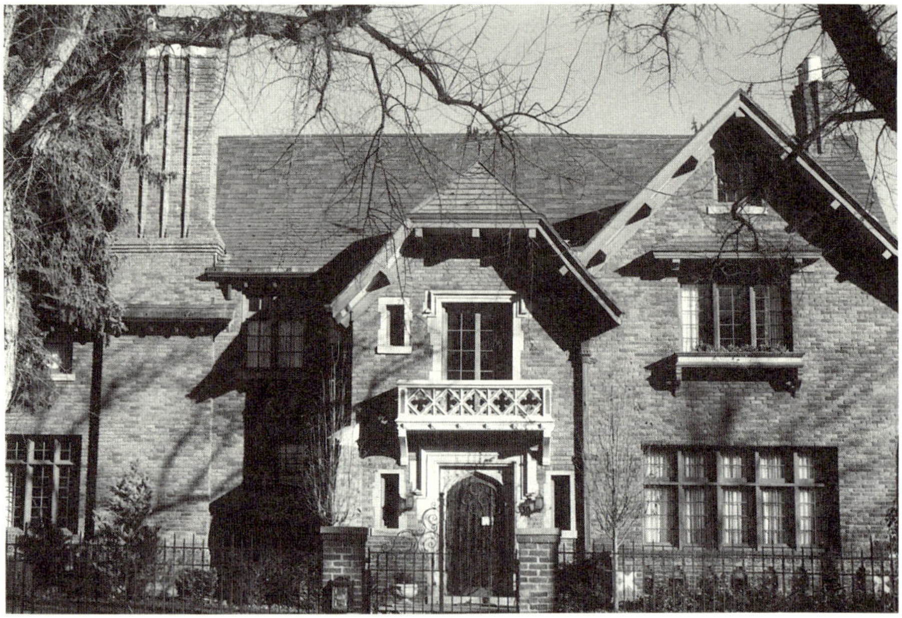

This English-style house at 330 Gilpin Street was the home of lawyer Clayton C. Dorsey, called "a man of Supreme Court caliber."

After Dorsey's wife, Marguerite, died, dentist Gerald P. Ivancie bought the house in 1960. The added bedrooms on the third floor housed eight Ivancie children.[52] The wall, spanned by brick pillars, leads to an arched door with ornate stone surround. Over the door a balcony, entered by French doors, lies under a truncated front gable. A large divided chimney balances the gable to the south. The house was purchased by Lynn and Floyd G. Nichols in 1996.

23
355 GILPIN STREET
Built: 1932
Architect: Jacques Benedict

This balanced Art Moderne, Benedict-designed house is elegant in its simplicity. The red brick, rectangular home is more than three times longer than its height. The low-pitched roof has wide Prairie style overhangs. The recessed entryway is surrounded by travertine marble, a typical Benedict touch. Spanning the strip of five windows and surrounded with decorative tile are two distinctive oriel windows. This brick $17,000 residence, built for Otis and Company manager Rex P. Arthur, had a three-car garage on the alley.

The Arthurs sold it to David and Virginia (Ballantine) Dunklee. David's grandfather, George F. Dunklee, was president of the Denver Bar Association in 1903 and became a district judge in 1923. His lawyer son, Edward V. Dunklee, was elected to both the Colorado House of Representatives and the state Senate. Of their four children, David is remembered as a mayor of Bow Mar and for his extensive community service, chairing committees of the Colorado Bar Association, Colorado Women's College, and Denver Symphony. He was a senior warden at St. John's Episcopal Cathedral, president of the Lions Club and Rocky Mountain Arthritis Foundation, and he received the National Volunteer Service Citation in 1979.

This Benedict-designed brick house at 355 Gilpin Street is elegant in its simplicity. It was the home of the David V. Dunklee family.

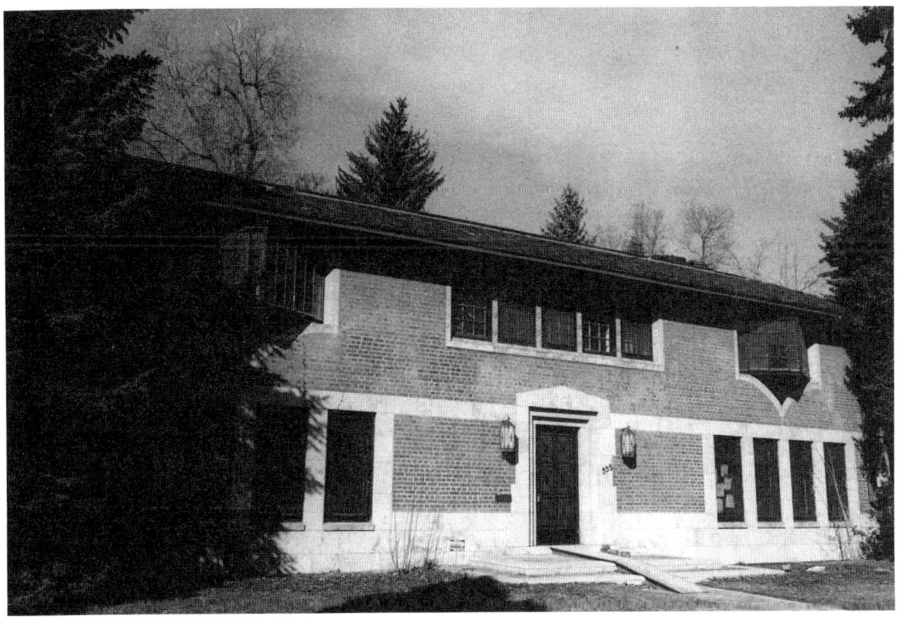

24
385 GILPIN STREET
Built: 1926
Architect: Burnham Hoyt

This cozy, little, L-shaped Spanish Mission-style house of tan stucco with a red tiled roof has a large, arched living-room window. The walled patio at the front entrance with a wrought-iron gate adds privacy. French doors open onto a second-story balcony. It was designed in 1925 by Burnham Hoyt for general manager of Mountain Motors O. Lewellyn Davis, Jr.; his wife Sally; and his daughter, Sally, a prominent and popular Denver photographer.

The garage was assimilated into the house and a three-car garage was built on the alley before the house was purchased by president of Van Schaack and Co. Thomas B. Knowles. After his wife, Eleanor Van Schaack, died in childbirth in 1947, he married the former Mary Kountze and lived there for 12 years.

When Claude and Anne (Waring) Maer bought the house during the seventies, they added some Mexican touches. "We flew in Claude's Bonanza to Guanajuato to buy some hand-painted, white-on-white fabric for the living-room curtains," Anne said. Later a friend brought back some six-inch, hand-painted Mexican tiles for the counter in the remodeled kitchen.

The next owners, Donald D. and Elizabeth Estey, added a glassed-in room to the south. "Elizabeth crafted a unique fireplace to give a Santa Fe appearance," said Don. "The tile floor is covered with a custom-made Portuguese woven rug and the walls are off-white, which sets off our modest art collection.

This is our favorite room. We could rent out our living room, we're there so seldom."

The Esteys added privacy to the entrance by planting an apple orchard in the small front yard. "Of 10 trees, six survive, and one is a good producer," Elizabeth said. Under the trees are 400 daffodil bulbs to herald the spring. Don is active in Country Club Historic Neighborhood, Inc.

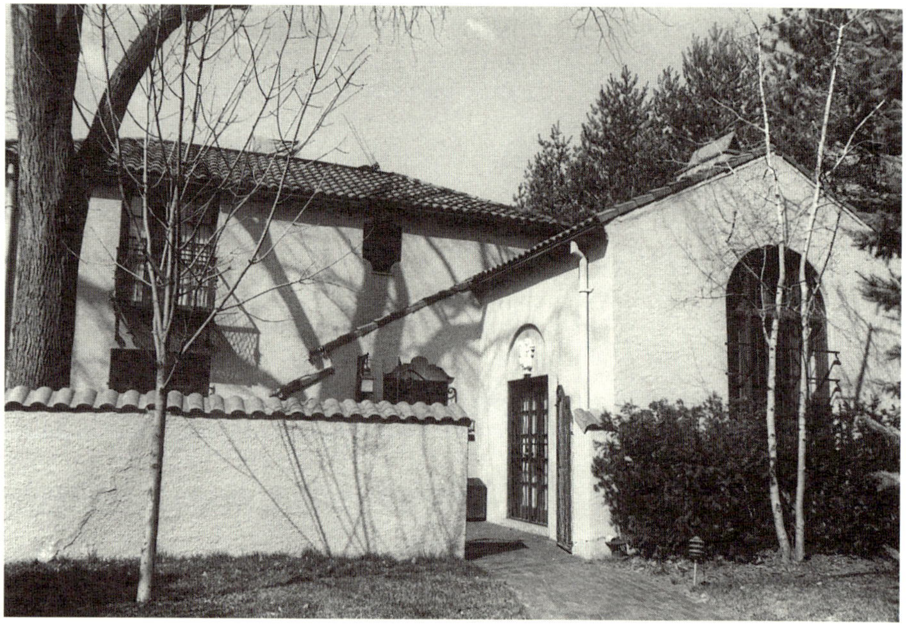

[ABOVE]
In 1926 Burnham Hoyt designed this Spanish Mission-style house at 385 Gilpin Street.

25
380 GILPIN STREET
Built: 1925
Architects:
Merrill and Burnham Hoyt

This is the second of four houses in the Country Club district built by the Sewell Thomases. While still living on High Street, they chose Merrill and Burnham Hoyt to design this two-story house on six lots at 380 Gilpin.[53] Like their former home at 360 High, this house has a porte cochere. The French Chateau-style farmhouse has a heavy slated roof, and an elegant travertine marble staircase is located in a tower. Worked into the leaded-glass tower

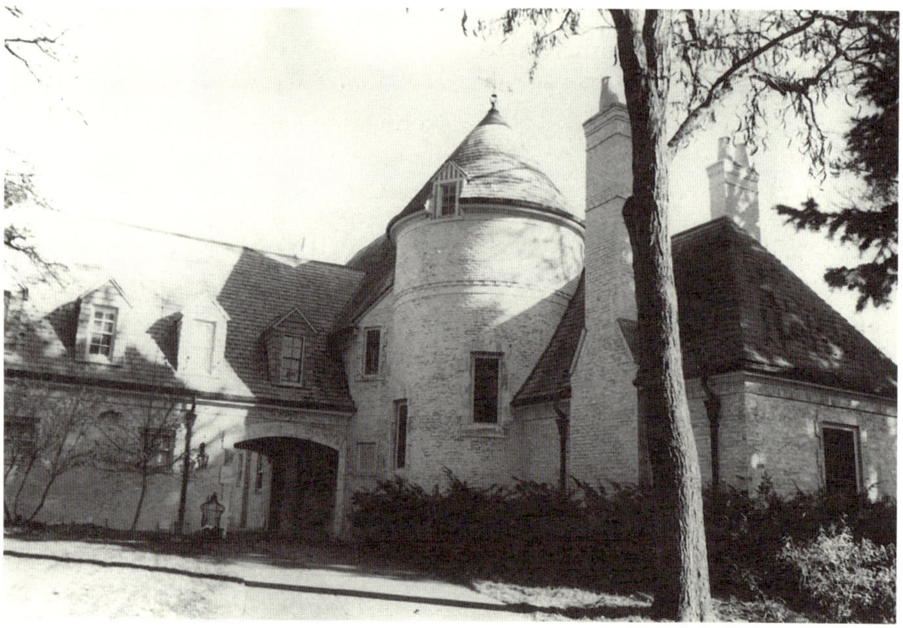

[RIGHT]
The French Chateau-style house at 380 Gilpin Street was a Junior Symphony Guild showhouse in 1996.

window are the initials of the owners, Mary Wade Thomas and Charles Sewell Thomas. The organ at the bottom of the tower had two sets of pipes. One was in the basement below the living room, and another "echo set" was in the tower so that the sound could filter down through the stairway. The organ was eventually given to St. John the Evangelist Church at 5th and Josephine, where their daughter, Lenore, was married. Thomas used the area with the little window at the top of the tower for his gun collection because the room could be locked up. The weather vane on top of the turret represents Thomas reading a book and was presented to the owners by one of their architects, Burnham Hoyt. An avid reader, Thomas had a large library lined with floor-to-ceiling bookshelves to accommodate his massive book collection of over 3,000 volumes.[54]

The kitchen's large pantry and commercial refrigerator reflected Marie Thomas's interest in cooking and entertaining. Known as a fabulous cook, Mrs. Thomas published a book on gourmet cuisine entitled *What to Eat and How to Cook It*. As one of Denver's top ten hostesses, she was famous for her formal entertaining, which was "mostly sit-down dinners with the simple elegance of beautiful china, silver and linens, and exquisite food," reported the *Denver Post* on May 10, 1959.

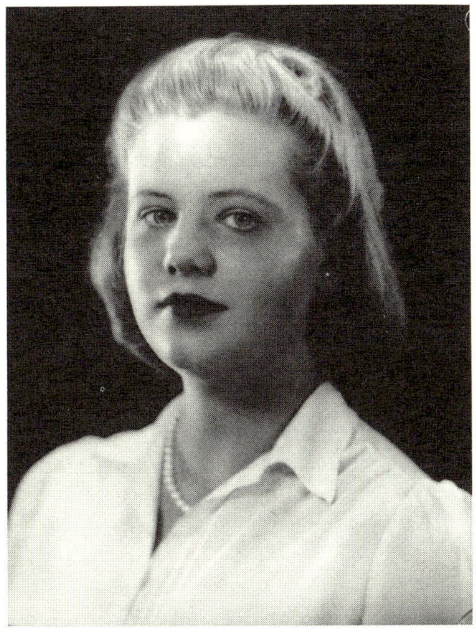

Lenore Thomas (Stoddart) grew up at 380 Gilpin Street during the time of the Lindburgh kidnapping in the early thirties. (Courtesy DPL Western History Department)

Their daughter, Lenore (Mrs. John Stoddart, Jr.), grew up in this house during the thirties. "I remember the trolley clickety-clacking up 4th Avenue. I used to take it to 1st and Steele to the Denver Riding Academy, where I rode with the Hot-n-tots," she said.

During the early thirties, there was a startling commotion on Gilpin Street. Marie Thomas opened her mailbox one day and found a note written in cold blood, demanding $10 or their daughter would be kidnapped. Terrified, she called the FBI to investigate, and trucks and police cars screamed through the Gilpin Street entrance gates. It seems that two neighbor boys, Jack Larson and Octave Chanute, Jr., inspired by the recent Lindbergh baby kidnapping, had decided to make some easy money. Lenore was indignant about the whole affair. "Was I only worth $10?" she demanded.

After being rescued, Lenore graduated from the Convent of the Sacred Heart and married 10th Mountain ski trooper John Stoddart from Buffalo, New York. The couple lived in Country Club Gardens apartments for five years before building a house at 280 Race Street in Country Club Annex.

After the Thomases sold the Gilpin Street house, the servants' quarters over the garage were converted into children's bedrooms, and an indoor swimming pool was added. A second tower was built at the southeast of the house.

Subsequent owners were the Clarence W. Kreiders, then the James R. Morrises. In 1996 the Junior Symphony Guild showed the house as "The Corner Chateau."

26
399 HIGH STREET
Built: 1924
Architect: unknown

This three-story, Georgian-style brick house with half basement was built in 1924 by Paul Loughridge, a partner with his neighbor, Arthur H. Bosworth, in the municipal and corporate securities firm of Bosworth, Chanute and Loughridge. A few years later he added a sleeping porch over the south veranda and three additions, one of which was designed by architect Temple H. Buell and Company in 1939.

The entrance portico, supported by two sets of fluted Corinthian columns, both with corresponding pilasters flanking the door, is covered with a balcony with white spindle-turned balusters. The white paneled door surround has a segmental arch and lead-pane sidelights. Keystones trim the windows of both the main house and the two symmetrical wings, which are set back from the front. A wrought-iron fence surrounds the house and 70-foot-wide south garden.

From 1986 until 1988 this corner house was owned by Shelley and Michael Wise, head of the former Silverado Savings and Loan. They had moved from 565 Circle Drive. While they lived on High Street the Wises remodeled extensively. "We watched them take down the [landmarked] original four-foot stone wall next to the Spanish gates," said neighbor Helen (Mrs. Gary) Christy, who then lived at 335 High Street. No building permit was found for this procedure. They replaced it with a five-foot wrought-iron fence.

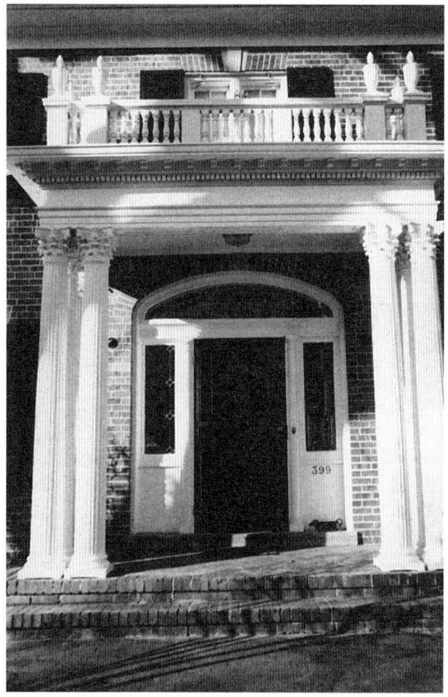

This red brick house with Corinthian columns on the portico at 399 High Street was owned by Silverado head, Michael Wise, during the eighties.

The Wises moved away in 1988 just before the catastrophic crash of Silverado Savings and Loans Company. Wise was accused of stealing nearly $6 million from investors, of defrauding 44 investors of $8.75 million, and of pocketing nearly $500,000 to remodel and landscape his Country Club home.[55] In 1999 he pleaded guilty to a charge of taking $9 million while he was president of Cornerstone Private Capital of Aspen, and he was sentenced to three and a half years in prison.

27
380 HIGH STREET
Built: 1924
Architects: Fisher and Fisher

This is an especially nice example of a large Spanish Colonial-style house with both simplicity and charm. "Architect Alan Fisher considered this his father's finest design in Country Club," wrote Sharon Elfenbein, who was given a personal tour of the area by Alan Fisher. The two-story projected entrance to this long rectilinear stucco house is striking. Over the recessed door is elaborate Baroque cast ornamentation, a casement window trimmed with pilasters, jambs, a decorative arched pediment, and a Mission-shaped curvilinear gable. Bedroom doors open onto second-floor wrought-iron balconies. Round arches surround the square heads of the windows.

John M. Kuykendall, the founder of Denver Omnibus and Cab Company and Master of Fox and Hounds at the Arapahoe Hunt Club, built the 30-by-109-foot house for $35,000. After his death his widow, Marjorie, lived there until 1945.

The next owner, George Robert Harris, added bathrooms, closed fireplaces, and remodeled bedrooms.

During the sixties and seventies the house was occupied by Clayton Glenville Dorn. The home was the setting for his daughter, Leslie's, wedding reception when she married

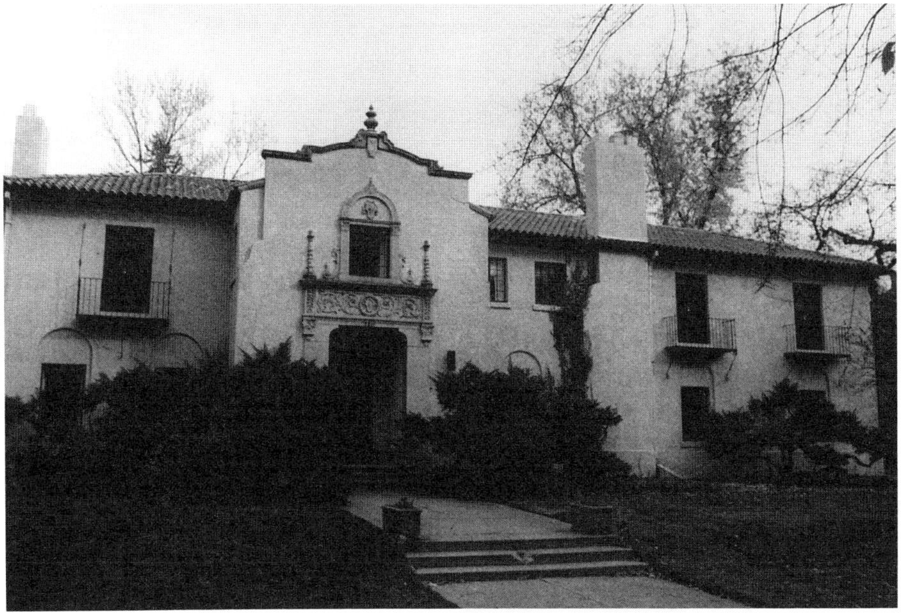

Elaborate Baroque ornmentation over the entry is a feature of this Spanish Colonial-style house at 380 High Street .

Robert Bruce Wilson, Jr. In 1964, Dorn became president of the Forest Oil Company after the death of his father, Forest D. Dorn, founder of the company. When the Dorns sold in the eighties, they divided the property and sold two lots at the east end of the 265-foot-deep property for houses that open onto Race Court, the original Race Street until 1920. Two houses were built, one at 1920 4th Avenue, occupied by John and Vivian Sweeney who had lived at 463 Race Street. The southern one was built by Keith and Carol Brown at 377 Race Court (although the official address is 377 Race Street).[56]

28
360 HIGH STREET
Built: 1920
Architect: Jacques Benedict

Sewell Thomas hired architect Jean Jacques Benois Benedict in 1920 to design the two-story, 39-by-98-foot, red brick residence at 360 High Street. The Tudor house has a half-timbered gable with lead-pane windows. On the north wall is a cantilevered oriel window and a porte cochere with a Tudor arch to welcome guests. The one-and-a-half-story garage and the iron and brick ornamental fence were built two years later. "There were only four houses on our side of the street when we lived there. The plots each had an acre of land," said daughter Lenore (Mrs. John) Stoddart.

Thomas, born Charles Sewell Thomas, was the son of Charles Spaulding Thomas, governor of Colorado from 1898 to 1901 and U.S. senator from 1913 to 1921.

Sewell Thomas, a mining engineer, married Marie Wade of St. Louis and built this comfortable house, not expecting they would have children. However, when their daughter, Lenore, arrived, they decided to move. "I was born there, but there were only two suites upstairs: theirs and a guest suite for Mother's many visitors from St. Louis," she said.

The sale of the house was easy. At a dinner party one night, Marie Thomas and her good friend Margaret Phipps were chatting. It seemed that her husband, Senator Lawrence C. Phipps, would be leaving Washington and moving back to Denver. Did anyone know of a house for sale?

However, the Phippses had a problem. They were to host Margaret's sister's wedding shortly after their move, and their belongings were still in transit from Washington. Mrs. Thomas stepped in. "Oh, I'll just leave all my furniture, silverware, and china for you to use," was her gracious offer.

Senator Phipps had three families. His children with his first wife, Ibrella Loomis[57] were Lawrence C. "Larry" Phipps, Jr., and Emma (Mrs. William White). His second set of children with Genevieve Chandler were Dorothy (Mrs. Van Holt Garrett) and Helen (Mrs. Donald Bromfield). General contractor Gerald Hughes Phipps and lawyer Allan Rogers Phipps were sons of his third wife, Margaret (Rogers) Phipps, and grew up in the High Street house. The brothers later collaborated to buy the Broncos football team. During the seventies, Gerald mentioned to Dr. Karl Arndt, "I'll bet you don't know anyone else who's searching for a football coach and a dean of the [Episcopal] cathedral at the same time." During the 1980s, Gerald Phipps lived in the house with his wife, Muriel Stokes Magarrell Phipps, until his death.

When Senator Phipps had built the mansion in Bel Caro, he gave 360 High to the University of Denver for its chancellor. Chester M. Alter lived there during his term from 1953 to 1966. Subsequent owners were Richard H. Shaw, son of George Hamlin Shaw (see 381 Franklin Street).

After some remodeling, the house had seven bedrooms and nine bathrooms in 1999. The doubly deep lot on East High Street allows room for a tennis court in back.

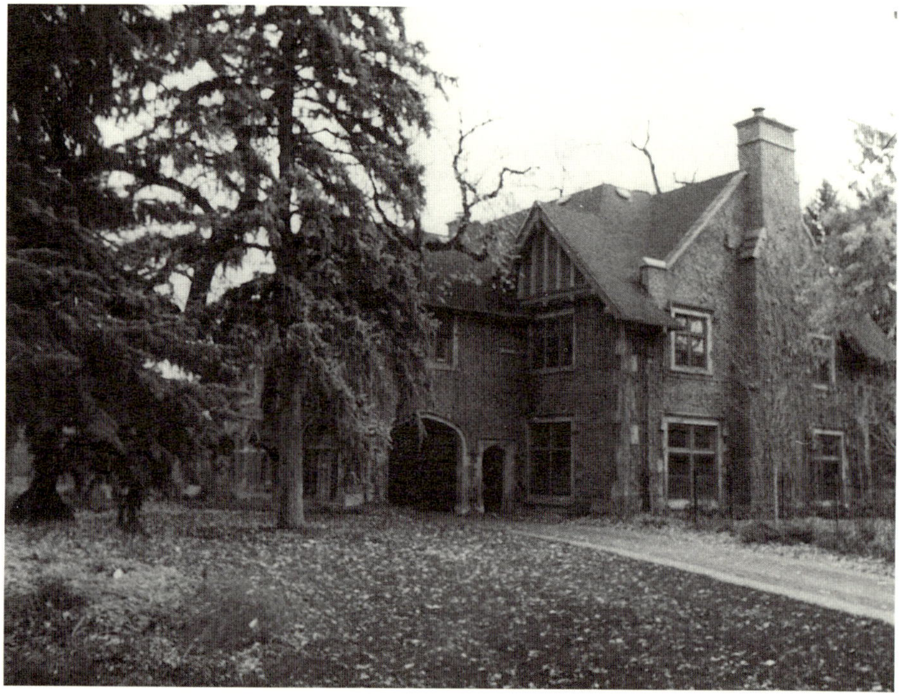

The Benedict-designed Tudor-style house at 360 High Street, built by Sewell Thomas, was sold to Senator Lawrence C. Phipps.

29
320 HIGH STREET
Built: 1914
Architects: Fisher and Fisher

The French Country home at 320 High Street was built by Colonel William E. Hughes a year after he built a house next door as a wedding present for his only living descendant, his granddaughter, Annie Clifton Springer.

Born in 1840, Colonel Hughes was a gifted and motivated pioneer, who made a success of each of the many ventures he attempted. In Texas he became a recognized authority on cattle breeding and banking. In St. Louis he became president of the Continental Land and Cattle Company, then moved the headquarters to Denver in 1896.[58]

In 1867 Hughes had married Annie C. Peete, who gave birth to a daughter, Eliza Clifton. Eliza's eventual marriage to John Springer produced a daughter, Annie Clifton, but Eliza's untimely death in 1904 and her widowed husband's outlandish behavior resulted in Annie living much of her life with her grandparents, the William Hugheses.

John Springer, who initiated the first national livestock association in Denver to slaughter and dress cattle for the markets, was a dashing, picturesque cattleman. The *Denver Post* wrote, "None who knew him . . . will forget his appearance, driving a coach and four horses thru [sic] Denver's streets. . . . He gave dignity to sportsmanship, which glorified the horse."[59] He helped manage much of his father-in-law's business. With all his wealth he later built a huge elaborate ranch in Littleton known as "Springer's Castle."

Springer was at home in politics and known as an orator. In 1904 he ran against Robert Speer for mayor and was later nominated by the Colorado Republicans for vice-president to run with William Howard Taft. Polly Pry wrote, "Nothing could squelch the titillating effervescence of Mr. Springer's speeches or induce him to modulate by half a note the appalling splendor of his clarion voice."[60]

After his wife, Eliza, died in 1904, John Springer then tarnished the Hughes reputation by marrying a "hussy" from St. Louis whom he had met while traveling on business. She toyed with drugs, posed nude for Bohemian artists, and carried on extramarital affairs, leading to the murder of one of her lovers at the Brown Palace Hotel.[61] In short, she

The Hughes family compound of 320 and 300 High Street was built out on the prairie during 1913 and 1914. Between the houses was a sunken garden. (Courtesy DPL Western History Department)

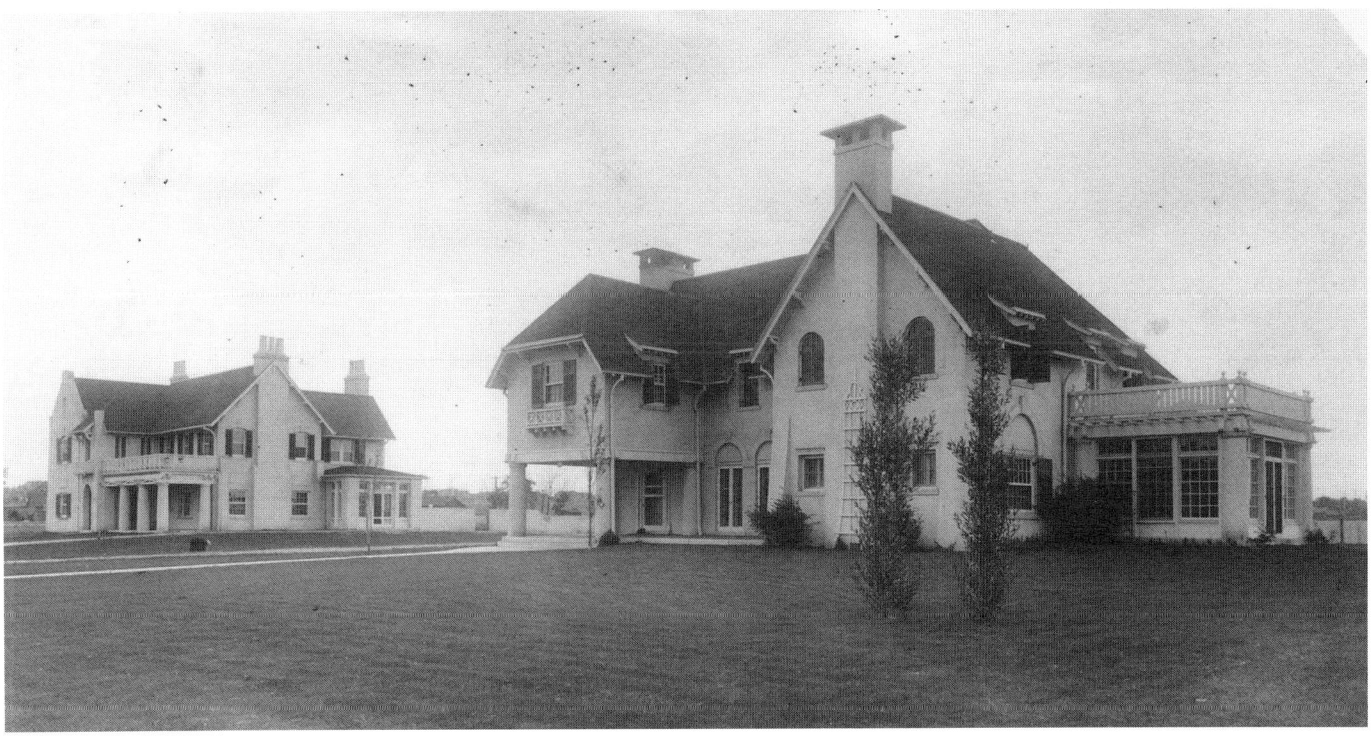

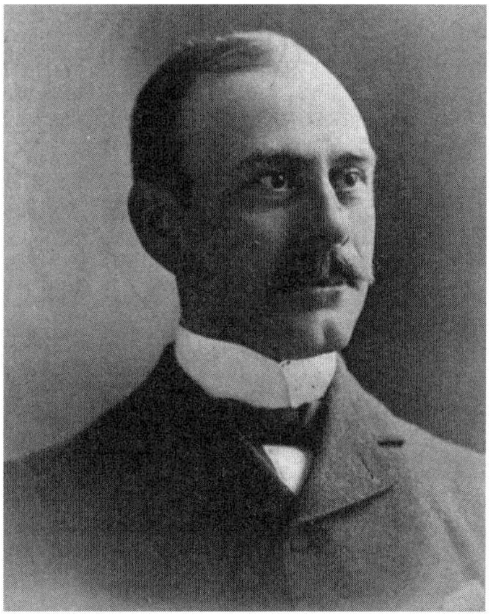

Dashing cattleman John Springer married into, then disgraced the Hughes family. (Courtesy DPL Western History Department)

was not a fit mother for Annie, who came to live with her grandparents.

The Colonel adored his granddaughter, and when she married Lafayette Hughes, he built the two houses side by side on High Street. After Hughes died, the house remained in the family, as Lafayette's brother, Gerald Hughes, moved into 320 High. Called "one of the smartest lawyers ever produced in the West,"[62] Hughes formed a partnership with his neighbor, Clayton C. Dorsey, who lived at 330 Gilpin Street. The firm of Hughes and Dorsey specialized in corporate and business law and handled only large cases. "The law partners Gerald Hughes and Clayton Dorsey operated in the thirties and forties . . . making sure the voice of big business was heeded at City Hall and the Capitol."[63]

Hughes, with his father, Senator Charles James Hughes, Jr., was among five men who incorporated the Fourth Avenue Realty Company, which developed Country Club Place and the Denver Country Club. Gerald Hughes, though a private person, served as a state senator from 1901 to 1905.

He is known for the huge political coup of implementing the plans of his friend, David Moffat, for completing a railroad tunnel through the Continental Divide. Seventeen years after Moffat's death, his widow presented Hughes with a cherished ring of Moffat's. "David wanted you to have this ring. He called me to his bedside the night before he died and said, 'Give this ring to Gerald. He's the one man among my associates who will see that the railroad is completed.' I waited to give you the ring to make sure David was right."[64]

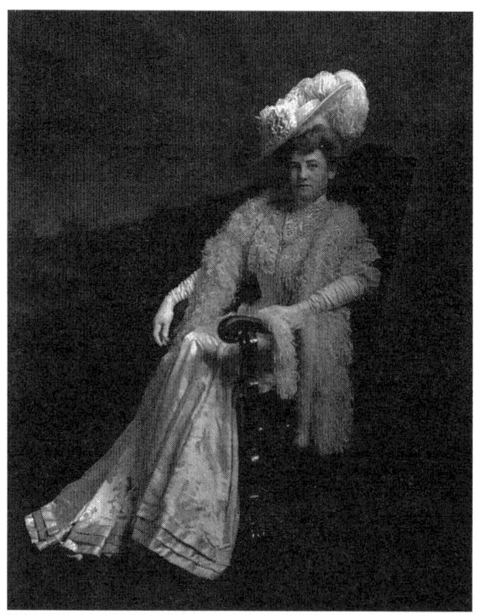

In 1907, Gerald Hughes married Mabel Y. Nagel, who was born on an Indian reservation in South Dakota where her father was the agent in charge of the reservation. As a founder of Children's Hospital, Mabel contributed much to the charitable and social life of Denver and died in 1969 as one of the wealthiest women in the city. They had no children.[65]

The asymmetrical Mediterranean house at 320 High is built of masonry with a steeply gabled tile roof. The off-center entry is protected by a glass arched canopy. North of the entry a second-story window and balconet is topped with a segmental keystone arch. To the south, the covered porch is supported by three massive round columns. The original Fisher plans

[LEFT]
After Colonel Hughes died, 320 High Street was sold to lawyer Gerald Hughes. His wife, the former Mabel Y. Nagel, was born on an Indian reservation in South Dakota. (Courtesy DPL Western History Department)

portray 320 and 300 High designed together as a family compound, at that time way out on the prairie.

During the sixties and seventies the Ferris H. Hamiltons lived in the house and installed a pool with a pool house. Rhonda and Robert Boswell bought it in 1989.

30
300 HIGH STREET
Built: 1913
Architects: Fisher and Fisher

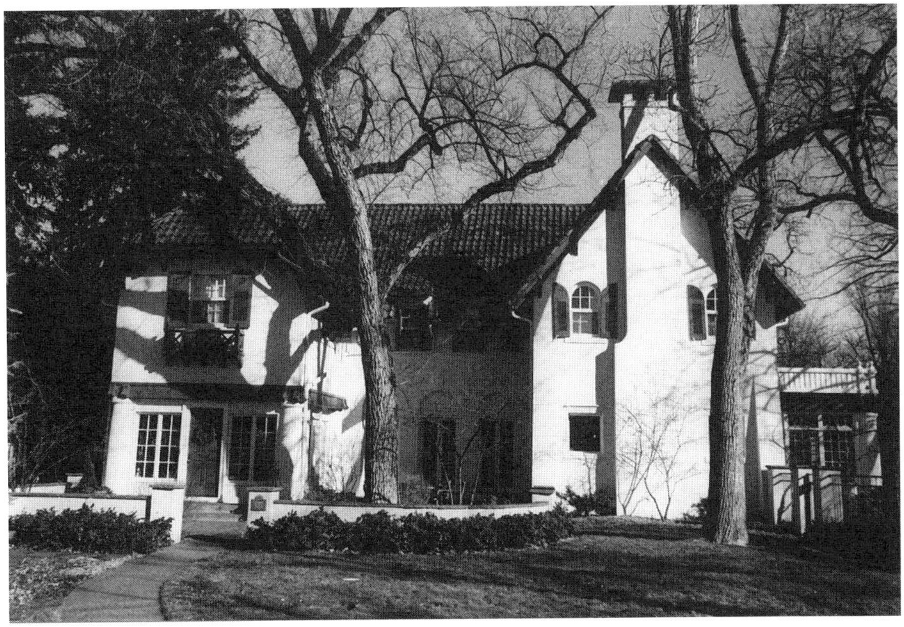

The house at 300 High Street, built for Lafayette Hughes, was later owned by both William V. Hodges and Carl Groos, Jr.

In 1913, Lafayette Hughes carried Annie Clinton Springer over the threshold of this two-story stucco house built for them by her grandfather, Colonel William E. Hughes. As long as they had just one son, the two-bedroom house was ample, but in 1919, twins Lafayette, Jr., and Charles H. were expected. A nursery, closet, kitchenette, and sleeping porch were added to the rear of the second floor, along with rooms for a nurse, maid, cook, and second maid.[66]

The entry and patio of this house are recessed between two steeply gabled wings. Dark shutters are curved to fit across the arched windows. The one-story completely glassed-in sunroom is topped by a wooden balustrade and opens onto the garden pool and fountain. Hughes landscaped and planted a sunken garden to the north.[67] The first-floor covered porch with a tile floor to the north was enclosed in 1924.[68] In 1938 he contracted with Elton S. Boerstler to build a two-car garage in back of the house. The two Hughes houses were designed by the Fishers to be complementary and form a family compound. However, during the eighties a house was built between them, replacing the sunken garden and lily pond.

When Colonel Hughes, of 320 High, died in 1918, lawyer and real estate investor Lafayette Hughes added to his own financial and real estate interests the large oil holdings and Texas ranches inherited by his wife, Colonel Hughes's granddaughter and only heir.

Lafayette Hughes was an ardent polo player. In 1923 he and Ira B. and Albert E. Humphreys, Jr., purchased 30 acres south of Alameda, from University Boulevard to Steele Street and between East Exposition and Alameda Avenues, for polo matches. The golfers at the Denver Country Club had finally objected to horses romping about their fairways and had expelled them from the premises. Hughes then commissioned Fisher and Fisher to build a three-story, 36-room Mediterranean home for himself on the new polo grounds.

A tragedy occurred in 1940 when his beautiful socialite wife, Annie, developed a tumor in her ear. Thinking it was caused by a malignancy, she shot herself in the bathroom. An autopsy report revealed that the lesion had been benign. She had been an excellent tennis player, golfer, and horsewoman and was a former president of the Children's Hospital board.

Gerald and Lafayette Hughes were two sons of U.S. Senator Charles James Hughes, a specialist in irrigation and mining law. The other son, Berrien, also a lawyer, was somewhat of a playboy. He loved sports and was especially fond of climbing up to ski the snowy slopes of Loveland Pass in the early days of Colorado skiing. However, in 1939, while slaloming through the trees with his friends, William V. Hodges, Jr.; Frank Ashley; and Charles Kendrick, he suffered a fatal accident.[69] Denver's new Winter Park commemorated this enthusiastic skier by naming the first groomed ski slope in his honor. As Dr. Giles Toll commented, "I'll bet more people are familiar with the Upper and Lower Hughes Trails at Winter Park [named after Berrien] than they are with his illustrious brothers, Gerald and Lafayette."

In 1959, the year after Lafayette Hughes died, the palatial Polo Club mansion was sold to Mrs. McIntosh Buell. His son, Lafayette, Jr., then developed the rest of the grounds into an exclusive residential subdivision of 35 building sites called the Polo Club.

After Lafayette Hughes moved from 300 High to the polo grounds, his friend, William V. Hodges, lived in the house for the next 40 years. Hodges graduated from East High School and attended Columbia University Law School, where he roomed with Senator Alva Adams of Pueblo. When he returned to Denver, he practiced law with his father before opening the firm of (Clayton C.) Dorsey and Hodges. With his first wife, Mabel Gilluly, he had two children, William, Jr., and Joseph G., before Mabel died in 1925. He then married Catherine Lowndes and moved to 300 High. When she died in 1933, he married Elizabeth Davis Berry.

A staunch Republican, Hodges was treasurer of the Republican National Committee from 1924 to 1928, campaigning for both Calvin Coolidge and Herbert Hoover.

Like many children raised in the older Country Club subdivisions, Hodges's sons, Joseph, and William, Jr., lived to the east in the newer subdivision, Country Club Annex. Lawyer Joseph, a Colorado junior golf champion in 1927, lived at 225 Vine, where his children grew up, before he moved to 150 Vine. His son, Joseph, Jr., a fifth generation of Hodges family lawyers, was instrumental in organizing the Cherry Creek Improvement Association. He and his wife, Jean, have lived at 2116 East 4th Avenue since 1979. The other son, William, Jr., a pioneer of the Colorado ski industry, lived next door to his brother at 235 Vine in a house that had been occupied by Colorado governor Dan Thornton.

During the seventies, 300 High was occupied by architect Carl Groos, Jr., and his wife, Marjorie "Mardi," a daughter of Temple and Mrs. McIntosh Buell. Groos came to Denver from San Antonio, Texas, in 1953 as one of the first representatives of I. M. Pei Associates in building the Denver U.S. Bank Center, the Hilton Hotel, and the adjoining May D & F store at Courthouse Square. While living there, Groos designed a contemporary house at the back of his lot for William V. Warren at 200 High Street. After Groos died, Mardi sold the house in the eighties to a developer who wanted to build five houses on those lots. With pressure from the neighbors and the Cherry Creek Improvement Association, the plan was reduced to building a house (312) between 300 and 320 on High Street. At the back of the lot, the horseless carriage house, which served both homes, was remodeled into 310 High Street. The original compound, therefore, now consists of five homes.

In 1988 the house was bought by Barbara and Ronald Miller. They enjoy the historic home and take great pride in retaining the original fixtures, such as the wall lamp and sconce in the master bedroom. The dark, paneled room that used to adjoin the dining room is labeled "Smoking Lounge," a nostalgic reminder of the days when men would retire after dinner to light up their cigars. "We use the whole house," Barbara said. "We have 10 nieces and nephews who really take over the nursery and sleeping porch when they come visit."

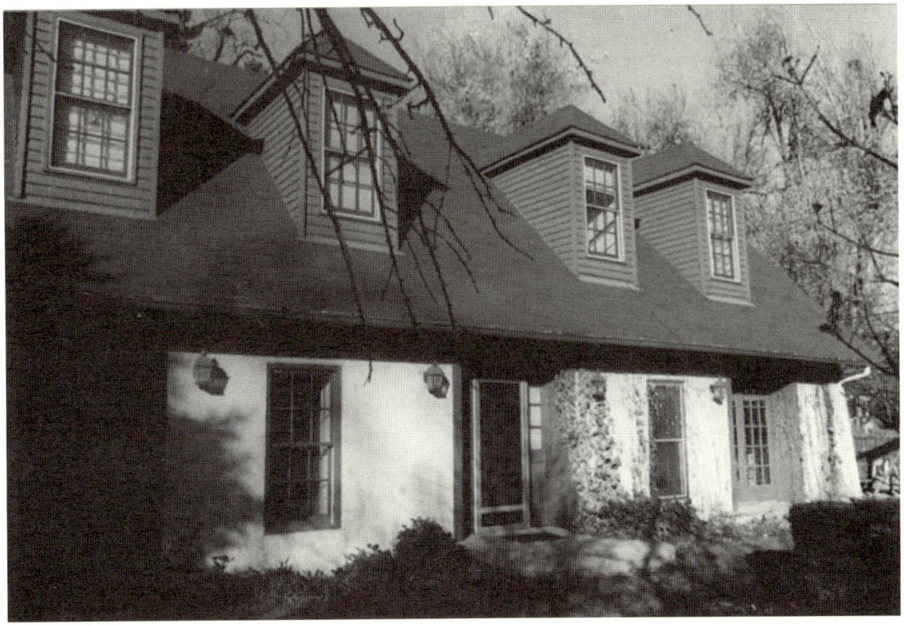

In 1985, the garage for the two Hughes houses was remodeled into this contemporary house at 310 High Street.

31
310 HIGH STREET
Built: 1914
Architects Fisher and Fisher
Remodeling: 1985
Designer Jerry Rossel

On the east of the deep lots in back of a sunken garden between 300 and 320 High Street, William Hughes had built a Fisher-designed garage for the two homes. It bordered on the original Race Street that was vacated by city ordinance in 1920. In 1985, Carl Groos sold his house at 300 High, including the lot to the north, to Jerry Rossel, president of Williamsburg Homes, Inc. Rossel sold the Groos house to the Ronald Millers, built and sold a traditional-style home on the street at 312 High, then remodeled the garage in back for his own family, leaving a 10-foot driveway between the two houses for access.

The remodeled garage echoes the French Country style created for the original Hughes compound. "This is a good example of adaptive preservation and remodeling," commented architect Edward D. White, Jr. "It's an interesting modern variation in the traditional buildings of the historic district. It is harmonious in character and unobtrusive in scale." The house was expanded to 5,000 square feet. Over the combination family-dining-kitchen area is a master suite and bedroom. The oversized fireplace was composed of cobblestones obtained from the old West Colfax Avenue viaduct. Two more bedrooms were added over the new garage that connects to the house through a breezeway. A formal living room and den complete the house.[70] "The study is paneled in oak with a corbelled ceiling. I guess this is Rossel's trademark," said current owner James Arkell. "Each of the three houses [300, 310 and 312 High] has a room completely paneled with either oak or cherry. Our house has no crawl space for pipes because it was built as a garage. The plumbing is in the walls of the first floor. . . . We can tell where the original garage was, as the walls are still there," Arkell said. "It was a squarish building, about 40 by 40 feet." The Arkells, who bought in 1991, are the fourth and longest owners of this 1985-remodeled house.

32
200 HIGH STREET
Built: 1966
Architect: Carl Groos, Jr.

Architect Carl Groos sold the back 17,000 square feet of his property at 300 High Street and designed a late International-style house for Marian and William V. Warren, Jr. The two-story, flat-roofed house has a tall entrance foyer with a grand piano that Warren played remarkably well. Architect Edward D. White, Jr., is impressed with the "large glass areas, generous interior spaces, fine materials, and freedom from the clutter of eclectic historical ornamentation of this house, while it harmonizes in scale and refinements with existing landmarks." Included are a living-room opening on to the south patio, an adjoining study, and a family room beside an outdoor lap pool to the north.

Warren, who operated a feed broker firm, had served as a trustee of the Denver Art Museum for six years and was vice-president of the board and co-chairman of their development fund campaign at the time of the purchase.

However, a scandal rocked the town in 1970. On October 20 the newspapers reported, "The FBI in New York announced the arrest of a man identified as the vice president of the Denver Art Museum after he allegedly attempted to sell two pieces of a $500,000 art collection stolen from a Larkspur, Colorado, rancher last Wednesday."[71] Warren, a friend of art collector Montgomery Ritchie, had absconded with 16 artworks shortly after visiting him at his ranch. Donning a wig and mustache he naively took off for a New York City art gallery to sell a Renoir painting and a Gauguin drawing. The proprietor, recognizing the works, reported the attempted sale to the FBI, who subsequently recovered 12 more pieces "from a residence in central Denver." The community was shocked and the art museum board felt the "charges were completely out of character with Mr. Warren's dedicated and efficient services to the museum over the past nine years."[72]

Anne Waring Maer had stopped by the Warrens' house once to pick up her son, Edward D. White, III, who was carpooling with the Warren children. Warren's wife, Marian, suggested she go find them in the attic. "I stood at the top of a ladder and watched Bill practicing a hand puppet show. He was phenomenal! He could change his voice and accent with such ease. He was a brilliant performer, and he used this to try to disguise himself."

Warren was convicted of transporting stolen artworks[73] three months later, fined $40,000,[74] given a suspended two-year prison term and sued for $50,000 by Ritchie. A month later his feed company was sued for $20,000 because he had failed to pay for delivered goods.[75] The family soon left town.

The house was sold to Howard and Priscilla Barnard Rea, who moved in with her two daughters, Ann and Phoebe Barnard and his children, Drayton, Kim, and Alison Rea.

In 1987, Bruce Ducker and his wife, Jaren, bought the house. Bruce is a lawyer-novelist with six books to his credit. Jaren has served as head of the Friends of the Denver Public Library, has served on the Civic Liberties Union board, and was appointed by the mayor to the Library Commission and the Board of Appeals for the City Building Department.

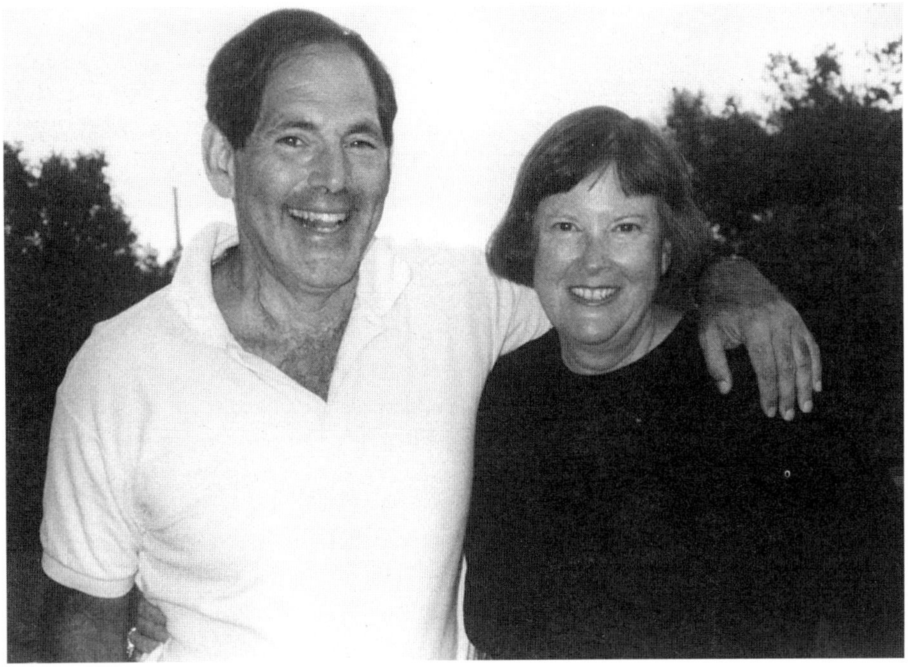

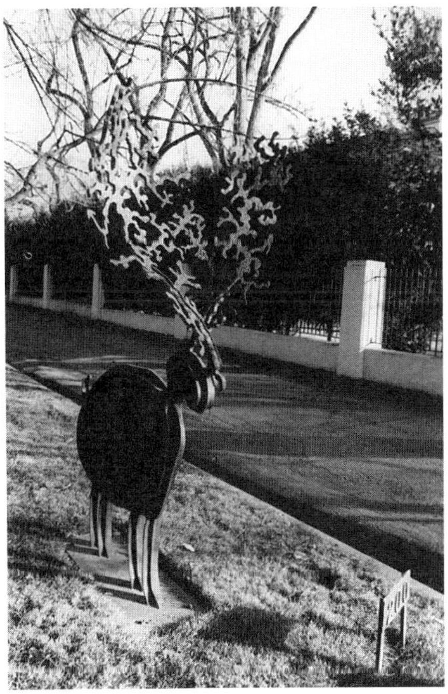

[ABOVE]
Behind his home at 300 High Street architect Carl Groos, Jr., built a house for vice-president of the Denver Art Museum, William V. Warren. The house at 200 High was later occupied by Jaren and Bruce Ducker.
(Courtesy the Bruce Duckers)

[LEFT]
The long driveway leading to the private house at 200 High Street is marked by a reindeer sculptured by Fred Myers.

The house is set back, so it is difficult for visitors to locate. "As a landmark we put a Fred Myers sculpture of a reindeer out on the street so people could find our house," Jaren said. "The house is very private, and it's like going away for the weekend to come home to this quiet spot, protected by the heavily wooded area to the east and the wide lawn at 190 High to the south."

33
301 HIGH STREET
Built: 1914
Architects: Marean and Norton

Financial expert Arthur H. Bosworth lived in this Mission-style stucco house at 301 High Street, two blocks from his brother, Robert G. Bosworth, at 314 Franklin Street. Both were sons of Mr. and Mrs. Joab Bosworth and were raised in a historic home at 1400 Josephine Street. Joab, a chemist, founded the Denver Fire Clay Company, but was killed during a laboratory experiment in 1890 when Arthur was only four years old. Joab's wife, Lenore, founded the Monday Literary Club and was active in the American Association of University Women (AAUW). She left her home, known as "the Bosworth house," to the AAUW to use as its headquarters when she died in 1947.

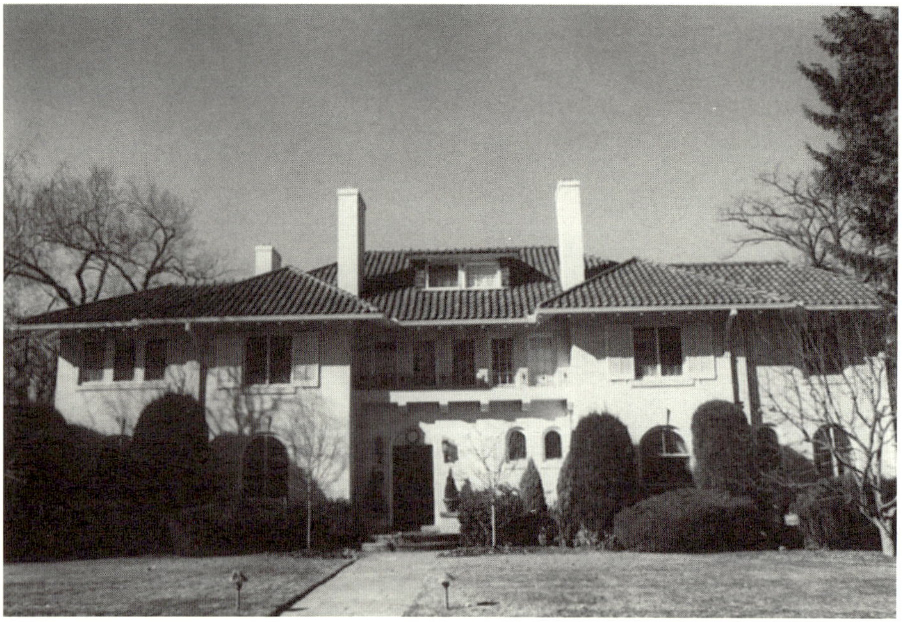

This Mission-style stucco house at the corner of 3rd and High was occupied by financial expert Arthur H. Bosworth.

Arthur Bosworth had always been interested in finance. After college he joined Governor William E. Sweet's investment firm, where he rose to president. Later he formed his own company with Octave Chanute and Paul Loughridge. In 1946, after his daughter, Betty, had married stockbroker Barry Sullivan, he merged with John J. Sullivan to form Bosworth, Sullivan and Company. It was said of Bosworth in 1925, before the age of computers that "he has a mind that works with the speed of lightning and the accuracy of controlled electricity." He was also described as a man who looked five years younger than his age, with a "round, jolly face and a wide, jolly mouth that lends itself to laughter."[76]

The two-and-a-half story stucco house is symmetrically designed in an H-plan with the side wings protruding, each with two arched keystone windows on the first floor and large double-hung windows above. The off-center front door is set in an arched opening balanced by two small arched windows in the recessed entryway to the north. Five glazed openings are located along the balcony above the entrance, and over the balcony are two dormer windows on the attic floor. The red tile roof is medium-pitched and hipped. The Denver Public Library publication *Lookout* of April 1928 stated, "At 301 High is an interesting yellow stucco house ornamented with Della Robbias," one over the front door in the recessed arch.

34
190 HIGH STREET
Built: 1917
Architect: Maurice Biscoe

Sidney Weil Sinsheimer came to Rocky Ford, Colorado, in 1900 as an engineer working for the first sugar beet factory in the Arkansas valley. He helped organize the Holly Sugar Company and was a popular socialite and resident of both Denver and Colorado Springs.

In 1917, Maurice Biscoe designed this Mediterranean home on six 265-foot deep lots. It features recessed moldings and arched windows with fanlights within the arch. Upstairs windows included transoms and recessed moldings. Exposed carved rafters lie under the eaves of the low-pitched, red tile roof. Over the south sunroom is a stone balustrade. A solid, six-foot stucco wall shields the garden. This house is one of the best examples of Biscoe's Mediterranean structures. It

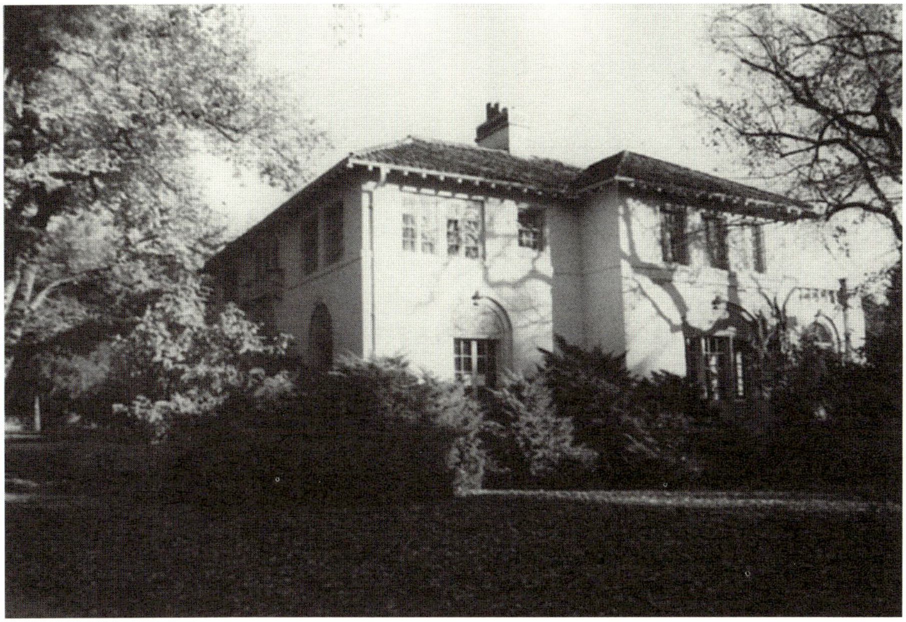

The large Mediterranea-style houe at 190 High Street was built for engineer Sidney W. Sinsheimer, who brought the first sugar beet factory to Colorado.

has classical, symmetrical lines and fine detailing around the doors and windows. A grand bay leads out to a patio and large garden in back.

Sinsheimer divorced his wife, Anna, in 1919. Shortly after his second marriage in 1926, Anna died, contributing $40,000 to his fortune seven years after their divorce. Sinsheimer was an active leader in the sugar industry until his fatal heart attack in 1933.[77]

After the divorce, the house was bought by a fun-loving oil and gas developer, Frank E. Kistler, who came to Colorado to manage his 14,000 acres of Wyoming oil leases. Eventually Kistler built his first-year profits of $1 million into $50 million. He took over Springer's Castle, the huge mansion John Springer had built in Littleton, and turned it into a 20,000-acre showplace, the Diamond K Ranch, later Highlands Ranch. This was a center for frequent dazzling social activities. He and his wife, Florence, hosted lavish parties in Paris, London, and Vienna. One of his favorites was a party he gave when he owned the Colorado Hotel in Glenwood Springs. Honored guest among the 385 dignitaries was ex-president Herbert Hoover, a long time friend of Kistler's.[78]

At 190 High Street, he and Florence raised three vivacious daughters and a son, Hughes E. Kistler. The teenaged daughters, too, were fond of entertaining. Robert "Robbie" McPhee and Philip Gates remembered those days in the twenties when they dressed up as pumpkins for Halloween and bunnies for Easter parties. "Seems like there was always an exotic car or two in the driveway," wrote Gates, "like a Pierce-Arrow with those strange headlights coming out of the fenders."

Medora Wilson (Mrs. Paul Douden, Jr.) watched a graduation party from her bedroom window at 140 High Street. "It was a circus party in the yard, but the only way you could get there was to climb to the second floor and slide down a two-story slide into the party. Little tents around the lawn had shooting galleries and other games and snacks."

After a January 1929 Mexican divorce, Florence Kistler stayed in the house. Frank then vacationed in Hawaii, met Leana Antonides in February, and married her in June.

Kistler's health and wealth were continually on a roller coaster. He lost his money and sold the Diamond K Ranch "We don't worry about the failures," he said, brushing aside the time he lost $12 million in a single day through the stock market.[79] With debilitating arthritis, Kistler turned

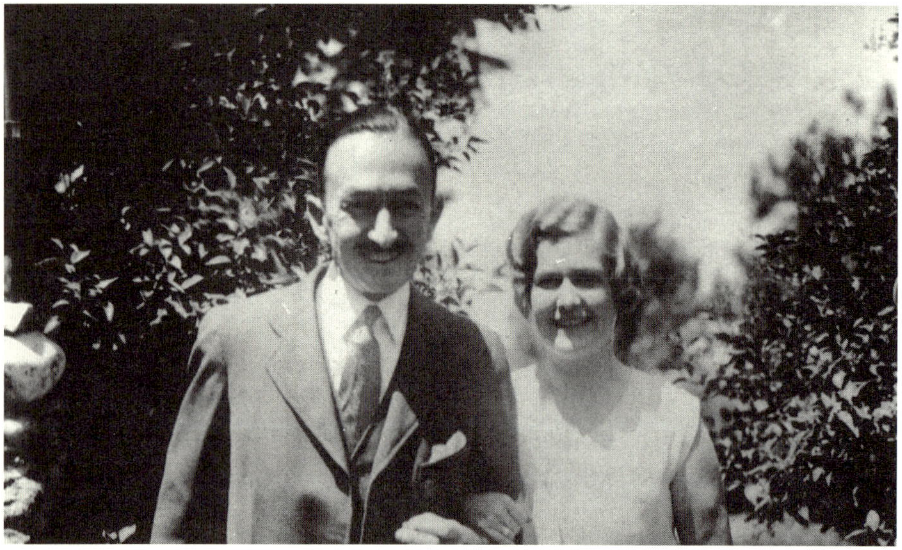

The house at 190 High Street, owned by Frank E. Kistler, was often the scene of lively parties. Later Kistler married the beautiful Leana Antionides and moved to Glenwood Springs. (Courtesy DPL Western History Department)

his attention to developing Glenwood Springs and its soothing hot mineral waters. He eventually moved there with his beautiful new wife, Leana.

In 1943, while Florence was staying in a house in the country, the house on High Street was burgled by some boys who made themselves at home for a few days, sleeping in the beds and emptying wine bottles. They ransacked every room, causing considerable damage and absconding with silverware, china, and a valuable Whistler oil painting.[80]

Charles A. Johnson, a neighbor at 230 Vine Street, had another story. "Both Mrs. Kistlers were shopping on Fifth Avenue in New York. They happened to be changing in adjacent fitting rooms, and both were charging clothes to Frank Kistler. The poor salesgirl was at her wit's end trying to keep the situation straight and confidential."

During the forties, lawyer Stanley T. Wallbank, president of the Denver Bar Association, the Chamber of Commerce, and the Legal Aid Society, and his wife, Nellie, raised their children, Elaine "Lainey" (Mrs. William Cable Jackson), Helen (Mrs. William Milliken), Elizabeth "B.J." (Mrs. James E. Stokes), and Lincoln Wallbank in this spacious mansion.

"The house had been abandoned and was a shambles when we moved in," said Lainey. "It has six bedrooms plus two porches, two rooms for servants in the back, and living quarters over the garage." Apparently, after the Lindbergh kidnapping, the bedrooms had all been connected by inside doors from the master bedroom to the nursery. These corridors were later turned into oddly shaped closets.[81]

During the sixties, cardiologist S. Gilbert Blount, Jr., and his wife, Jean, raised five daughters in the house. Blount is a Professor Emeritus of Medicine at the University of Colorado Health Sciences Center and was involved in the care of President Dwight D. Eisenhower when he suffered a heart attack while visiting his wife's family in Denver.

When the girls left the big house, the Blounts moved across the street to a smaller but similar Mediterranean house at 363 High Street.

Later occupants of the house at 190 High Street were Lon Schreur; his wife, Christine; and her son, Julian Wassenaar. Wassenaar said, "Just for the fun of it we made a secret passage from the study to the wine cellar with a spiral staircase. The entrance was behind a painting." Christine Schreur Smith loved the big house but wanted something less spacious. In 1996 she, like the Blounts, moved to the similar, but smaller house across the street at 363 High.

35
195 HIGH STREET
Built: 1912
Architect: Frederick Harnois

In 1912, houses were built side by side at 195 and 149 High Street by Tyson Swinney Dines, a partner of the law firm of Dines, (Orville) Dines and (Peter Hagner) Holme. Dines chose the corner lot at 195 High Street for a two-story, Spanish Colonial Revival house designed by architect Frederick Harnois, who was then living nearby at the home he designed for himself at 164 Lafayette Street. A tiled portico with arched openings marks the entrance. The semicircular bay window off the living room, flanked by decorative cartouches, is echoed on a smaller scale on the north facade. A covered porch to the south is closed with a patterned screen. While he was building this house, Harnois designed a stucco, Mission-style house next door at 149 High Street for his son, Tyson, Jr.

Tyson S. Dines came from Missouri to Denver in 1892 and opened a law office specializing in mining law. He was a humble man who lent his abilities to the community by heading the Chamber of Commerce, serving on the Denver School Board, and teaching at the University of Denver law school. He was also a thrifty and conservative member of the Old Guard of the Denver Country Club.

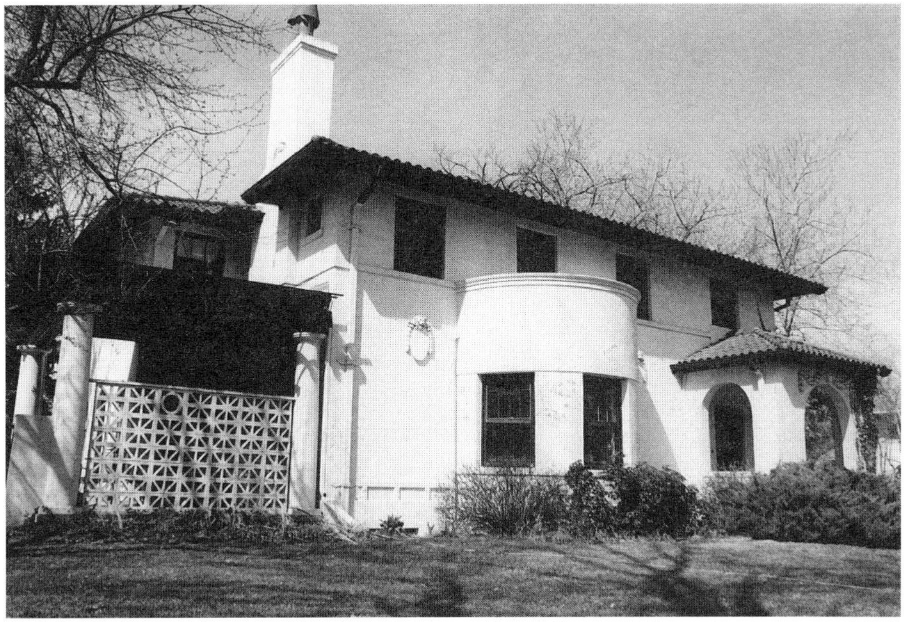

This 1912 Spanish Colonial Revival house at 195 High Street was designed by Frederick Harnois.

His granddaughter, Marcia (Strickland), tells a story about his dog: "Each day he would give his springer spaniel, Lord Chesterfield, a pail to carry to the Denver Country Club. When the pail was brimming over with a rejected gourmet repast, he would carry it home to enjoy on the front steps."

The Dines family had a unique habit of "name-dropping." Tyson Swinney Dines changed his middle name to Tyson "S." Dines. His son, Tyson Mauzey Dines, changed his middle name to "M," then Tyson M. Dines, Jr., dropped the "M." Therefore, Tyson S. Dines's son is Tyson M. Dines, and his son and grandson are Tyson Dines, Jr., and Tyson Dines, III. Son Eugene, has no middle name or initial.

The family populated the Country Club Historic Neighborhood: Two of the four sons, Courtland and Eugene, lived at 195 High Street when they were students at Yale, the traditional family alma mater. When first married, Eugene stayed at the family home with his bride, Marie Eaton, before moving to a house of their own. Their children, Eugene, David, Bruce, and Marcia, all lived in the neighborhood. Eugene, Jr., and his wife, Winston "Winkie,"

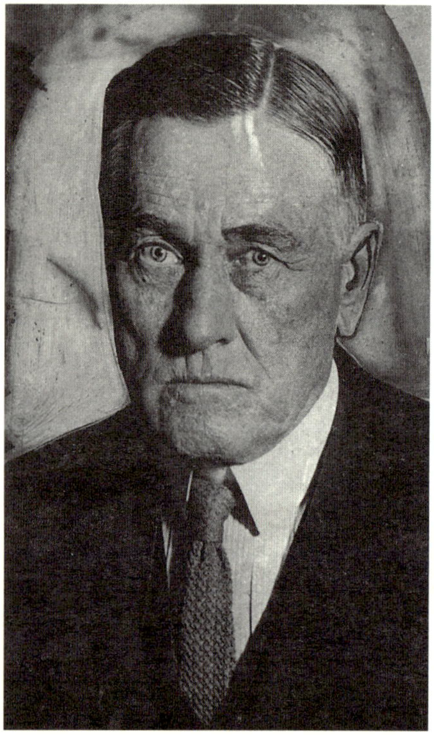

Many of the descendants of lawyer Tyson S. Dines spent their childhoods at 195 High Street and still live in the neighborhood. (Courtesy DPL Western History Department)

bought a house at 2022 East 4th Avenue. Dave and Bette, then Bruce and his wife, Dorothy, lived at 350 Gaylord. After she married Jerome Strickland, Marcia moved to the spacious house at 360 Gilpin Street to accommodate their combined families. After Eugene died in 1962, his widow, Marie, moved to 1953 East 3rd Avenue.

Tyson S. Dines's dashing son, Courtland, was a broker, an avid golfer, and one of the first Denverites to own an airplane. A fun-loving playboy, he was adored by his niece, Marcia (Strickland), who said, "Uncle Court was an absolute delight. He had no children, but he had a place in Estes Park that was the greatest fun for us." Three of his four marriages ended in divorce. He died at the age of 56 of his third heart attack.

The house at 195 High became "Annapolis Annex" soon after 1925, when Captain Mary Parker Converse moved to Denver from Boston after the death of her husband, wealthy shoe manufacturer and yachtsman Harry E. Converse. Having raised five children, socialite Converse relocated to a spot where she could run over and play tennis every day at the Denver Country Club. During a Colorado open tennis tournament there, she invited some of the players to stay at her home. She became good friends with Don Budge, whom she later saw play at Wimbledon. Missing her old pleasure of exercising her license as a yachting pilot, she booked passage, at age 66, on a freighter to Africa with the understanding that she would do her own navigating. After three years of diligent study, she became a licensed ship's captain in 1940. She was the only female four-striped captain in the Merchant Marine. One evening, as she was dressing for the symphony, she was called by a naval recruiting officer who wanted to know if she would help teach a navigation program for new officers. Two days a week her dining room became the Annapolis Annex, from which she graduated 200 officers in navigation. On other days she practiced singing and piano, attended the symphony, and graciously hostessed open houses for acquaintances, friends, and neighbors every Wednesday. "She had an electric car and used to give us all a

During World War II 195 High Street became "Annapolis Annex" as Captain Mary Converse taught navigation for the Merchant Marine. (Courtesy DPL Western History Department)

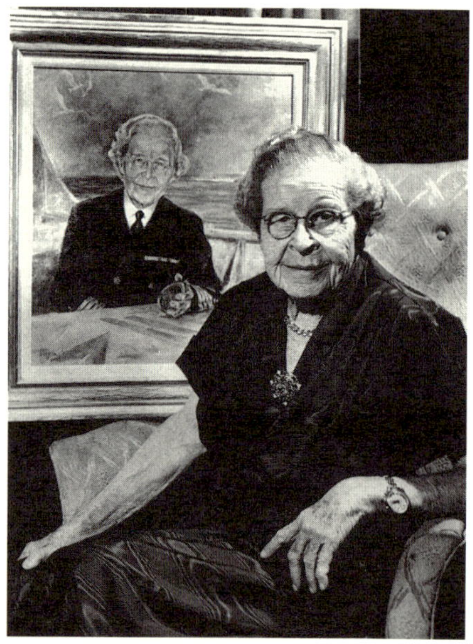

ride around the neighborhood," said Medora Wilson (Mrs. Paul A. Douden, Jr.) of 140 High Street.

Converse remodeled the basement in 1936 and built a masonry addition to the west in 1950. At the age of 83, she moved to California to be near her 47 grandchildren.

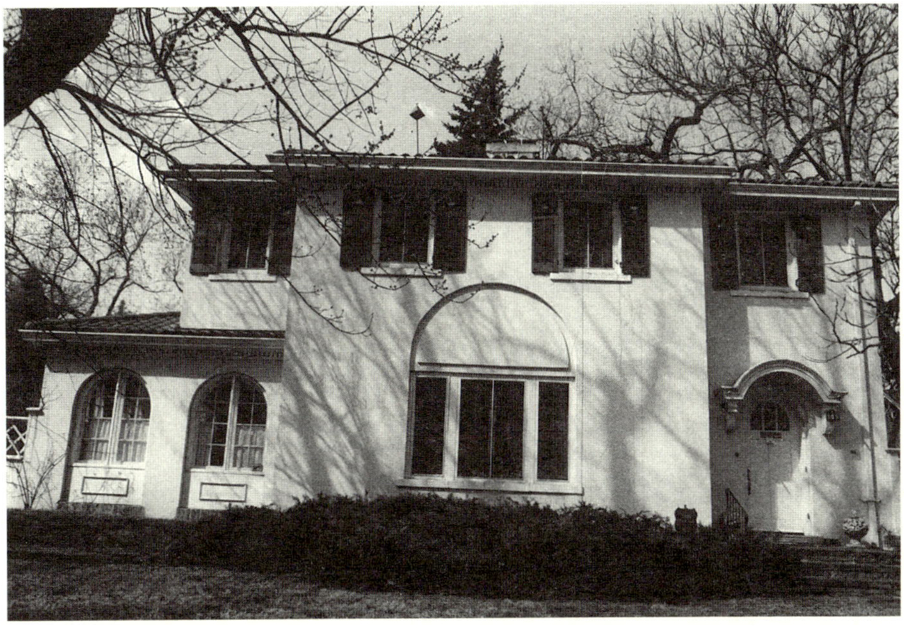

Tyson S. Dines built a house for his son, Tyson M. Dines at 149 High Street.

36
149 HIGH STREET
Built 1912
Architect: Frederick Harnois

Tyson M. "Tice" Dines entered his father's law firm after graduating from Yale. Some time after he married Isabel Allen he moved into the house at 149 High Street, which, at the time, was next door to his parents' house at 195 High.

The home was designed by Frederick Harnois, an architect who arrived in Denver in 1893 and formed a partnership with Theodore Boal, designer of the original clubhouse for the Denver Country Club. Like 195 High, the house is asymmetrical, is Mediterranean in style, and has a patterned screen shielding the garden. A decorative arched canopy over the entrance is repeated by a large semi-circular arch recessed in the wall above the casement windows in the adjacent living room. To the south is a sunroom with arched windows.

Dines was the essence of respectable conservatism: formal, responsible, Ivy League. In 1923 he moved to Logan Street, where he died at age 80 after months of ill health.

The older son, Tyson, Jr., who was born in the High Street house, was suave and dashing, and enjoyed sailing, traveling, and square dancing. He followed his Yale education with a law degree at the University of Denver. He had a special interest in languages, spoke German, and studied the classics. Dines taught languages at the private Colorado Academy, for a number of years. His three children are Sherman (Mrs. Stephen Waite); Tyson, III; and Marian.

The younger son, Allen, following an education at Yale and a stint in the Navy, went to Harvard Law School, then spent five years in Washington with the State Department. He returned to Denver, practicing in the law firm of Holme, Roberts, Moore and Owen. After five terms in the Colorado House of Representatives, where he was speaker, he served two terms in the state Senate.

In the early sixties another state senator, Frank A. Kemp, Jr., bought

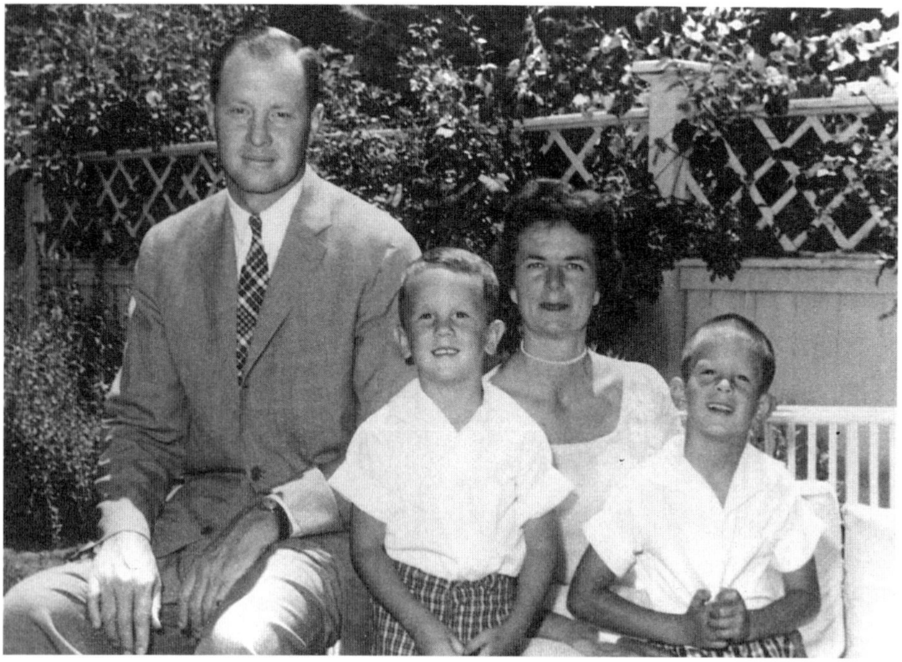

State senator Frank A. Kemp, Jr.; his wife, Polly; and their two sons, Frank A "Alec," and J. Hovey Kemp have lived at 149 High Street since the early sixties. (Courtesy Frank A. Kemps)

the house with his award-winning, freelance journalist wife, Polly. After serving in the Marines in the Pacific in World War II, where he earned at least six medals including two Purple Hearts, Kemp became a self-employed ranch businessman and real estate appraiser. As a Republican he served four terms in the Colorado House and Senate. Helping with his campaigns were his wife and his two sons, Frank A. "Alec" Kemp, IV, and J. Hovey Kemp. In 1968, after Kemp's unsuccessful bid for the U.S. Senate, Tom Gavin wrote in the *Denver Post*,[82] "Kemp's got an open mind, and he listens. You've now lost a good and decent man."

37
170 AND 180 HIGH STREET
Built: 1977
Architect: James S. Sudler, II

"These two houses should be discussed as a unit," said Barbara Sudler Hornby, whose late husband, James Stewart Sudler, II's firm, designed the two contemporary houses. The houses are on the east end of the deep lots on High Street. Sudler's own house at 180 High complements the house designed by Joal Cronenwett of James Sudler Associates at 170 High for the Karl Arndts.

As an architect, Sudler was influenced by International style concepts of clean horizontal lines, sparse ornamentation, and purpose for each element of a house. As he said on tape in 1975, he was "concerned with function primarily, then proportion and design."[83] Barbara said, "While Jim was designing our house I had no idea what it would really look like. Jim arranged the functional elements, then put walls around it." The same modus operandi was used in building the Denver Art Museum.

His own house was one of the first to use solar energy for heat, collected on the south side of a 60 degree gable roof and stored in a rock room in the basement. The compound was designed so that the Arndt's house to the south is low and would not obstruct the solar collectors. "Solar design is ten percent more expensive, but we both were environmentally minded. We haven't really been able to tell if it saves money," Barbara said.

The house at 180 High is U-shaped, enclosing a courtyard edged with a historic frieze from the top of the old International Trust building. Sudler, a devout preservationist and

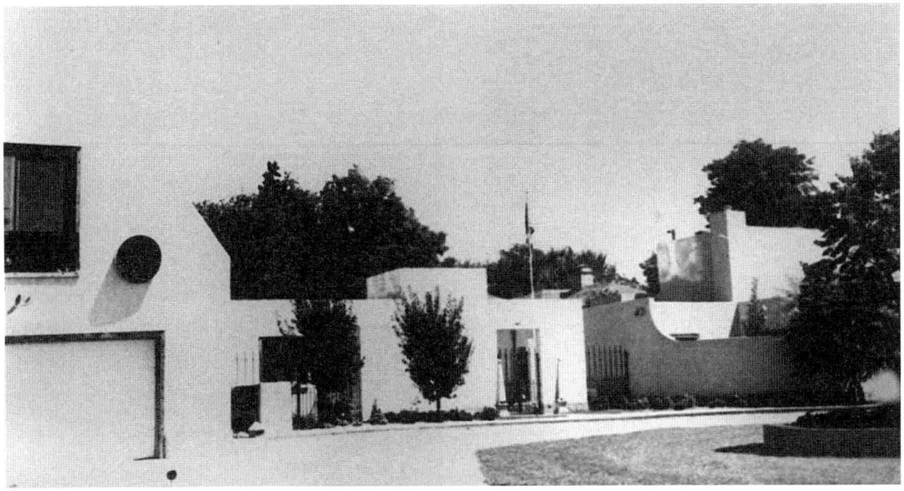

During the seventies the houses at 180 and 170 High Street were designed as a unit by James Sudler, II, for himself and the Karl Arndts. (Courtesy Denver Planning Office)

member of the Denver Landmark Commission, incorporated original sculptures into his buildings, such as the Federal Building at 19th and Stout streets. Barbara had wanted a courtyard that was totally enclosed, but Sudler felt that this would make too large a house and that the trees in the eastern vacated alley would shade it enough. Unfortunately the trees were taken down during the late nineties. The house offers utmost privacy and great outdoor living with a minimum of upkeep.

Sudler's favorite and best-known building is the Denver Art Museum, which he designed with Gio Ponti of Milan, Italy. Of it he said, "We came up with a beautifully functioning building, but it looked like two awful refrigerators stuck next to each other. . . . Then we worked for a year and a half to proportion it and make that look good."[84] In 1974 Sudler became the first architect to receive the Governor's Award for the Arts and Humanities. Other of his buildings, designed in collaboration with architect Rodney Davis of 315 Franklin Street, are the dramatic Church of the Risen Christ on South Monaco Parkway, the United States Courthouse, and the Federal Building.

Sudler was also dedicated to historic preservation and open space in downtown areas. As journalist Joanne Ditmer, who served with him on the Urban Environment Subcommittee of the Planning Board, wrote, "He would push anyone and everyone connected with the city into making it a livelier, more attractive and better place to live."[85]

In 1974, Sudler's wife, Barbara, became Executive Director of Historic Denver, Inc., then moved in 1979 to the presidency of the Colorado Historical Society. "First I preserved a city, then a state. What about a country?" she asks. She still lives in the house with her well-known husband, journalist William H. Hornby, former editor of the *Denver Post.*

Barbara Sudler (Hornby) was president of the Colorado Historical Society in 1984 when the organization sponsored the renovation of the Georgetown Loop railway between Georgetown and Silver Plume. (Courtesy Stephen Hart Library, Colorado Historical Society)

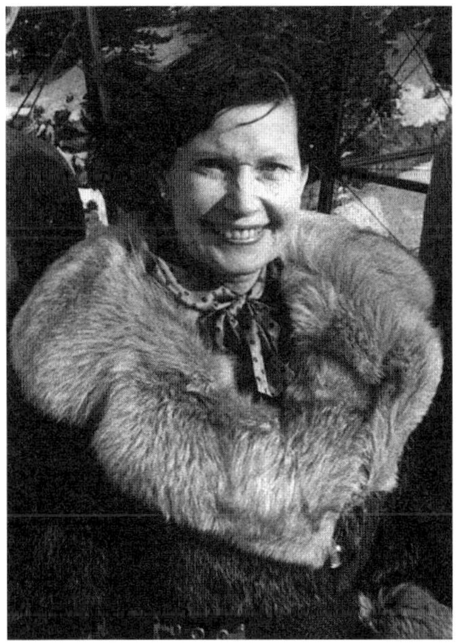

170 HIGH STREET

Joal Cronenwett of James Sudler Associates designed the other house across the courtyard as a retirement home for the Sudlers' long-time friends and associates, physician Karl F. Arndt and his wife, Helen Millett Arndt. Helen had worked on the Art and Architecture Committee of the Episcopal Diocese of Colorado with Sudler for many years.

During the sixties, with emphasis on renovating the downtown area, citizens became upset at the devastation of historic buildings. Helen had been appointed the first woman member of the Denver Planning Board in 1959. One of her accomplishments was launching a Mountain View Preservation Ordinance, passed by City Council in 1968. As a former member of the Denver Planning Board and good friend of Arndt's, historian Thomas J. Noel, wrote of her: "While protecting the mountainous backdrop that is Denver's greatest landmark, Arndt also tried to save manmade landmarks."[86]

Together with Sudler she spearheaded the Denver Landmark Commission in 1967 and worked to identify buildings of historic and/or architectural significance that should be saved. The task was not always easy, but Arndt was persuasive and persistent. Edward D. White, Jr., an early and long-time member of the Landmark Commission said, "Helen loved it when Commission member Bob (Dr. Robert L.) Stearns, then president of the University of Colorado, would go to the mayor's office with her. He may not have understood exactly what Helen was after, but he had a lot of clout and helped her accomplish her goals." The Urban Renewal Authority found it much easier to wipe out whole blocks of downtown buildings rather than shuffle their bulldozers between historic treasures.

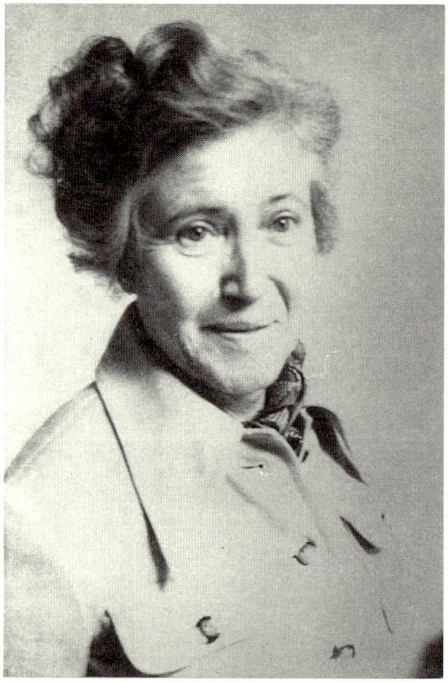

Helen Millett Arndt was a founder of the Denver Landmark Commission. (Courtesy St. John's Cathedral)

For her extraordinary efforts, Arndt was one of 66 people honored by receiving the Award of Merit, presented by the American Association for State and Local History. For her accomplishments her name is engraved on a memorial wall at the amphitheater at Denver's Civic Center.

Both of the High Street houses are made of DriVit, a plaster-over-foam material that insulates exceptionally well and is less expensive than stucco. The house at 170 High includes a hallway or "art gallery" for paintings, including those by their son, Burnham, who majored in Fine Arts at the University of Colorado. He is named for a former friend and next-door neighbor, architect Burnham Hoyt. The entrance is marked with stone sculptures made by Burnham. Porch furniture was built by another son, iron designer Karl Dickson Arndt, who lives in the house. In the garden is a statue executed by a friend, Marian Buchan. Helen and Karl Arndt, a former chairman of the board of trustees of the Denver Art Museum, collected paintings, sculptures by Edgar Britton, and tapestries by Herbert Bayer.

In his youth, Dr. Arndt had been an avid mountain climber and skier, and was pictured in the ski museum at Vail, Colorado. Another son,

Nicholas, is an accomplished fisherman and an owner of Anglers All, a popular store of fishing equipment in Littleton. A daughter, Sarah Millett "Milly" Arndt (Mrs. Matthew Gale), died at age 49. She had attended Kent School, and an art sale is held in her memory at the school each year.

Dr. Arndt, who practiced medicine with his father, Dr. Rudolph Arndt, received the Gold-Headed Cane award from the University of Colorado School of Medicine as an "outstanding practitioner of internal medicine." Arndt joked about the inception of the houses: "I take total credit for Jim Sudler selling us this property," he said. "I told him the butcher's family goes hungry, the doctor's family gets sick, and the architect's wife has no house of her own. Barbara needed a house!"

Property for a third house in the complex on the street at 160 High Street was eventually sold to Donald Newman, who built a contemporary house there.

38
140 HIGH STREET
Built: 1914
Architect: Maurice Biscoe

This stucco Mediterranean-inspired house, with its large arched windows, massive masonry walls and chimney, and expansive, tiled hipped roof, was shifted among family and friends for several decades. It was owned by president of the Interstate Trust Company Valdo F. Wilson in 1917. He sold it to a friend, state Senator Christopher F. Cusack. "Chris was a friend of my father's who taught me everything I know about riding horses and polo ponies," said Medora Wilson (Mrs. Paul Douden, Jr.), whose father, realtor Arthur D. Wilson, bought the house from his uncle in 1928. The property included the nearly-acre-sized lot to the north that was later owned by Henri de Compeigne and sold to Barbara and James S. Sudler, II, in the 1960s. Maurice Biscoe designed oak paneling, a massive fireplace, and an intricate plaster ceiling in the dining room for this meticulously detailed home.[87] The wide entry porch is decorated with a molded garland of fruit over the door.

Realtor Wilson, president of A.D. Wilson and Company, moved into the house with his wife and two daughters, Medora and Elaine. It was like country then. Pets were common and the girls had a monkey, "Tippy-Tin"; a pig; and a lamb. "When our handyman built a go-cart, the lamb pulled all the neighborhood children around the block," said Medora. "Groceries were delivered then. The vegetable man and the egg and chicken man came around, and Royal Crest delivered milk."

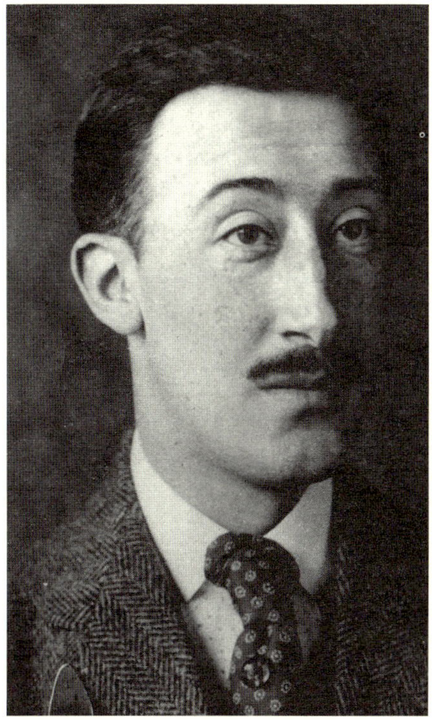

The house at 140 High Street was occupied during the fifties and sixties by French nobleman Henri de Compiegne. (Courtesy DPL Western History Department)

A constant playmate of Medora's, Patsy White (Mrs. Walter A. "Bill" Steele) lived next door at 124 High in a 1916 Spanish Colonial house, the only design of architect Eugene Groves in the Country Club district. It was one of the few examples in Denver of the Pueblo Revival style with its characteristic flat-roofed combination of blocks with vigas. The Lowell White family lived there for 55 years. When they sold, it was torn down in 1989. The house is described in Noel and Norgren's *Denver: The City Beautiful.*[88] "We had a stucco chicken house to match our house," Patsy said.

The next owner of 140 High was French nobleman Henri de Compiegne, who lived there with his wife, Anne Lewis, and namesake son. Born the Marquis de Compiegne, he renounced his title to become an American citizen in 1936. After twice receiving the Croix de Guerre in World War I, de Compiegne came to Denver in 1922 representing French oil interests and helped develop the Salt Creek oil field in Wyoming.

De Compiegne, who lived in the house until he died in 1971, had saved the nearly-acre lot to the north, hoping his son would return to Denver. He was a good friend of Myron Blackmer, grandfather of the James Sudlers' oldest child, Eleanor "Leli." One day in the late sixties, Barbara Sudler (Hornby) went to see him about selling this land. He had always been very close to the family and liked the idea of Jamie [James S. Sudler, III] living there. He sold the land at a bargain two percent interest! "When I told Jim, he sent me out to find some more two percent land," Barbara said.

39
101 HIGH STREET
Built: 1920
Architects:
Merrill and Burnham Hoyt

Gano-Downs was one of the most popular men's clothing stores in downtown Denver. The founder of the store, George W. Gano, came to Denver as a boy and opened shop in 1886. The store grew from a tiny cubbyhole in the Windsor Hotel Building to one of the most widely known stores in the West. One of the store's most distinctive features was its shadow-box display windows, which were installed in 1917. The business was sold in 1936, but successors carried on the tradition, opening a branch in Cherry Creek North when it became a shopping center during the fifties.

Gano's son, Merritt W., built this Mediterranean L-shaped house during the twenties, adding an attached garage in 1929. The side entry on the north has a small balcony with an arched window above. A French door on the east is topped with an arched lunette and is flanked by long, narrow sidelights. Windows, flush with the wall, are unadorned. A row of casement windows on the south

The wide garden and Mediterranean, L-shaped house at 101 High Street were built in 1929 by Merritt W. Gano of Gano-Downs men's clothing store.

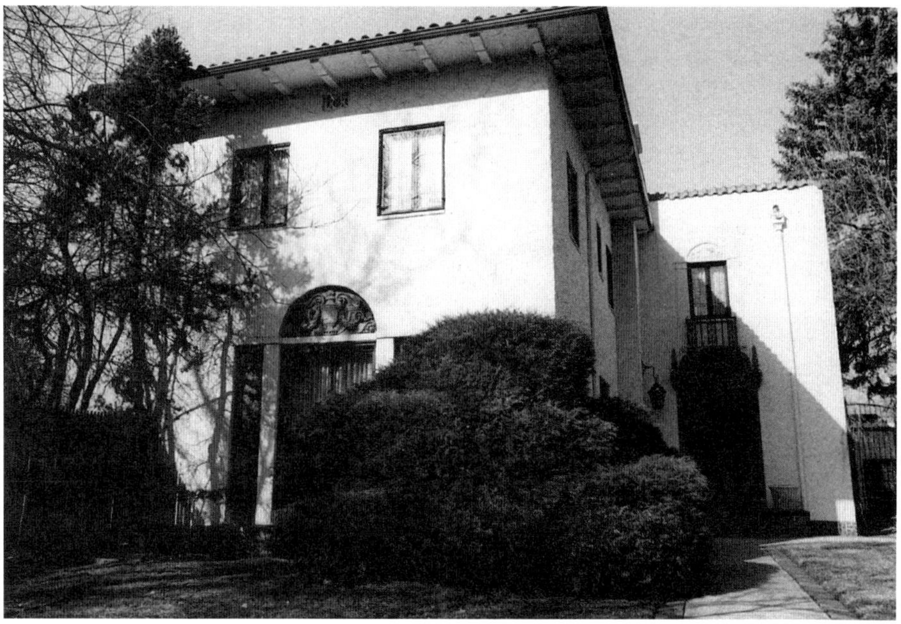

overlooks the wide 100-foot side lawn on the south across from the Denver Country Club. The hipped roof is red tile over the front section, and a tile-capped parapet encloses the flat roof beyond the entrance.

During the twenties and thirties this countrylike, open yard was a great gathering spot for Merritt, Jr., and his neighborhood friends, such as Charles and Lafayette Hughes, Jr., of 300 High; Robbie Wilson at 180 Franklin, Quentin Mitchell of 1640 East 3rd Avenue; Dan O'Rourke at 2012 East 4th Avenue; and Philip Gates at 140 Gilpin. Gates, whose Gilpin Street house backed up to this house, dated those nostalgic days by writing, "I can remember the day in May of 1927 when Merritt Gano came running out of his kitchen door yelling 'Lindy made it!'"[89]

During the sixties and early seventies, Ann and cattle feedlot owner David Cudahay Wilhelm lived there with their three children, Jean, David, Jr., and Andrew.

Carol and George G. Shaw, an eminent contractor, then bought 101 High, a house they had always admired. For over 25 years they have enjoyed the elegant home and spacious side lawn.

Before 1923, spectators could cheer on the Denver Country Club polo team from graveled 1st Avenue. (Courtesy DPL Western History Department)

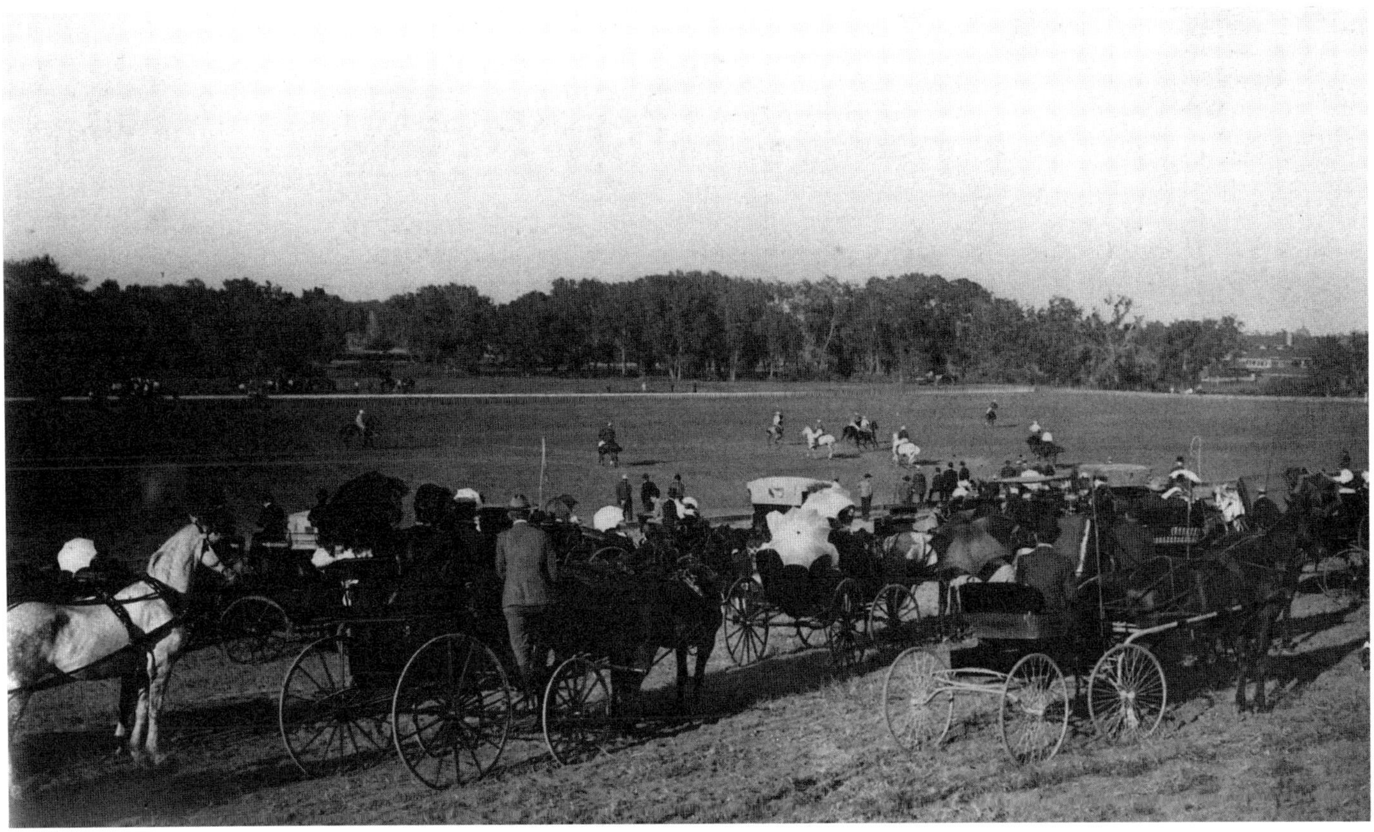

TOUR 3: COUNTRY CLUB ANNEX

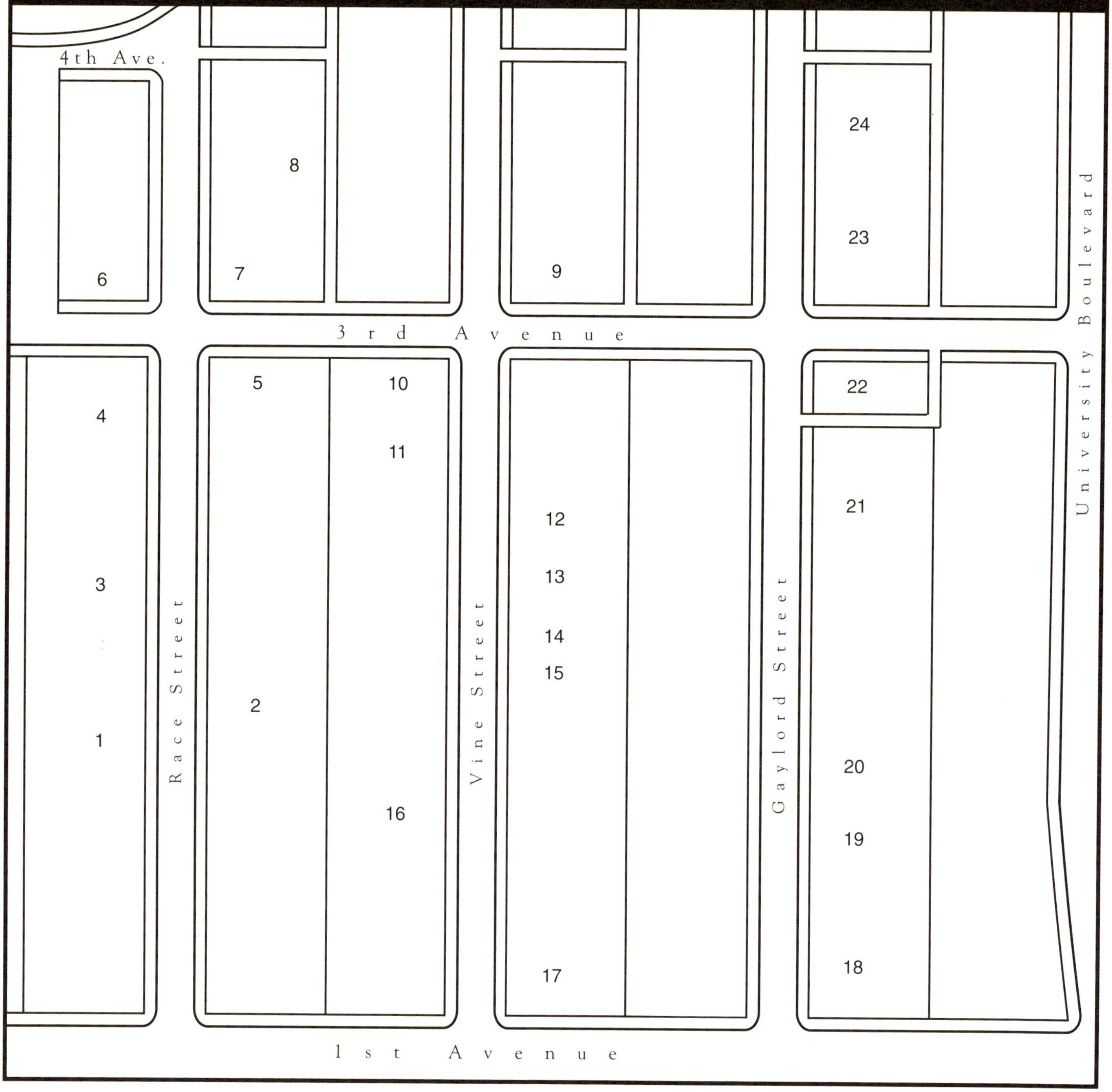

TOUR #3

1. 161 Race Street
2. 160 Race Street
3. 191 Race Street
4. 245 Race Street
5. 280 Race Street
6. 1953 3rd Avenue
7. 300 Race Street
8. Unplatted block at Race Street and East 3rd Avenue (including 338, 344, and 358 Race and 2011 and 2019 3rd Avenue)
9. 300 Vine Street
10. 275 Vine Streeet
11. 265 Vine Street
12. 230 Vine Street
13. 210 Vine Street
14. 160 Vine Street
15. 150 Vine Street
16. 127 Vine Street
17. 100 Vine Street
18. 100 Gaylord Street
19. 130 Gaylord Street
20. 140 Gaylord Street
21. 240 Gaylord Street
22. 2300-2320 East 3rd Avenue
23. 316 Gaylord Street
24. 350 Gaylord Street

[OPPOSITE PAGE]
The third tour of Country Club Annex includes Race, Vine, and Gaylord Streets and the 1889 Capitol Annex subdivision.

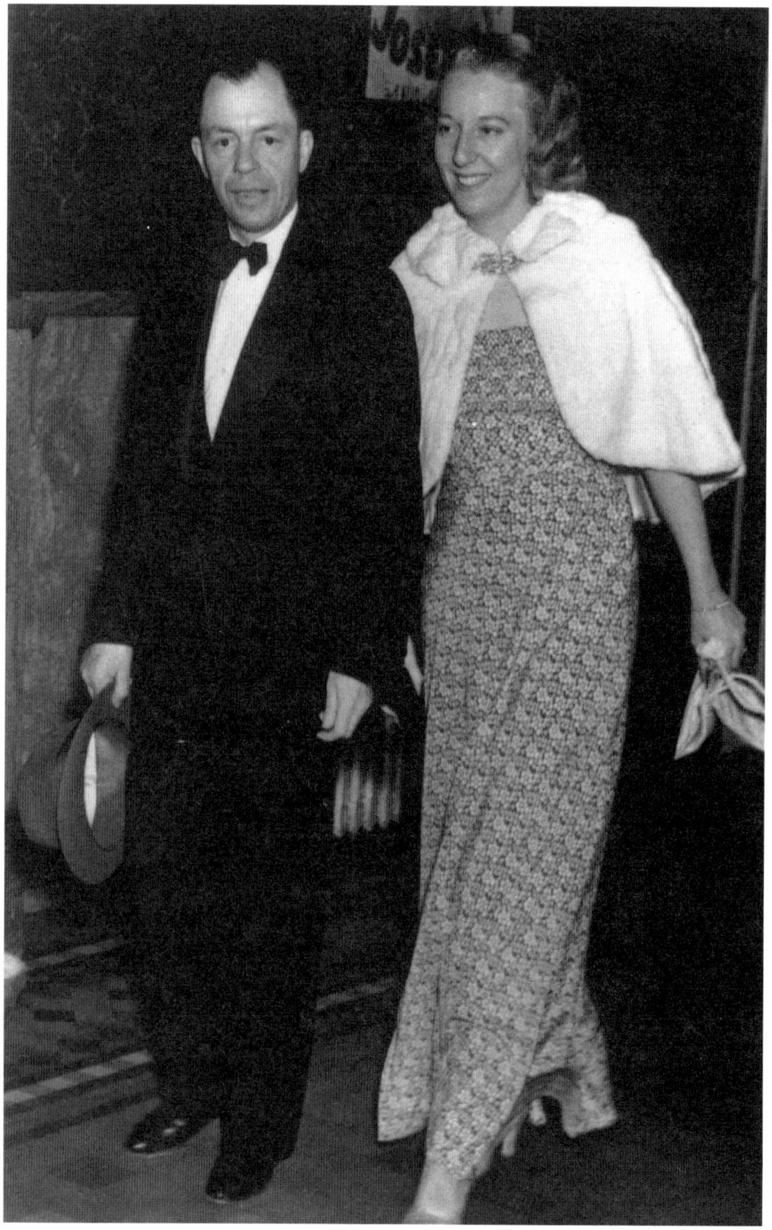

Lawrence Phipps, Jr., who, with his father, planned the Country Club Annex subdivision, lived at 161 Race Street with his second wife, Bertha, before moving to Diamond K Ranch. (Courtesy DPL Western History Department)

~ Tour 3 ~

1
161 RACE STREET
Built: 1919
Architect: Jacques Benedict

During the twenties, while Senator Lawrence C. Phipps was fulfilling two terms in Washington, D.C., lawyer Lawrence C. "Larry" Phipps, Jr., acted as his father's lawyer in buying up property to form the Country Club Annex subdivision.

In 1919, Larry Phipps and his wife, Gladys (Hart) Phipps, built a house on 1.48 acres of untouched, unplatted land on the northwest corner of Race and 1st Avenue. The alley, which was the original Race Street between 1st and 3rd Avenues just west of his property, was vacated in 1920, enlarging his land by 28.8 feet. Ordinance 36 of that year reads, "For an ordinance vacating the present location of Race Street between 1st and 3rd avenues . . . and the relocation of this portion of Race Street as dedicated by Lawrence C. Phipps and Louise Iliff," both of whom owned pieces of property adjacent to this alley. "The vacated property reverts severally to the owners of property abutting on said vacated street up to and as far as the center line," the ordinance reads. The property adjoined deep lots on High Street of the subdivision, Country Club Place. Race Street was relocated to the east of his property where it is now, leaving 265 feet of property unbroken by street or alley. The west side of Race Street remains unplatted.

The Spanish, buff brick house on this corner is a symmetrical, rectangular structure with a low-pitched, red tile roof and overhanging eaves. It is notable for its large scale, structural clarity, and absence of ornamentation. Decorative enrichment is reserved for the north entrance, framed by an eclectic arrangement of a wood door surround within a Gothic stone arch flanked by round pilasters with floral capitals. Above is a stone frieze and balconet within a segmented, round arched casement with a curvilinear, stone arched head. The 4,467 square-foot house has six bedrooms, five-and-a-half baths, four fireplaces, and a heated four-car garage. The Phippses put an addition on the rear and side of the house in 1933.

Larry Phipps's first marriage resulted in three daughters, Mary (Mrs. Chapman Young), Joan (Pechman), and Diana (Braden), but ended in divorce. Five years

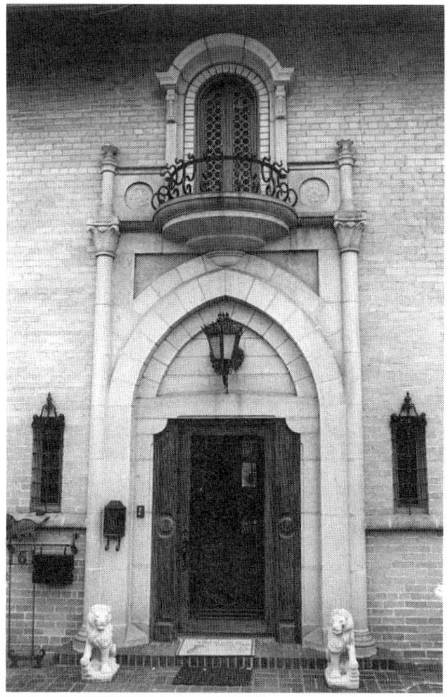

Lawrence C. Phipps, Jr., built the Spanish house at 161 Race Street when he planned the Country Club Annex subdivision.

later he married Bertha Richmond. After living in the house for a few years, they moved their family, after three more children: Lawrence, III; Richmond; and Henry, to the Tudor castle on the Diamond K Ranch that he had purchased in 1937 from Frank E. Kistler of 190 High Street.

A dedicated horseman and polo player, Larry changed the name of the estate to Highlands Ranch and instituted the Arapahoe Hunt, which was formalized in 1929 with John F. Kuykendall as Master of Fox and Hounds. Kuykendall served until his death three years later, when Larry Phipps assumed the role for 22 years. Charles A. Johnson, Jr., lived on the adjoining ranch. He participated in the first hunt at the age of seven: "It was pretty disorganized. No one was dressed properly. They chased a rabbit instead of a hound or coyote. My horse took off like a rocket and kept galloping in front of the master, which put me in immediate disgrace," he said.

After a second divorce, Phipps married Swiss-born Elaine Oakes. Following his death in 1976, the ranch property was bought by oil billionaire Marvin Davis for $13.7 million. Three days later, Davis sold the property to the Mission Viejo Corporation for $28.1 million, resulting in a vicious family feud, with daughter Richmond Phipps suing the estate executors—her brother, Lawrence, III, and her uncle, Gerald Phipps, for mismanagement of the estate.[1] Meanwhile, during the next eight years, Mission Viejo converted its investment into a community of 4,000 homes with 10,000 residents that was known as the Highlands Ranch residential area near Littleton.[2]

The house at 161 Race Street was purchased by prominent businessman and civic leader Clarence J. Daly during the forties. Daly was president of the Capitol Life Insurance Company, founded by his father. He also served on the boards of the Denver Symphony Association, Children's Hospital, and Kent Denver Country Day School. He retired at the age of 84, three years before his death in 1976. His wife, Marie, a leader of the Junior League and Debutante Ball, died nine days later, also in their home at 161 Race.

Daly's sister, Imogene Daly, who lived at 125 Gaylord Street, had been a dedicated volunteer for Rocky Mountain Planned Parenthood since 1916. In 1967 she was awarded the first Margaret Sanger Medallion for her outstanding service to the Colorado organization.

2
160 RACE STREET
Built: 1925
Architects: Varian and Varian

Fords were among the most popular automobiles of the thirties when Robert Gentry Stovall, of Stovall-Irwin Motor Company at Broadway and Alameda, moved into the house where his family has lived since

The Robert Stovall family has lived at 160 Race Street since 1935.

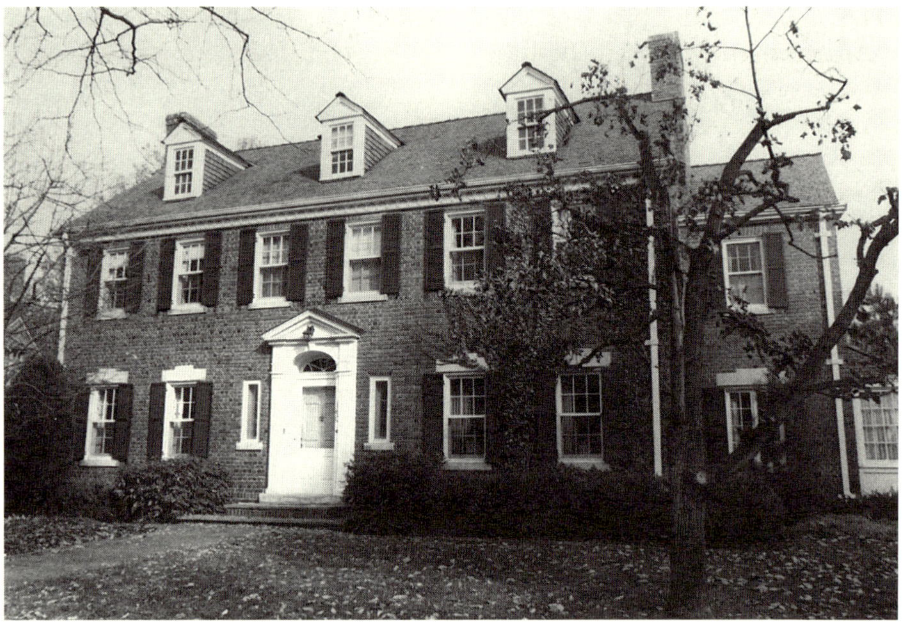

1935. Stovall's success as a Ford dealer for 43 years earned him the presidency of the Denver Automobile Dealers Association in 1944.

The Stovalls raised three children in this house: Barbara, who married Denver & Rio Grande Railroad treasurer Willett Moore; Robert, Jr., who married Ann Bates and was president of Stovall Motors for 18 years before opening his own law practice; and Marjorie "Mardie."

Mardie remembers the plethora of children in the neighborhood while she was growing up in this house, including an enclave of black families living in Capitol Annex across 3rd Avenue during the thirties. "There was a row of little houses between Race and Vine. I used to go down and play with a little boy named Willie," she recalled.

After the senior Stovall's death in 1968, the house reverted to Mardie and her husband, Ralph Sargent, Jr., vice-president for Public Affairs of the Public Service Company of Colorado. Sargent was a founder of the Rocky Mountain Center on Environment (ROMCOE). For his dedication he received the Edward Hobbs Hilliard Memorial Award after his premature death at age 53 in 1976. Their five children, Crispin, founder of CS Advocare, a personal accounting service; business consultant Ralph, III, "Topper; sculptor William Frederik "Rik;" Dorothy Dyer "DeDe" (Mrs. Frederick Long); and Barbara Ann "Bambi" were nearly grown by the time the Sargents moved back into the house. In 1980 Mardie married lawyer John B. Tweedy, who was instrumental in organizing the ski development of Vail during the fifties and sixties.

In 1925 the three-story, red brick Georgian Colonial house had been built by lawyer Thomas Keely, of the law firm of Hughes and Dorsey and legal counsel for the First National Bank. The house has a white pilastered entrance with a triangular pediment that is repeated by three pedimented dormers on the third floor. Medium-pitched gabled roofs cover both the main house and the two-story addition to the south. Shaped rafters trim the roofline between paired end chimneys.

3
191 RACE STREET
Built: 1928
Architect: unknown

"There must have been 50 kids in those two blocks," said Horace "Jack" Phelps, Jr., who grew up at 191 Race Street during the twenties and thirties. "Race Street was all gravel and we'd shut off the street at both ends.

West of this house at 191 Race Street was the original Race Street, vacated in 1920.

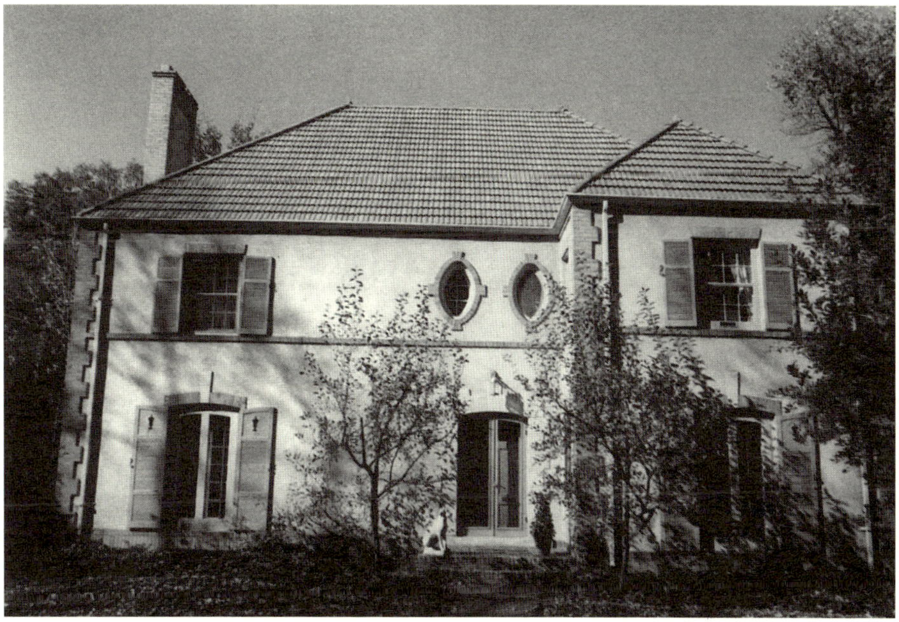

Nothing could interfere with our wonderful big marble games."

His father, Horace Ferguson Phelps, was a Denver-born, fourth-generation lawyer who served two terms as a state representative. He had followed in the footsteps of his father, Horace Phelps, a member of the first state legislature. In 1923, Horace Ferguson Phelps married Dorothy H. Eaton, granddaughter of Colorado governor Benjamin Harrison Eaton. They moved into 191 Race near the Denver Country Club tennis courts. Phelps was a Denver, Colorado, and Rocky Mountain tennis champion. Their sons, Horace, Jr., "Jack" Phelps, who married Joan Stapp, and William Eaton Phelps, who married Dorothy "Dody" Thomas of 315 Humboldt Street, both settled in the Denver Country Club area at 319 Gaylord and 246 Race, respectively.

To the west of their property was the original Race Street, vacated by city ordinance in 1920 when Race Street was moved to its present location. The Phelpses simply fenced off this vacated alley, but their neighbors used it in other ways. "Mel Schlesinger, to the south, incorporated the land into his yard. To the north, the Sullivans used it for a vegetable garden. Stanley Wallbank, behind us at 190 High Street, just surreptitiously appropriated the land by plowing it up. No one really ever knew what happened to it," said Jack Phelps.

In the early thirties the former chancellor of the University of Denver (DU), English-born Heber Harper, moved into the L-shaped, stucco Mediterranean house with blue French doors, red brick quoins, and a simple arched entry centered under two distinctive oeil-de-boeuf second-story windows.

An ordained Methodist minister, Dr. Harper served as a pastor for six years before coming to Denver in 1922. After he left DU in 1927, he became regional director of the Federal Security Administration. During World War II he consulted with the State Department in creating the United Nations Relief and Rehabilitation Administration (UNRRA) and the UN Educational, Scientific and Cultural Organization (UNESCO). Shortly after the Harpers sold this home, Harper, at the age of 84, drowned while swimming near his summer home in Rhode Island in 1969. His widow, Rachel, was popular in social circles and an avid skater at the Denver Country Club.

4
245 RACE STREET
Built: 1929
Designer-Builders: Writer Brothers, Inc.

By the second quarter of the century more people were buying "spec" houses—houses already built by designer-contractor firms before they were sold—rather than custom-designing them from scratch with an architect.

This 2,500-square-foot, red brick, steeply-gabled Tudor house was built on six lots as a "spec" house at the corner of 3rd and Race for $13,000 in 1929. The residence has since doubled in size. The north side of this cross-gabled home extends forward, forming an L shape, while two gabled dormers break the roofline.

In 1948, Continental Airlines president Robert Six lived there with his first wife, Pfizer Corporation heiress Henrietta Erhart. They put in a swimming pool, made the garage into a dining room, and then built a new garage and breezeway. After their divorce, Henrietta moved to 300 Vine Street. Six married Broadway star Ethel Merman, moved to Cherry Hills, and sold the Race Street house to Ellen and mining lawyer J. Ramsay Harris in 1954. "When we bought the house from them, it was in terrible repair. There were termites and the roof leaked," said Ellen.

At that time, Ellen was running for Congress against incumbent Byron Rogers. To run as the first Denver female congressional candidate, she resigned her chairmanship of the National Citizens for Eisenhower Congressional Committee. The "Ellen Harris for Congress Committee" was chaired by her friend and

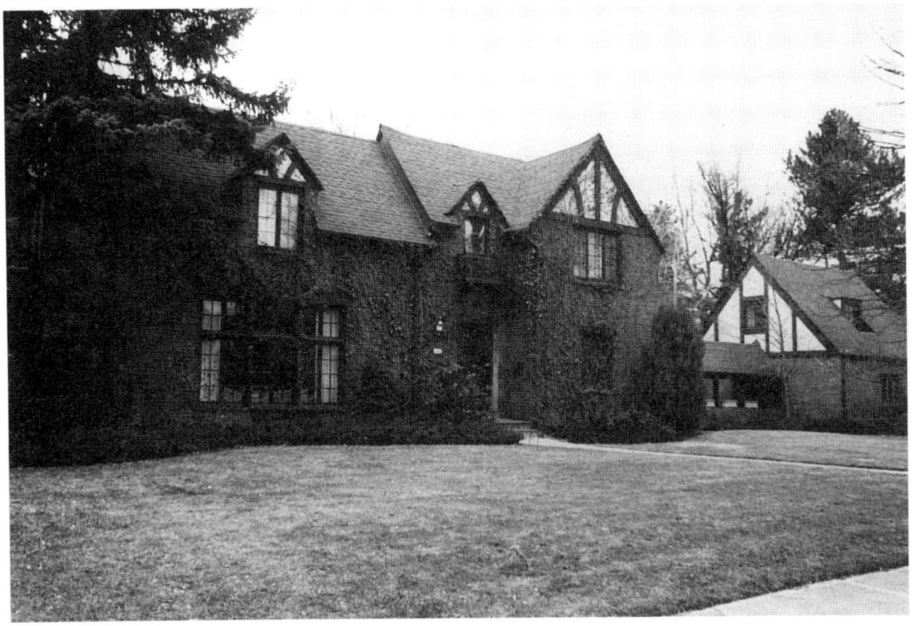

[Above]
The house at 245 Race Street has had many additions since Writers Brothers, Inc. built it in 1929.

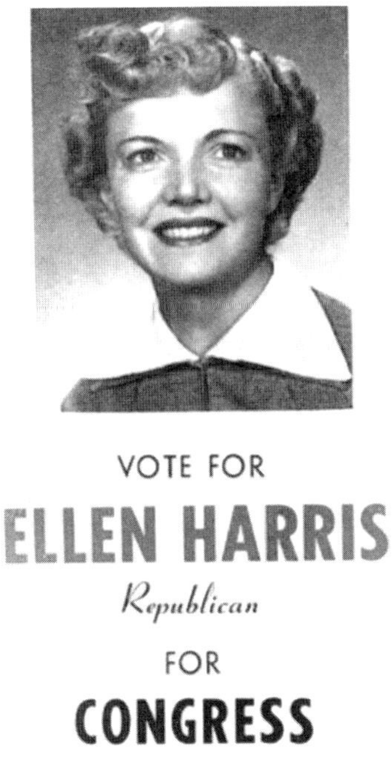

[Left]
Ellen (Mrs. J. Ramsay) Harris lived at 245 Race Street when she ran for Congress in 1954. (Courtesy Ellen Harris)

Country Club neighbor, Jane Kennedy Garnsey (O'Donnell). After a three-to-one-victory in the Republican primary, she lost to Democrat Rogers. "Eisenhower didn't directly support me," Ellen said, "but every morning about 8 o'clock the doorbell would ring and a carrier would be there with Eisenhower's golf winnings from the day before. Sometimes they would be as high as $500."

Ellen was a founder of the first Denver Symphony Ball and a leader in many community projects. At one time she was on 22 boards or committees.

The Harrises enjoyed their swimming pool and so did the whole neighborhood. "My one rule was that they had to bring their own towels. People would go over to the Country Club, but they didn't want to pay to swim there, so they brought towels to our house and left them. Every week or so, I would go over to return armloads of towels."

During the early seventies the house was bought by Ann and Austin Marquis, president of Pella Products of Colorado. During the nineties, owners Margaret "Margy" and attorney Michael Anderson added a master bedroom and new kitchen on the back of the house. They remodeled the family room, a haven for their three children. Margy is active in Historic Denver, Inc., and the chair of their 2000 house tour.

5
280 RACE STREET
Built: 1950
Designer: Sewell Thomas

This red brick house, based on Georgian Colonial features, was designed and built in 1950. Mining engineer Sewell Thomas, who had already built two houses in the Country Club neighborhood (360 High and 380 Gilpin), lent his expertise to his daughter, Lenore, and her husband, John Stoddart. They built this home at the same time Thomas was building a one-story California house nearby for himself and his wife at 2101 East 4th Avenue. "Daddy designed the houses and we all helped. The houses were close, so Daddy could order a joint load of lumber and the workmen could work at one house, then finish up the day at the other one," Lenore said.

The two-story masonry residence had three bedrooms and two baths, a full basement, and a two-car attached garage. "We wanted three bedrooms and two baths, but when the twins arrived in 1959, we added a sunroom and another bedroom, then built another garage," Lenore said.

While raising their three children in this house, Lenore Stoddart spent many years on the boards of the Denver Museum of Natural History and Children's Hospital. In 1982 she started a consignment store at 4th and Downing for the benefit of the hospital. By 1999 La Cache had netted over a million dollars for the hospital.

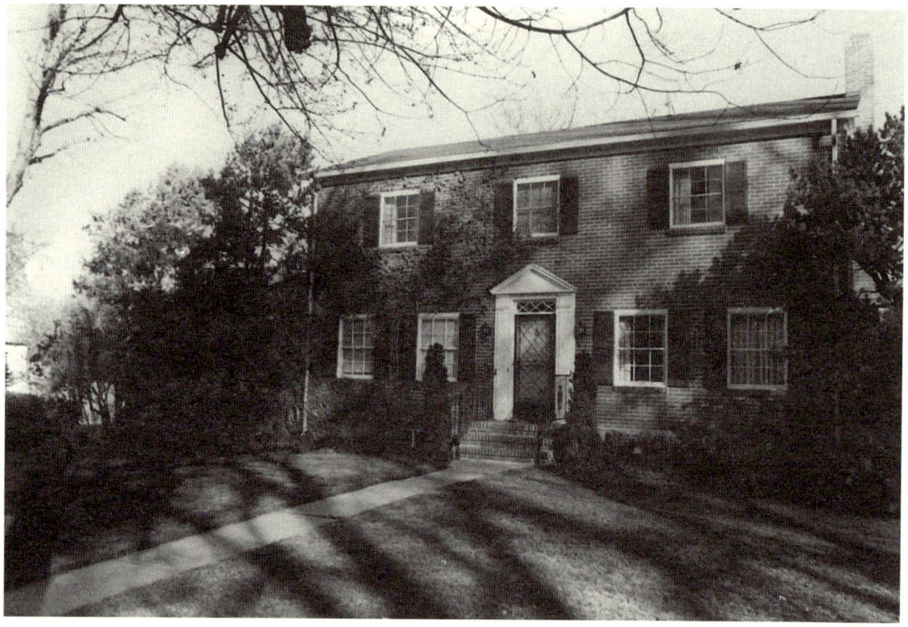

Sewell Thomas built the house at 280 Race Street for his daughter, Lenore, and her husband, John Stoddart.

After graduating from Yale, John Stoddart served with the 10th Mountain Division at Camp Hale, then opted to stay in Denver to work at Capitol Life Insurance Company, then as a consultant for Van Schaack and Company. For many years he chaired the Metropolitan Mental Health Association, also serving on the national board.

"When mother died, John and I moved over to their house on 4th Avenue," said Lenore, "but selling our Race Street house was like selling one of the children. We'd given birth to it."

6
1953 3RD AVENUE
Built: 1953
Architect: unknown

This small, 2,149-square-foot "builder's house" was constructed in 1953. Although the Assessor's Office records the date as 1954, next-door neighbor Mary Lee (Mrs. Martin) Anderson said, "I remember that the people who built the house [the Lawrence C. Kellogs] set the address at 1953 to reflect the year they built it."

After prominent investor and business leader Eugene Dines died in 1962, his widow, Marie Eaton Dines, moved into this retirement house to be near her children, all living in the Country Club district. Bruce and Dorothy Dines were at 350 Gaylord. Eugene, Jr., and his wife, Winston, lived at 2022 East 4th Avenue, and Marcia moved into 360 Gilpin when she married Jerome Strickland in 1969.

Marie Eaton Dines and Dorothy Eaton (Mrs. Horace F.) Phelps, whose grandfather, Benjamin H. Eaton, was governor from 1885 to 1887, were raised on the Eaton Ranch near Greeley. "We loved to go out there," said Marcia (Dines) Strickland. "They had a nine-hole golf course and a lake with peacocks running around."

The charming, white Colonial Revival house on 3rd Avenue has a simple recessed entry. Large dormers give light to two bedrooms and bath on the second floor. In the basement is another little bedroom. A small patio on the east reduces the upkeep of the 6,890-square-foot plot.

Until about 1989, the bus went right by the house, which lies at the end of the island between Race Court and Race Street.

The small house at 1953 East 3rd Avenue was built between Race Street and Race Court.

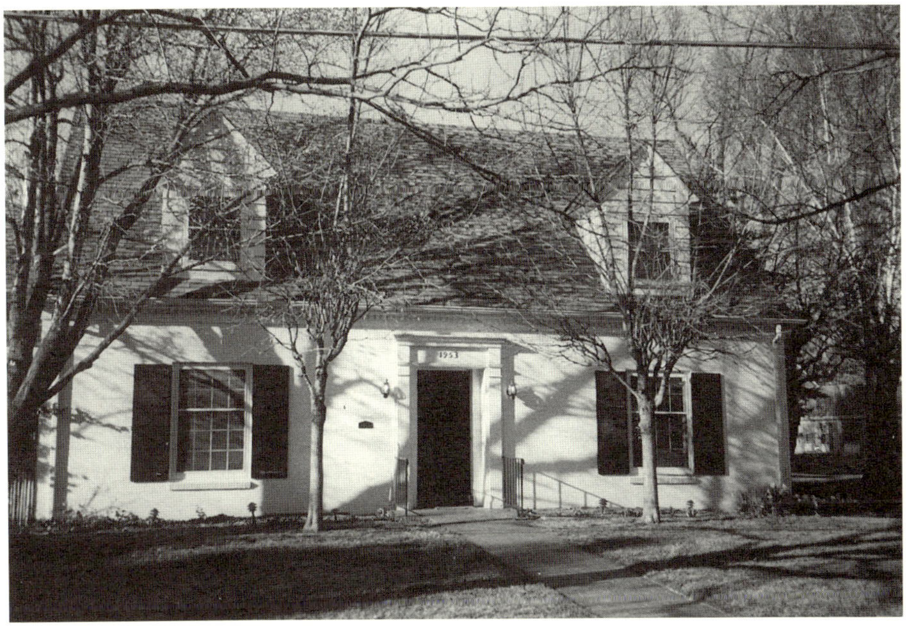

7
300 RACE STREET
Built: 1954
Architect: unknown

This 2,148-square-foot, red brick, one-story house was built by *Rocky Mountain News* editor Jack Foster and his wife, Frances "Frankie," while he was at the height of his career. Foster had been sent to Denver by Scripps-Howard in 1926 as a reporter for three years while the faltering newspaper suffered bitter competition with the *Denver Post*. "At that time we used all manner of stunts to attract attention. We gave away five gallons of gas with one want ad and exploded bombs on the roof of the building with the opening of the Moffat Tunnel,"[3] he said. When the tunnel opened in 1927, Foster entered from the west portal and reporter Mary Coyle from the east. When the last few feet were blasted aside, Foster grabbed her, gave her a big kiss and ran for a telephone. Coyle, later Mrs. Robert Chase, was awarded Denver's first Pulitzer Prize as author of the play *Harvey*.

In 1940, Foster returned to the *Rocky Mountain News* to begin 30 years as editor and doubled its circulation during the first six years. One of the first and most popular columns was "Molly Mayfield's" advice to the lovelorn. Although the author was anonymous, the

"Race Street bunch," as Ellen (Mrs. J. Ramsay) Harris of 245 Race called the close-knit residents along her block, were aware that Frances Foster was the author. "We all used to write letters for her to answer," she said.

Foster retired in 1970 and Mary and Marmaduke Holt moved in. "My dressmaker was the same one as Frankie Foster," Mary Holt (Joyce) said. "She came to my house one day and mentioned, 'I've just been over to the Fosters' and they're going to sell their house.' There was a courtyard and a greenhouse and Marmy loved to garden."

Holt was a prominent and respected lawyer, and both he and Mary were loyal members of St. John's Episcopal Cathedral. Holt died in 1976. Five years later Mary married Robert Joyce. After he died in 1985, the house was sold and remodeled by Gerald and interior designer Jaculine Harrier-Coss.

The brown one-story house is a vernacular design of the 1950s. It was efficiently laid out with a low-pitched roof and well-proportioned rooms. Harrier-Coss redecorated it, skillfully blending contemporary design with primitive furnishings. Low living-room and library ceilings were angled and raised "to cathedral them," as Gerald said. The wood-paneled walls are now white. Glass bricks are used for walls and ceilings. Modern stained-glass doors and windows throughout the house were created by Harrier-Coss.

"When I looked at the house, I didn't like the outside at all, but the inside intrigued me. I liked the space. There are few rooms, but they're big," said Harrier-Coss. She remodeled a basement room into an office for her husband, pushing out the west wall to form an atrium with shelves of plants and light coming from the glass-brick roof. This area is shut off from the street by a concrete wall, matching the new single-car garage on 3rd Avenue that replaced the rose garden and trees. Both garages have bright copper doors as a "signature to the house," as Harrier-Coss expressed it.

"The house looks quite different," was Mary Joyce's understatement, "but I guess they were trying to get light into the basement."

Two copper garage doors are featured at the remodeled one-story house at 300 Race Street.

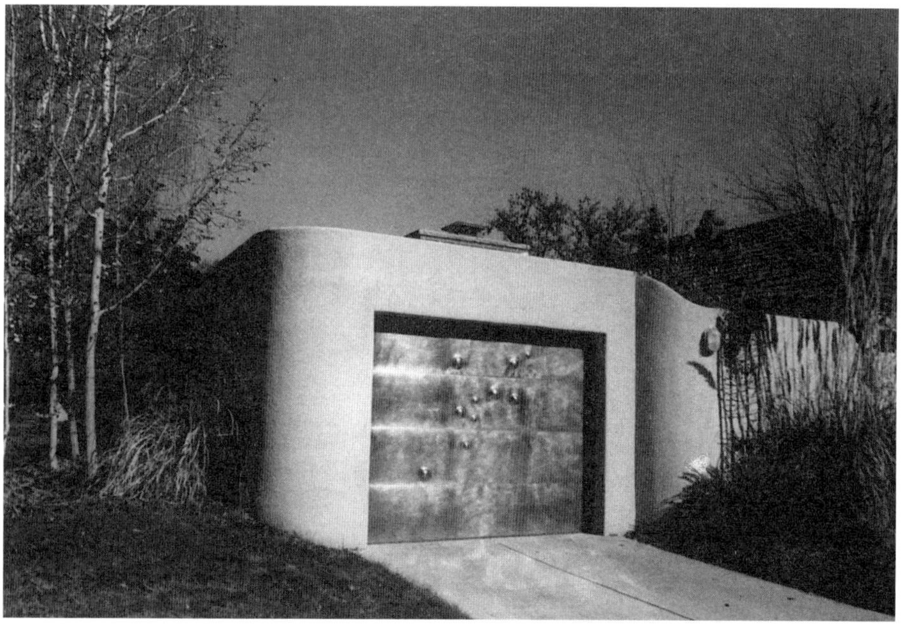

8
UNPLATTED BLOCK AT RACE STREET AND EAST 3RD AVENUE

The rest of this unplatted block between Race Street and the alley, and 3rd Avenue and the northern alley, was once a quiet little farming community where odd-shaped plots were grandfathered in before zoning laws, creating odd-shaped houses. A number of people mentioned that blacks were very much in evidence. By 1905 this isolated property was in the name of Elizabeth Iliff Warren, widow of cattle king John Wesley Iliff, who had died in 1878. It was later transferred to her daughter, Louise Iliff, then sold piecemeal to home owners as Country Club Annex developed. These houses are described below to demonstrate the haphazard development of this unplatted land.

338 RACE STREET
Built: 1951
Architect: unknown

During the fifties, a one-story, two-bedroom house with a single-car garage was built by Jack Haliburton on a lot that is 110 feet wide and only 60 feet deep. The house was sold to a widow, Lulu J. Simson, who, with her late husband, George, had raised their family at 150 Vine Street. After she died the house was taken over by her daughter's family, the Kevin Crokes.

In 1979, contractors Charles R. Walker and Mitchell Wright wanted to enlarge the house to sell, but had trouble conforming to zoning laws on a lot only 60 feet deep. The Board of Adjustment was more sympathetic when Walker told them he planned to live in the house. Apparently he later changed his mind. Walker and Wright then added a 19-foot addition, a second floor, and a sweeping staircase.[4] The brownish-grey-painted brick house has a dramatic mansard roof. The middle section of the house is three feet lower than the main section, so the mansard roof extends both higher and lower than the main roof. It is centered by a white panel window flanked by two smaller windows. The front garage is on the south.

344 RACE STREET
Remodeled: 1986
Architect: Richard E. Henry

Just north of 338 Race is another greatly enlarged house. "When we moved across the street in 1954, there was just a little one-story, brick ranch house owned by Ruby and Bill [William F.] Clements, who started the White Spot restaurants in Denver," said Mary Lee (Mrs. Martin) Anderson of 361 Race Street.

Architect Richard E. Henry remodeled the house from 1986 to 1988 for owner Lou Jahde: "The lot

On unplatted land at 344 Race Street, a new house was built in the late 1980s on a lot only 60 feet deep.

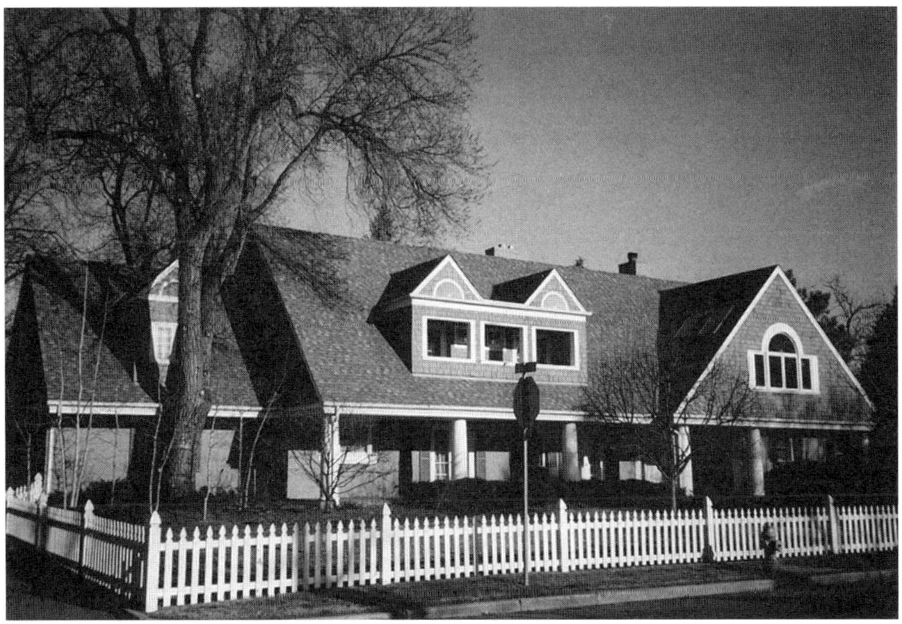

size was so skinny and narrow [60 feet] that we couldn't scrape off and build a new house because of the setback requirements. We therefore kept the footprint of the house that was there but added a second floor, disguising the height by using dormers and gables. The first floor was concrete block with brick. For the second floor I put shingles on the gables and porch," Henry said. The entry has a long veranda supported by large, white, round tapered columns. "I made the columns extra fat because the roof was so large and the proportions were better," explained the architect. The prominent front gable has a strip of four windows. A roundel is over the recessed front entry.

During the early nineties, the Robert Jarretts added the white picket fence. When they sold the house to Jacquie Hellenbeck for $1.2 million in 1998, she also bought the tiny house on the alley, 358 Race, and "Weedy Patch," (described below) for a total of over 18,000 square feet of property.

At 390 Race Street between 1936 and 1949 was a little shack with a bright light on top that was run by the Guardian Signal Company. This rather unreliable guard service (described below) was managed by the Victor Simers, who lived at 1921 East 4th Avenue.

358 RACE STREET

Built: 1907
Architect: unknown

Down the alley, this little 700-square-foot house is the original farmhouse on the block. It is behind 344 Race Street, and nestles up to the alley that borders both the Park Lane Square (Circle Drive) and Capitol Annex subdivisions. "In 1953, Tom O'Rourke [who lived across the alley at 2012 East 4th Avenue] bought the house and farmland south of it from an elderly black gentleman who had raised his corn and beans there for generations. O'Rourke then gave the farmer life tenancy in the tiny house," said Sidney (Mrs. Caleb) Gates. O'Rourke's sister, Patsy Monaghan, said she remembers a Mrs. Porter who lived there and was very generous with the vegetables she grew.

When Peter and Betsy (Gates) Cosgriff owned the land and their children lived in the little house, they wanted to build a larger house there, but the fire department refused a permit because the alleys were too narrow for fire trucks. They

On the alley bordering Park Lane Square is a 700-square-foot farmhouse that was built in 1907, two decades before Country Club Annex was developed.

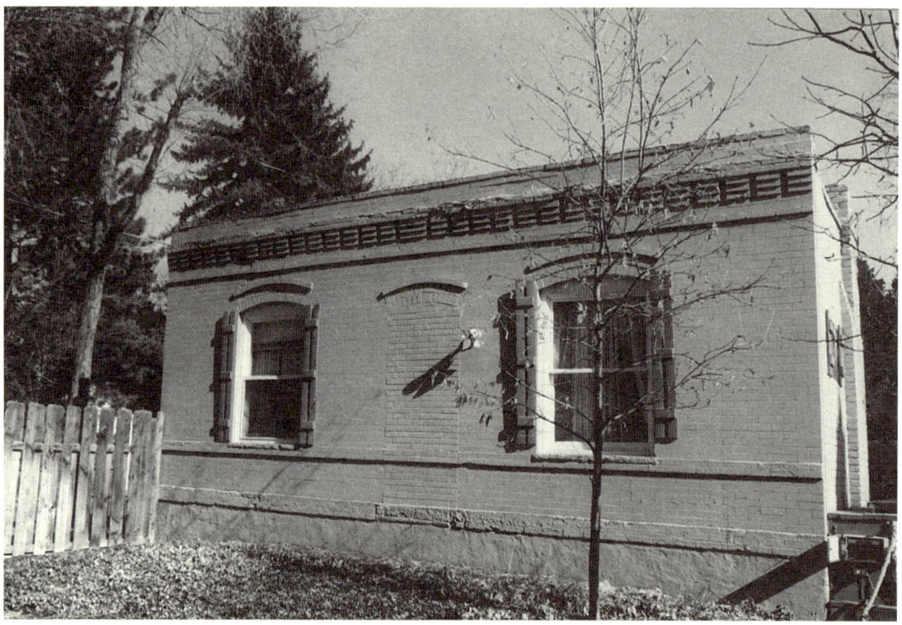

allowed some relatives to use the 156-by-65-foot farm land along the alley for a vegetable garden.

"WEEDY PATCH"

During the seventies and eighties, three young matrons plowed up and cultivated this farmland on the west side of the alley between Race and Vine to plant vegetables. The land, owned by Peter Cosgriff who lived in Leadville, was occupied by his father, Stewart, who was called "Farmer Cosgriff" by these gardeners. As Knobby (Mrs. Macintosh) Brown said, "We put so much nourishment into that soil you could practically eat it." The other women were Sidney Gates and Elaine (Mrs. William Cable) Jackson, who fertilized, planted, and pulled up weeds that were knee-high. They grew plum and apple trees as well as all kinds of fruits and vegetables. "It was our own secret garden," Jackson said. The small house in the corner, the original farmhouse, was their only source of water to grow the plants.

"At that time Race Street just had little farm houses," Gates added, speaking of the era just before the expansion of the Cherry Creek North shopping center.

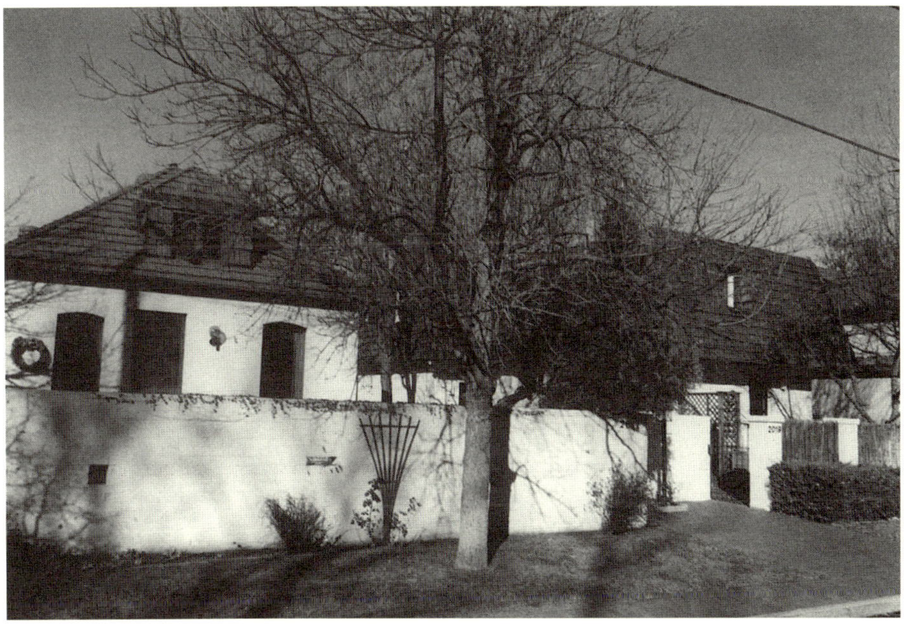

[LEFT]
These two white homes on 3rd Avenue were originally tiny brick houses with a frontage of only 32.5 feet.

2011 EAST 3RD AVENUE
Built: 1906, and
2019 EAST 3RD AVENUE
Built: 1912
Architects: unknown

Another house, approached only from the alley, was 326 Race Street (now 2019 East 3rd), just south of Weedy Patch. This, and the house at 2011 3rd, set on lots with only 32.5 feet frontage and 182 feet along the alley, are remodels of nineteenth-century, red brick bungalows. They are now painted white and have shingle roofs. To the west, 2011 is built of rough stucco with a hipped roof and two hipped dormers. The house at 2019 is white-painted brick with a dormered mansard roof. Both have front sitting decks, protected from 3rd Avenue by six-foot fences.

This unplatted block gives an idea of the informal, countrylike farm life of this area during the first three quarters of the twentieth century. The alley marks the western border of the Capitol Annex subdivision that was platted in 1889.

9
300 VINE STREET
Built: 1911
Remodeled: 1954
Architect: Alfred Watts Grant

Typical of the houses in Capitol Annex, the one-block subdivision platted in 1889 just west of the town of Harman, was the original of this one-story brick cottage and farm built in 1911 for R. W. Smith[5] at 300 Vine Street. These tiny houses were often occupied by black families who worked, either in Harman or in the Country Club district.

When Marion C. James owned the property during the forties, a gigantic vegetable garden dwarfed the tiny house on the three deep, 25-foot lots between the street and the alley.

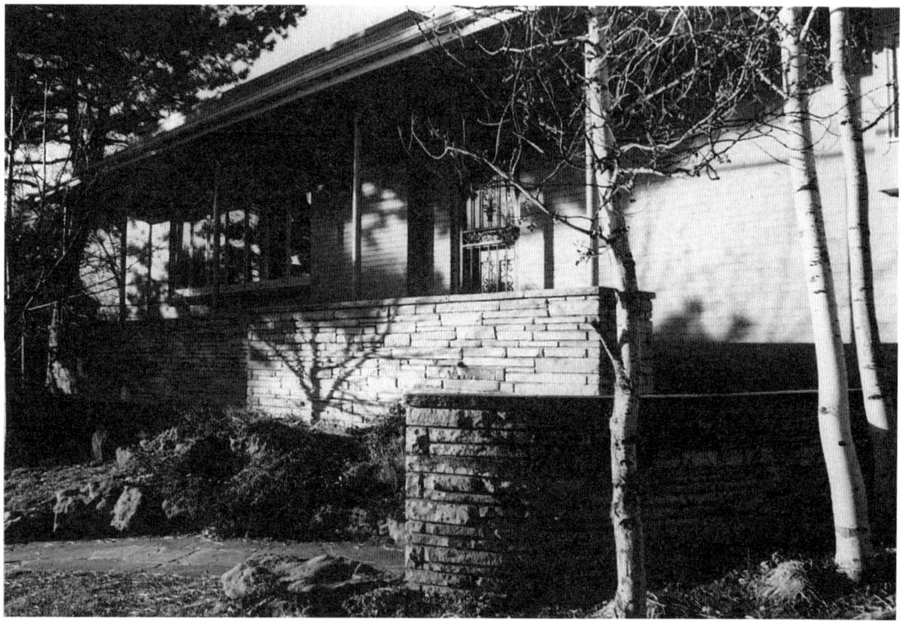

The 1911 house at 300 Vine Street was remodeled by owner-architect Alfred Watts Grant during the 1950s.

Architect Alfred Watts Grant bought the property in the early fifties from Henrietta Six, who had just divorced Continental Airline president Robert Six and moved from 245 Race Street. Grant engaged Kappel Brierly as the contractor and enlarged the house to over 3,154 square feet by extending each end to form an L shape. The modernistic, painted brick house has a flat roof, sleek lines, and three rows of five projected casement windows along 3rd Avenue. Grant built an L-shaped living room with two fireplaces and a kitchen and guest room along 3rd Avenue. On Vine Street he added a three-room suite for his father, connecting the house to the garage. "Every room has a view of the garden," said their son, Hugh "Sandy" Grant. Notable is the patterned masonry wall along 3rd Avenue and the alley.

The remainder of the 11,800 square feet of property at 300 Vine was devoted to a Japanese garden. "My father had Stanley K. Yoshimura come from San Francisco to design the first residential Japanese garden in Denver. He had three concrete lanterns, and recycled water to maintain a pool with a curved bamboo bridge, a river running the entire length of the yard, and a waterfall at one end. Denver local Japanese landscape gardener George Fukuma helped with the bonsai trees," Grant said.

Hugh Grant grew up in this house while his father was designing over 100 buildings, including the Ross University Hills Library and Arvada West High School. His mother, Beatrice, was active in the Denver Art Museum, Central City Opera, and the Friends of the Denver Public Library. Close friends of the Grant family were Anne and artist Vance Kirkland, who was a professor at the University of Denver. He painted from 1932 until his death in 1981.[6] "My mother dated Vance before they each were married, and they always remained close friends. As a child I used to stay with the Kirklands when my parents were away. It was my second home," said Grant, who currently heads the Vance Kirkland Foundation.

Started in 1996, the foundation, initiated to increase the appreciation of Kirkland's paintings, achieved phenomenal success by sponsoring exhibitions in 13 museums in Europe by 1999. "The popularity of his paintings is spreading like a domino effect, especially in eastern Europe," Grant said.

During the seventies when stockbroker William C. Dabney, Jr., owned the house, he combined the rooms of the grandfather suite to make a Trophy Room. "It was a very private house and well built," he said. "It had a great yard and an unusual Japanese garden with bonsai trees."

In 1988 another 120-square-foot addition to the east wing was built for owner John Cormey by Gordon E. Lewis Construction Company.[7]

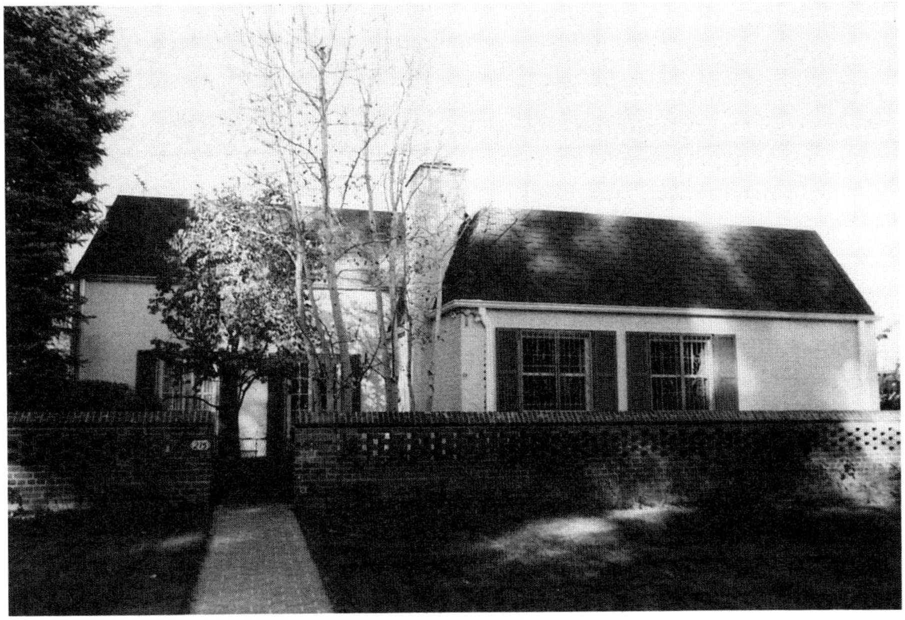

This small brick house at 275 Vine Street was built in the garden of the house to the south. Originally the property was part of the Capitol Annex subdivision.

10
275 VINE STREET
Built: 1968
Architect: Stuart Olson

The garden north of Mrs. Davis Moore's brick Tudor house at 265 Vine was sold to Dorothy "Dolly" and E. T. H. Talmage, Jr., who engaged architect Stuart Olson to build a small retirement home. The decorative brick wall surrounding the garden was retained, bordering this house and lending continuity and privacy to the entry patio.

"We used every inch of the lot," Ed said. The master bedroom and spacious living room of this compact house are on the first floor. On the second floor are two bedrooms and a bath "for our children when they come home from college."

The white brick house is located on property originally included in the small Capitol Annex subdivision, which extended 75 feet south of 3rd Avenue. This land was bought by Lawrence Phipps in 1925 as an addition to Country Club Annex.

The Talmages sold the house to Clara (Mrs. Henry C.) Van Schaack after her husband died. Living there by herself, she installed double locks and security doors and windows. "If there were a fire I don't think we'd ever get out," said current owner Phyllis "Chick" Alexander. Mrs. Van Schaack remained there after she married Albert E. Humphreys, Jr. The Bruce Alexanders moved from the Hilltop neighborhood to this house during the eighties. Bruce had been raised at 140 Humboldt Street, so was returning to the Country Club Historic Neighborhood. "We did not remodel the house, just redecorated," Chick said.

11
265 VINE STREET
Built: 1936
Architects: Varian and Varian

Banker Davis Willett Moore carried his young bride, Elsie "Wigsie" Bailey Moore, over the threshold of this house on July 11, 1936. The couple had received the $9,000, 30-by-56-foot home[8] from Elsie's mother, Mrs. Dewey C. Bailey, widow of the mayor of Denver from 1919 to 1923.

The red brick, L-shaped house was designed by architects Ernest P. and his son, Lester E. Varian. The house has Tudor elements with opposing steep gables. One has a large oriel window in the front. A patterned brick chimney tapers as it reaches its full height. A dormer of three small windows is above the inconspicuous entrance, approached by a curved walkway. In 1950 a den, with second-floor guest room and bath, was added to the north, and a formal garden beyond was designed by landscape architect Jack Harenberg. Striking is the decorative brick wall surrounding the garden, retained when the garden was later replaced by the house to the north.

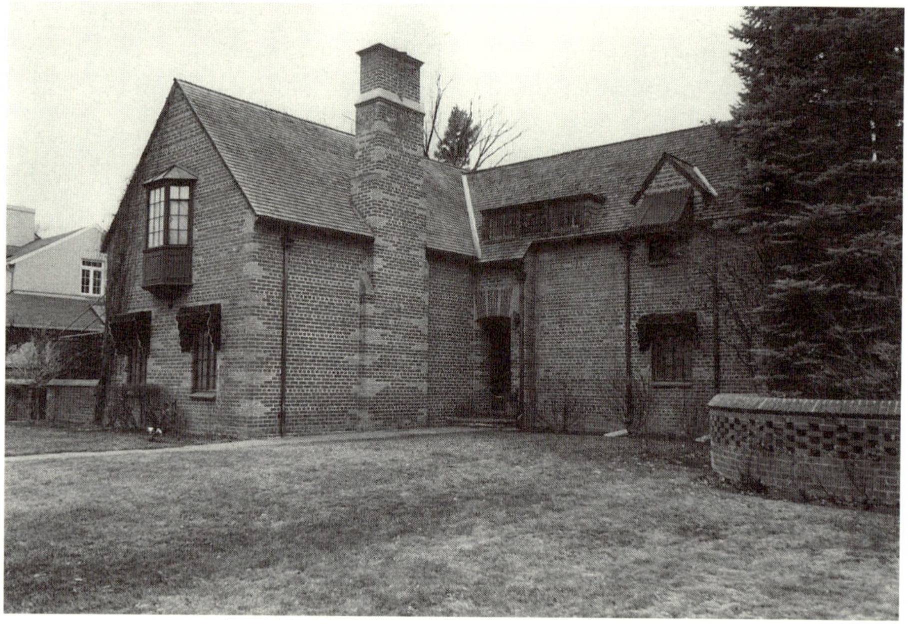

The L-shaped house at 265 Vine Street was built for banker Davis Willett Moore when he married "Wigsie" Bailey, daughter of the mayor of Denver from 1919 until 1923.

Moore, executive senior vice-president of the First National Bank, was a community leader in the Central City Opera Association and the University of Denver Associates, and a generous supporter of the Denver Art Museum. He lived in the house until his divorce in 1957.[9] "Wigsie" remained in the house for several more years.

During the eighties and nineties, John and Nora Kimball lived in the home.

The house was bought in 1998 by commercial realtor Richard A. and freelance writer Anne O'Brien. Anne and "Rick" take great pride in owning a historic home and are preserving its original charm. They have remodeled the kitchen to include a sunny family room. The dining room, previously used as a pool room, is restored to its former elegance and opens onto the garden to the south.

12
230 VINE STREET
Built: 1937
Designer-Builder: Elton S. Boerstler

In 1939, real estate and mining investor Charles Alfred Johnson, Sr., bought this two-story "spec" house built by Elton S. Boerstler, a contractor who built many homes in both Park Hill and Hilltop.

Thirteen years before, the Johnsons had finished a Merrill and Burnham Hoyt-designed summer castle near Sedalia, Colorado, named Charlford after the Johnsons' two sons, Charles, Jr., and his half-brother Gifford Phillips. The 2,400-acre estate included a two-bedroom guesthouse, a heated swimming pool, a picnic house, a tennis court, and a six-car garage.[10] At one time, the senior Johnson hosted the Arapahoe Hunt there.[11] The family continued to spend their summers there after they bought the house in town at 230 Vine. In 1954 they sold Charlford to Mildred "Tweet" Ruddock (Walker) Kimball, who changed the name to Cherokee Ranch.

The home on Vine Street was made of blonde brick. Arched dormer windows break the line of the steep hipped roof and echo the Queen Anne arched door surround of the entrance porch. The tall south chimney is typical of Boerstler's ornate signature brickwork. Beige concrete blocks form both the door surround and quoins. The Johnsons added a one-story brick sunroom designed by Burnham Hoyt to the rear of the house in 1940.

The Charles Alfred Johnson family lived at 230 Vine Street while they summered at their castle, Charlford, near Sedalia, Colorado. (Courtesy Charles A. Johnson)

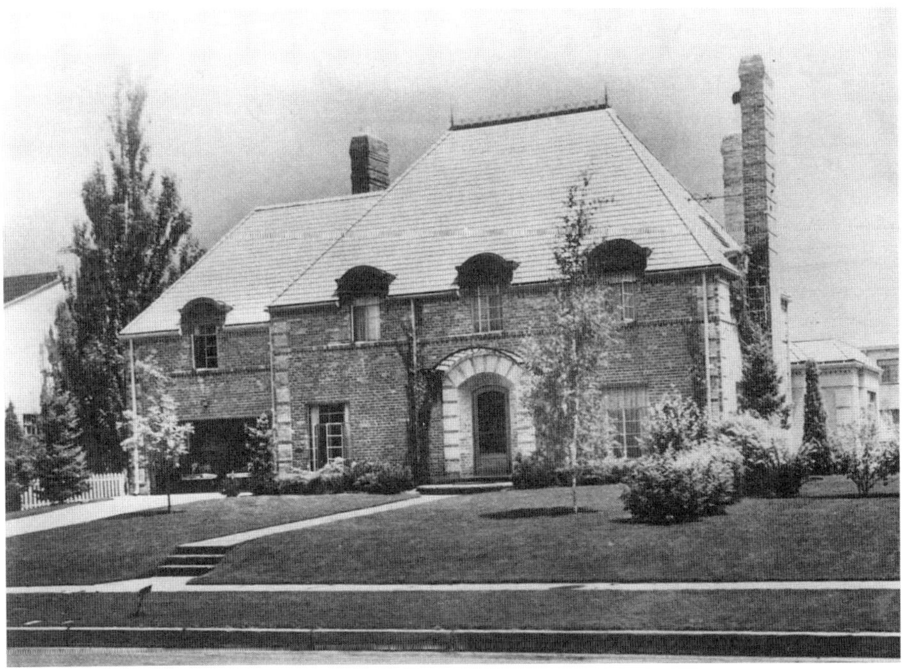

Gifford Phillips became a publisher and television producer. Charles, Jr., developed an enviable reputation as a talented watercolor landscape painter, holding a one-man show in 1957 at Mile High Center.[12] His interest in history led to the publication of such books as *Denver's Mayor Speer* in 1970, *Stages Along Cherry Creek* in 1980, and *Opera in the Rockies: The History of the Central City Opera* in 1992. Journalist Lee Olson said of the Speer book, "Johnson does a good job of rounding up the facts. . . . There's a lot of work in the book and it is a valuable addition to the Denver bookshelf."[13]

In 1948 Charles Johnson, Sr., sold the Vine Street house to his friend, George Bart Berger, Jr., who had married Laurene Porter Walker in 1932. Nephew W. Bart Berger said, "It was like living in the country when Lornie and George moved out to Vine Street. Who was going to visit them *that* far out?"

George Berger returned from Yale to enter the family-run Colorado National Bank, becoming its fifth president in 1955. As a community leader he served as president of the Denver Art Museum, a trustee of the Denver Museum of Natural History, director of the Aspen Ski Corporation, and a member of the Denver Chamber of Commerce. A born

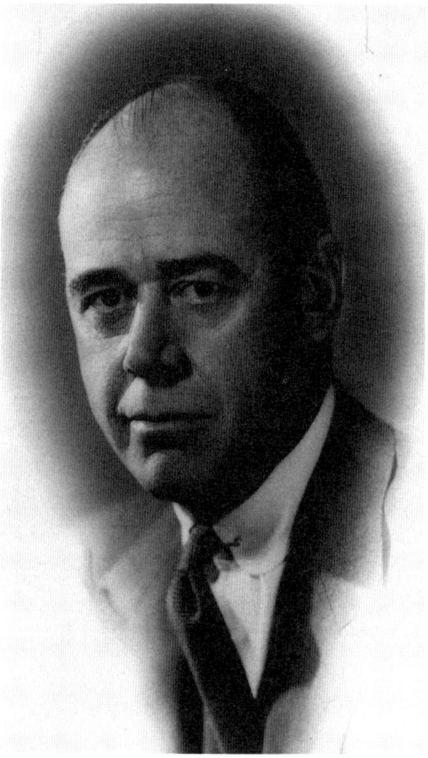

In 1948, the C. A. Johnsons sold the house at 230 Vine Street to George Bart Berger, Jr.

athlete, he once held the state junior golf championship, and was an avid fisherman and duck hunter. Of their three daughters, two live in the Country Club district. Susan (Mrs. Warren) Sheridan lives at 181 Race. Laurene "Baba" Berger (Mrs. John) Brooks lived at 401 Gilpin before moving to 155 Gilpin, where they lived for 31 years. The other daughter, Caroline, married Kent Rickenbaugh.

When the Johnsons bought the property from W. Oscar Temple in 1939, they also bought the lot to the south where Boerstler had started a house at 220 Vine. They filled in the existing foundation to make a garden. The Berger girls loved "playing house" on the old abandoned house foundation. "At that time Gaylord had big vacant lots, and we had fun pitching snow fights and building forts and caves," Baba said.

The girls grew up in this house, half a block from the Denver Country Club. Baba and her friend, Sidney Brock (Gates) of 130 Gaylord, acquired business acumen during their childhood. "Mr. Brock built us a pop stand. We got cases of pop delivered from Charlie's [Market on 4th Avenue] and set up shop on one of the golf fairways. All Daddy's friend would come by, playing golf, and feel they had to patronize us. We then took the empty bottles back to Charley's and collected the refund on the bottles."

The George Bergers lived here from 1948 to 1987.

13, 14, 15
210, 160, AND 150 VINE STREET

When the subdivision, Country Club Annex, was first pieced together by Lawrence C. Phipps, new president of Denver Brick and Pipe (formerly Denver Sewer Pipe and Clay Company and later Denver Brick and Tile), William John Geddes put the family business to good use by helping build a brick house for his widowed mother, Susan (Mrs. William F.) Geddes, and flanking houses for his two sisters, Jean (Mrs. William Oscar) Temple and Ethel (Mrs. George, Jr.) Simson.

Geddes, who lived at 2155 Hawthorne Place, had taken over the presidency of the company from his father, William F. Geddes, in 1925. His brother-in-law, W. Oscar Temple, was secretary-treasurer of the business at that time.

The three Tudor-style homes are outstanding examples of the fine brick and stonework for which the family business was noted. Denver Brick and Tile grew out of William F. Geddes's early work in stone quarrying and contracting (see 2155 Hawthorne Place).

210 VINE STREET
Built: 1928
Architect: Gordon E. White

The asymmetrical eclectic Tudor house at 210 Vine, built between 1926 and 1928, is of diamond-shaped patterned brick with three dormer windows and half timbering on the prominent steep gable. Beside the entry with arched tan door surround are four leaded windows and a small sidelight. On the two front gutters are stone plaques engraved

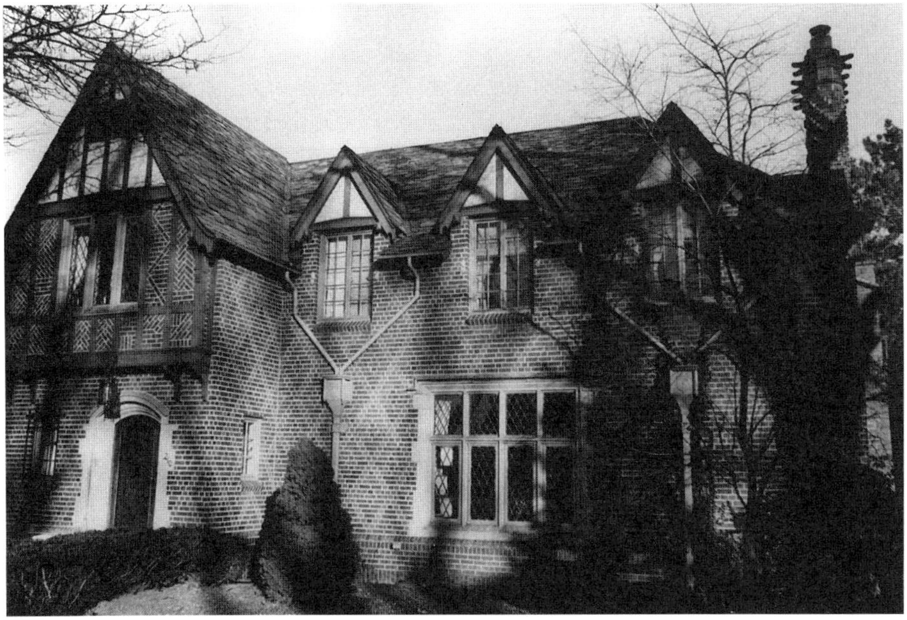

William John Geddes, president of Denver Sewer Pipe and Clay Company, built three houses side by side on Vine street for his family. The house at 210 Vine Street was occupied by his sister's family, the W. Oscar Temples.

with a "T" (for Temple). The roof is of slate.[14] The attached garage, built in 1937 by Temple, matches the house with a half-timbered gable and steeply pitched slate roof. The old garage was remodeled into a maid's room and another garage was built. The see-through, wrought-iron gate is separated by matching brick pillars. A nostalgic hitching post remains on the sidewalk lawn. A double chimney with ornate pots vents the fireplaces to the south. Jean Temple stayed at 210 Vine after her husband died in 1949. After her death in 1971, her son, William Geddes Temple; wife Marjorie; and four teenaged "in and out" children lived there.

Current owners Andrea and Dr. Lawrence Ketch, a plastic surgeon at the University of Colorado Health Sciences Center, added to and restored the back of the house to reflect the original residence. "It's difficult to obtain the same materials, but we were able to match the brick and will try to copy the original plans, which are in the [Denver Public] library," Ketch said. The house forms an L shape around an extensive sunny pool and patio.

160 VINE STREET
Built 1928
Architect: unknown

At 160 Vine, the 1928 house for Susan Geddes is of lighter brick with two stories, a full basement, and a garage. The house has steep front and side gables with tall ribbon windows of leaded square panes and designs of stained glass. On the wall next to the side entrance is a coat of arms with two crowned lions and the inscription "JE MAINTIENDRAI," loosely translated as "I will maintain [this house]."

150 VINE STREET
Built: 1928
Architect: Henry James Manning

Architect Henry Manning designed the red brick, two-story house with full basement at 150 Vine for Ethel and George Simson, Jr., in 1926. Distinctive features are the cantilevered bay windows, the octagonal entrance tower, the stone door moldings, and the rusticated oriel windows.

"We always thought it was the best-looking house in Denver— still do," said Peggy (Simson) Mason. The four Simson daughters are Jean (Mrs. William E. Bradford), Suzanne (Mrs. James Philpott, Jr.), Peggy (Mrs. Gordon Mason), and Emmy Lou (Mrs. Kevin Croke). Three of

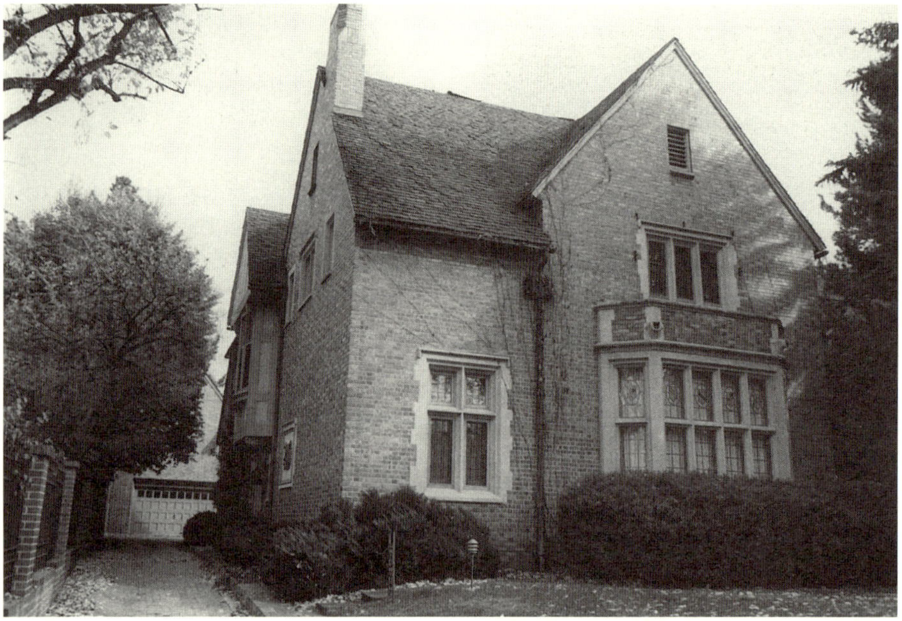

the daughters lived in the Country Club district: the Bradfords at 150 Race, the Philpotts at 142 Marion, and the Crokes at 338 Race Street.

Seven years after Simson died at the age of 49, his widow moved across the street to a smaller house at 211 Vine in 1952, then two years later to 338 Race. When she left, the Crokes moved into the Race Street house.

In 1959 the presidency of Denver Brick and Tile turned to William John Geddes's nephew, William Geddes Temple. The Dartmouth graduate was a 17-year member of the mayoral-appointed Denver Water Board, a president of the

[ABOVE]:
William J. Geddes built the house at 160 Vine Street for his widowed mother, Mrs. William F. Geddes.

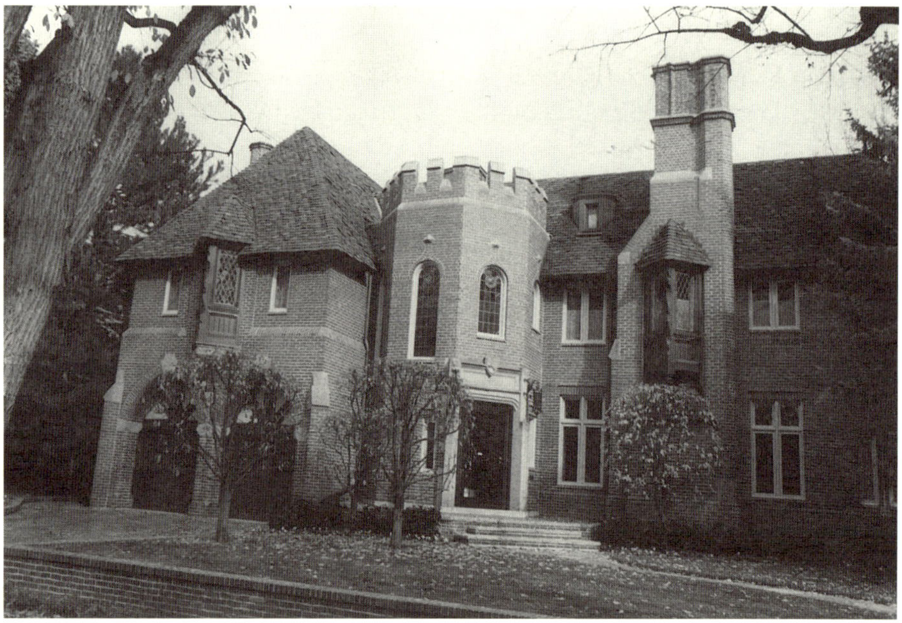

[RIGHT]
The house at 150 Vine Street was designed by Henry James Manning for William Geddes's sister's family, the George Simsons.

board of Presbyterian Medical Center, a trustee of the University of Denver, and a director of the Boys Club of Denver. His premature death occurred in 1978.

William Temple's sister, Jean Ann, and her husband, William Mead Davis, lived in the neighborhood at 540 Circle Drive.

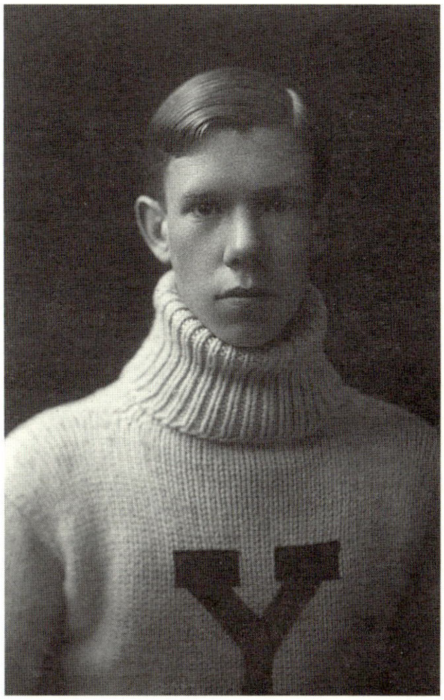

[LEFT]
After rooming with Lawrence C. Phipps, Jr., at Yale, Denise Barkalow took the job of managing the business affairs of Senator Lawrence C. Phipps.

16
127 VINE STREET
Built: 1930
Designers-Builders: Writer Brothers

In 1930, Russell and Harold Writer took out building permits to construct several "spec" houses in Country Club Annex (1st to 3rd; Race to Gaylord). One of these was a brick residence with a front-drive garage at 127 Vine Street. The house was bought in 1931 by Denise Barkalow, son of one of the four brothers whose pioneer Barkalow Brothers news agency, based in Omaha, Nebraska, had branches in railway centers in the western United States.

[BELOW]
The Denise Barkalow family lived at 127 Vine Street near the Lawrence Phippses.

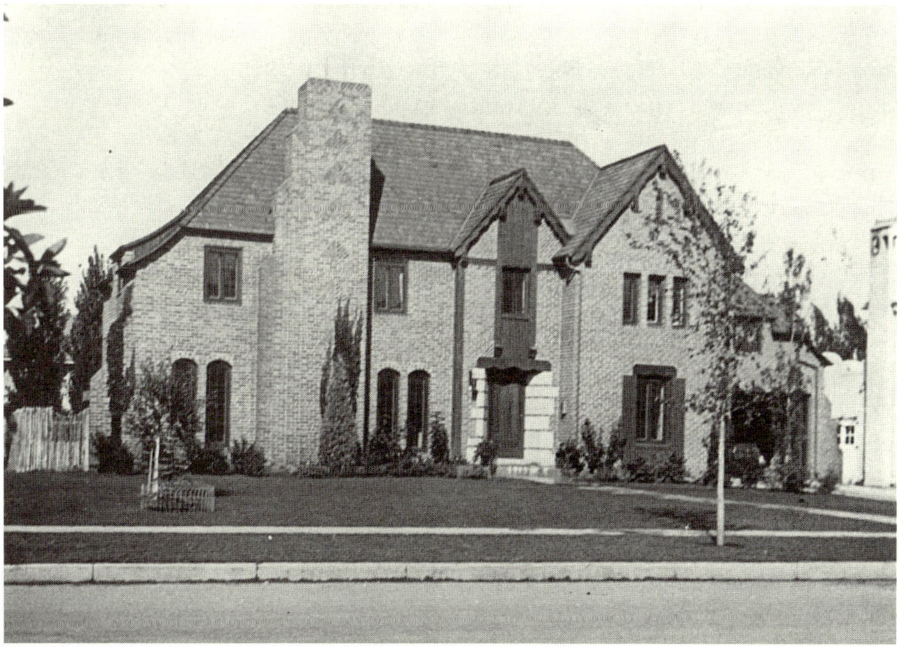

Denise went east to St. Paul's Preparatory School, then to college, serving for three years as coxswain (1905-1907) on the Yale rowing crew, "my only important claim to achievement," he wrote.[15] He then returned to Omaha, married Louise Porter Peck, and took over the Barkalow Brothers agency for a couple of years after his father died. However, his old college friend, Lawrence C. "Larry" Phipps, Jr., offered him the job of managing the business affairs of his father, Senator Lawrence C. Phipps.

Barkalow moved his wife and three daughters, Mary (Mrs. Samuel Sherman), Caroline "Celby" (Mrs. Wilbur Lakas) and Gladys (Mrs. Philip Alexander, Jr.) to Washington, D.C., for the 12 years of Senator Phipps' two terms in office. Barkalow's daughter Gladys was named after Larry's first wife, Gladys Hart. The family then returned to Denver and moved into 127 Vine, near the Larry Phipps family who lived at 161 Race Street.

The eclectic Tudor house has a hipped main roof and two front gables. The curved ornamental bargeboards and decorative door surround, originally brown, have been painted beige. The brickwork in the chimney features a triangular or vertical pattern. The red brick contrasts with the door trim and narrow panel above the entry of light beige. "The house has tall windows and Norman features of heavy beams to accent the ornamental plaster ceilings, an Art Deco design often installed by the Writers [Brothers Construction Company]," said Gladys Barkalow Alexander, who grew up in the house. Virginia and Lee McAlester in their book *A Field Guide to American Houses*, wrote: "Informal domestic building in northwestern France (particularly Normandy and Brittany) shares much with Medieval English tradition. The use of half-timbering with a variety of different wall materials, as well as roofs of flat tile, slate, stone, or thatch, are common to both."

17
100 VINE STREET
Built: 1929
Architect: Temple Buell

Architect Temple Hoyne Buell, who later developed the Cherry Creek Shopping Center, designed this distinctive house for his brother-in-law, Donald M. McIntosh, and his wife, the former Ruth Hollister. The pyramidal-shaped steep roofs of this chateauesque brick house are covered with polychromatic slates that taper to smaller ones as they reach the pinnacle. The attached garage was later incorporated into the house. An addition on the north and a new garage with tool shed were added in 1932. Arched windows were added and a well was drilled in the backyard for irrigation of the extensive garden.

The house was built when the McIntoshes returned to Denver from Chicago. After a divorce, Ruth remained there with their two children, then married a childhood friend, architect Dudley Tyler Smith, in 1941. Their son, Dudley, Jr., now owner of West Southwest Gallery in Cherry Creek North, grew up in that house playing tennis and golf at the Denver Country Club. "Of course there were no walls or fences on the two-lane road separating us from the Country Club fairways. I took up golf because we had a yard full of golf balls, and we could wander across the street and play a few holes now and then," said Dudley Smith, Jr.

The elder Smith formed the architectural firm of Smith, (Casper) Hegner and (Thomas) Moore in 1945, that designed the University of Denver Law School, at that time located at 14th Avenue and Bannock Street, and consulted on the Air Force Academy chapel. Smith's real love was the outdoors. He climbed Longs Peak 18 times, skied, and took up white-water rafting.

Subsequent owners of the house were president of Holly Sugar Company John Bunker and his wife, Emily, an expert and consultant on Asian art for the Denver Art Museum.

18
100 GAYLORD STREET
Built: 1928
Architects:
Merrill and Burnham Hoyt

Two of Denver's most prominent designer firms created this gracious home. The Donald Bromfields hired Merrill and Burnham Hoyt to design the eclectic Tudor mansion, while

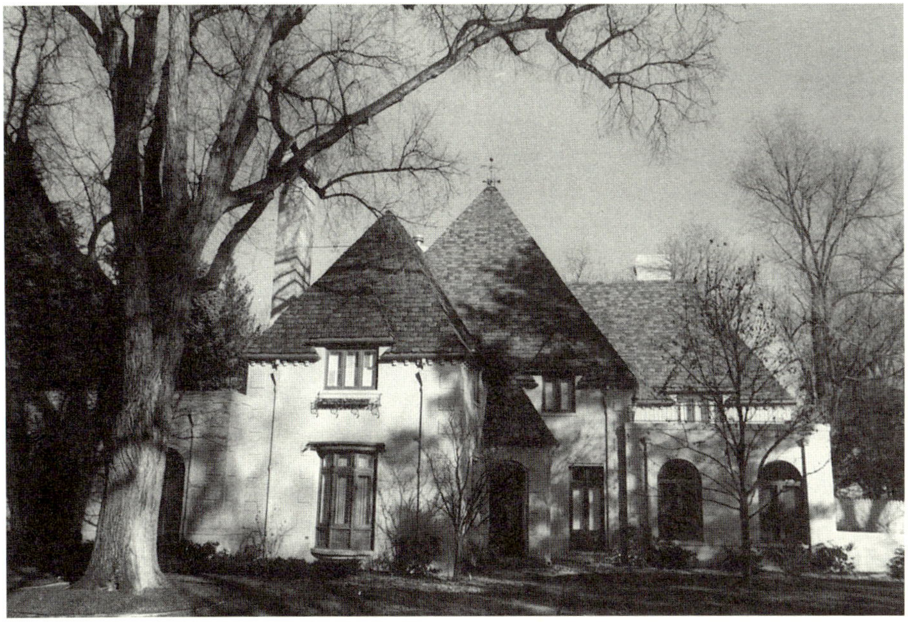

landscape architect Saco DeBoer planned the grounds with a barbecue and swimming pool. DeBoer divided the yard into several separate gardens, as explained in the Botanic Gardens' *Green Thumb* magazine: "The reasonable complexity of the garden makes it inviting."[16]

Bromfield had arrived in Denver from New Jersey in 1905. In 1920 he married Helen Phipps, daughter of Senator Lawrence C. Phipps. He then joined forces with his brother-in-law, Van Holt Garrett, who had married Helen's sister, Dorothy Phipps, to form the prominent real estate firm Garrett-Bromfield. Helen Bromfield was a tireless community

[ABOVE]
Temple Hoyne Buell designed the house at 100 Vine Street for his brother-in-law, Donald McIntosh. The roofs of the pyramids are covered with polychromatic slate.

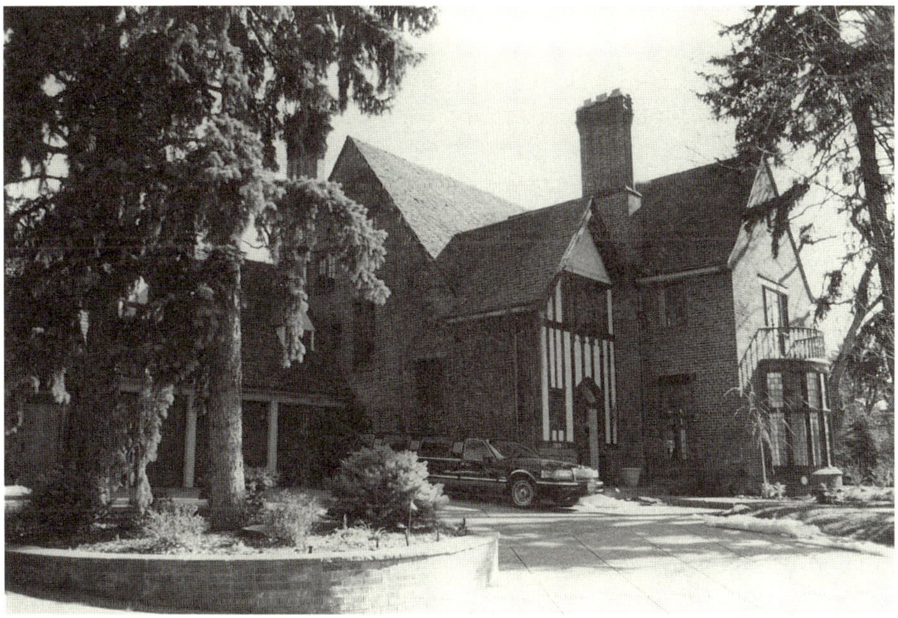

[RIGHT]
The eclectic Tudor house at 100 Gaylord Street was built by Donald Bromfield. A 12-foot wall separates the property from the commercial area on University Boulevard.

worker, heading the Junior League and the Colorado Association for Mental Health, making good use of the spacious home for meetings and entertaining.

The 17-room brick mansion has a full basement and attached garage. The front entrance gable is half-timbered, which complements the brick walls and large decorative chimneys. The magnificent 14-foot-high living room is paneled in wood decorated with elaborate carving. The property was later extended east to University Boulevard, which provided jobs for workmen during the Depression era. In 1937, Burnham Hoyt designed a greenhouse and upstairs sunporch on the third floor to add to the rear of the property. The Bromfields also added a billiard table and shooting gallery. Of the 11 bedrooms, six were for servants: a cook, nursemaid, second maid, laundress, chauffeur, and handyman. The Bromfields' initials and family crest are carved above the front door. In 1929 they built a "Writers' Cottage," later used as a playhouse for their two daughters, Genevieve (Mrs. William H. Roberts), and Edith (Mrs. James Struthers).

Later, as commercial interests moved west from Cherry Creek North, the land east of the alley was rezoned for business and part of the spacious garden disappeared. It seems that late one night, furious at the noise and lack of privacy, owner Joe. P. Paine hired a convoy of bricklayers to start erecting an illegal 12-foot wall to protect the property. Denver Landmark Commissioner Edward D. White, Jr., said, "They counted the existing wall as a retaining wall and built on top of that." The wall, once erected, was never condemned and removed.

This house was the site of a Junior Symphony Guild Designer Home in 1977.

19
130 GAYLORD STREET
Built: 1928
Architect: Burnham Hoyt

When Genevieve Kassler married Sidney L. Brock, Jr., the couple retained architect Burnham Hoyt to design an asymmetrical, two-story French Normandy home that was completed two years later. The brick house was painted white at that time and has a steep hipped roof with rusticated shingles. The stone door surround of the recessed front entry has a flattened arch with a small Gothic arched window beside it and a gabled dormer above. Square-headed dormers face west and south. The wide chimney, with double pots, dominates the front facade of the house. "Hoyt designed it to look like a French provincial house, but now the white paint has been removed and it looks quite different," said Sidney Brock Gates, who grew up in the house.

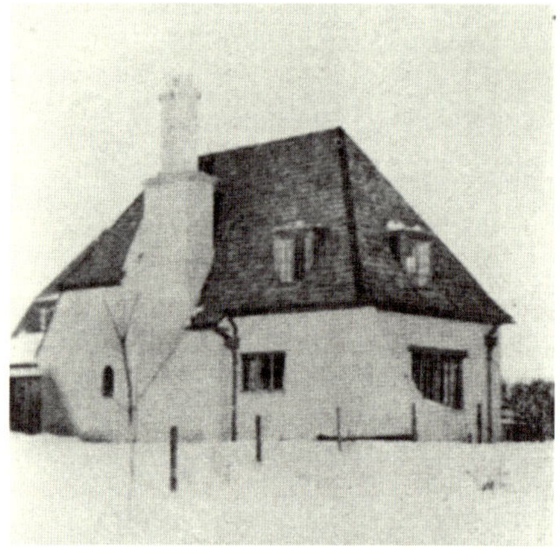

The house at 130 Gaylord was originally painted white, as shown on this 1928 Christmas card. (Courtesy Sidney Brook Gates)

It was here, a half block from the farming community of Harman, that the Brocks raised their children, Olivia, Jonathan, and Sidney. "While I was growing up, there was a barn with horses in back of us and small farmhouses with chickens and roosters to wake us up," Sidney said.

Sidney L. Brock, Jr., started a career at the First National Bank in 1927. He was senior vice-president when he retired in 1968, then became a consultant for the Continental Investment Company. Although many hours were spent at the Wigwam Fishing and Denver Country Clubs, his special interest was serving as a longtime trustee of the Mt. Airy Psychiatric Foundation.

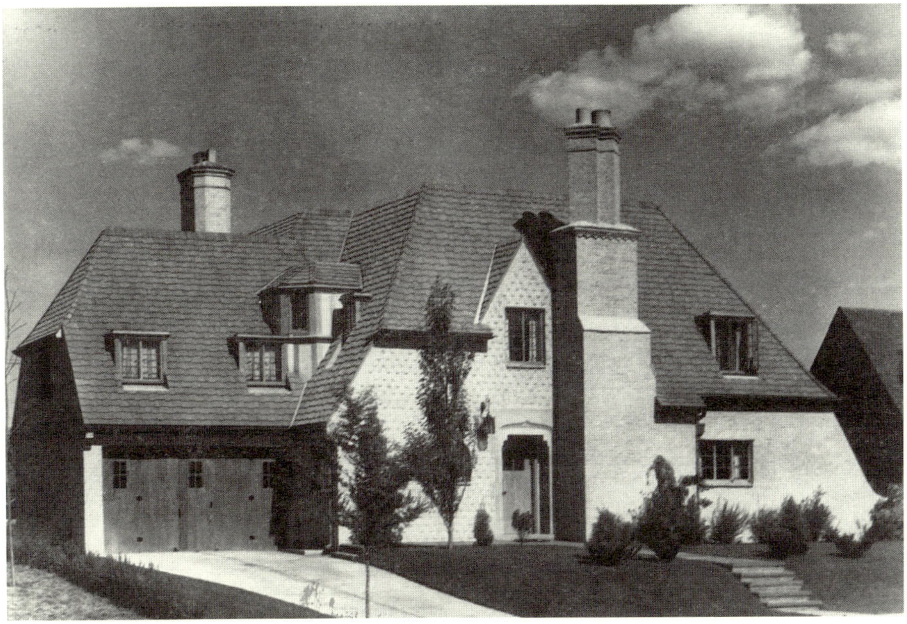

The 1928 French Normandy house, designed by Burnham Hoyt at 130 Gaylord Street, was the home of the Sidney L. Brock, Jr., family.

The Brocks daughter, Sidney, married investment banker Caleb F. Gates, Jr., and raised their children, Caleb, III "Chief", Lindsay, and Jonathan at 100 Franklin Street.

20
140 GAYLORD STREET
Built: 1923
Architect: unknown

This house has always been a center of activity for the Country Club Historic Neighborhood, Inc. (CCHN), nee the Cherry Creek Improvement Association (CCIA), the organization of home owners that has protected and preserved the area. During the sixties and seventies, Charles Lyon-Campbell "Chuck" Warren was its president for six years and continues to be a dominant figure in the organization. As soon as Chris and Kathleen Economos moved into the house in 1983, Kathleen came on board, serving on many committees as well as chairing the group.

Chuck Warren is a fourth-generation Coloradan and great grandson of Captain Charles Warren, a Civil War veteran, who established his family in Fort Collins in 1872 while starting a lumber business. The elder Warren built the first reservoir on the Cache la Poudre River, the Warren Lake Reservoir, and was described as a "worthy pioneer . . . of high ideals."[17] His son, Nathan C. Warren, a GOP leader, served 12 years in the state Senate. "Senator Nate" was also a director of the Denver Grain Exchange, the National Livestock Show, and the Denver Union Stockyards. His son, Charles P. Warren, a cashier at the First National Bank of Fort Collins,[18] sired a son, Charles L. Warren who, after a stint in the U.S. Navy, went to the University of Colorado, where he met and married Emma Josephine "E.J." Palmer from Sterling. They moved to Denver, and he became a vice-president of Merrill Lynch, specializing in institutional business. The Warren legacy of community service led him to the presidency of the Denver Zoological Foundation, The Park People, the Colorado Wildlife Heritage Foundation, and the University of Denver Humanities Institute. He also served several terms as president of the CCIA and helped with the Greater Cherry Creek Steering Committee and the Cherry Creek Foundation and Parkway Study. Both he and "E.J.," a founder of Tumbleweed Bookstore in Hilltop, have served on the vestry of St. John's Episcopal Cathedral. Their children, Diana; Charles, Jr.; and Robin, comprise a

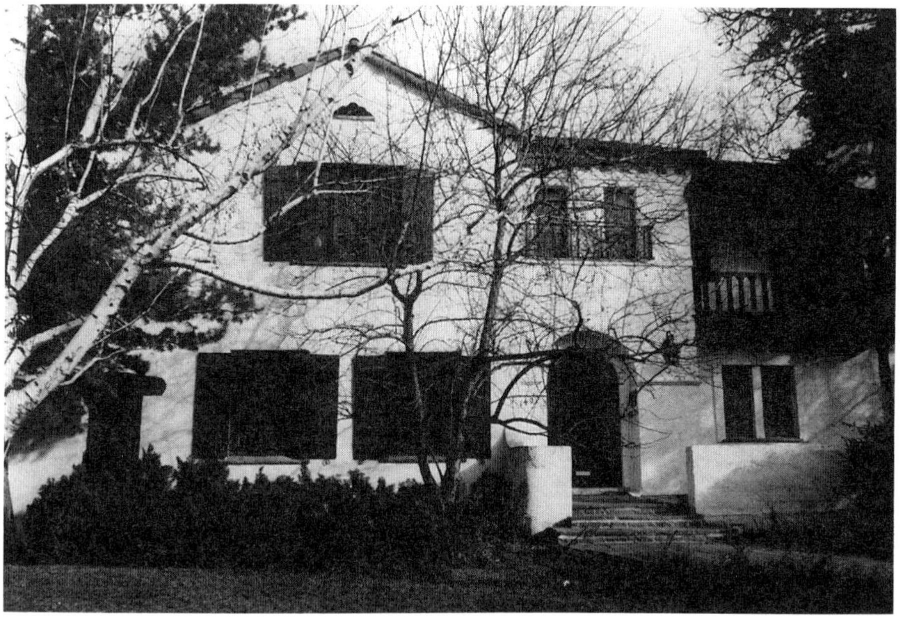

When the Monterey Spanish house 140 Gaylord Street was built in 1923, the area was a small farming community.

Describing herself as a community activist, Kathleen jumped right into CCIA activities, volunteering for their newsletter, for the Landmark Committee, and as treasurer and president of the organization. "I think traffic is our biggest problem," she said. "The Cherry Creek shopping development has attracted thousands more cars, and there are more problems like the traffic at 4th Avenue and Race."

One reason the Economoses like this Monterey Spanish house is the stability of the neighborhood. "Most of the houses are only on their third owners," Kathleen said. Over the recessed arched entry of this asymmetrical stucco house is an ornate wrought-iron balconet spanning two floor-length windows. A decorative

fifth generation of loyal Colorado Warrens.

Chuck and E.J. lived at 140 Gaylord for 23 years, moving to 2101 4th Avenue when the John Stoddarts left in 1983. At that time, Kathleen and Financial Planner Chris Economos moved into the house with their three daughters. "My husband adored the house," said Kathleen. Although there is a strip of stores directly behind their house, "there is no real problem as Alfalfa's built a uniform 10-foot fence to the corner. As part of the agreement, no restaurant will be allowed," she said.

For many years the house at 140 Gaylord Street was occupied by the Charles Warren family: Charles; Robin; Diana; Charles, Jr.; and E. J.

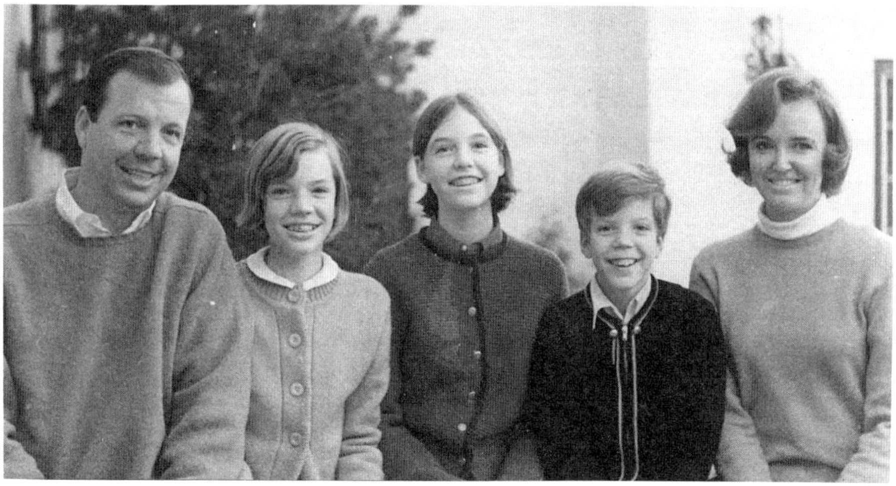

frieze trims the line of the red tile roof. The most striking feature is the cantilevered second-floor balcony with a brown wood balustrade that opens off of a bedroom. On a hot summer night, this is a great place to sleep.

21
240 GAYLORD STREET
Built: 1958
Architect: unknown

Two of the rare ranch-style houses in the district were built side by side on Gaylord Street, just south of the alley that divides Country Club Annex from Capitol Annex.

The small, low, white brick 1950s house at 240 Gaylord has a low-pitched roof with a side gable. Wings project at each side of the recessed entry porch. Three chimney pots trim the wide front chimney. Because the house is level with the ground, not raised like many Country Club homes, it has heavily guarded windows.

Although the house backs up on the commercial shops on the west side of University Boulevard, this area was quiet when it was built. The street had only a few small houses and the Blue Parrot Restaurant, where a live parrot would greet each guest with a cackling "Hello."

"Uncle Ed built 240 Gaylord for his divorced wife, Ruth. We called her 'Auntie Rae,'" said Gladys (Mrs. Philip, Jr.) Alexander, speaking of Edwin Kassler, Jr., who had lived at 369 Humboldt Street. During the late fifties, Ed's sister, Ruth Kassler Alexander, and her husband, Philip K. "P. K." Alexander, moved there from their larger home at 140 Humboldt Street. Ruth's sister, Genevieve Kassler Brock, lived at 130 Gaylord Street. After P. K. died in 1970, F. George "Porie" Robinson of Robinson Brick Company and his wife, Marybelle "Merbie," found this an excellent retirement home.

At 240 Gaylord is one of the few ranch-style houses in the area.

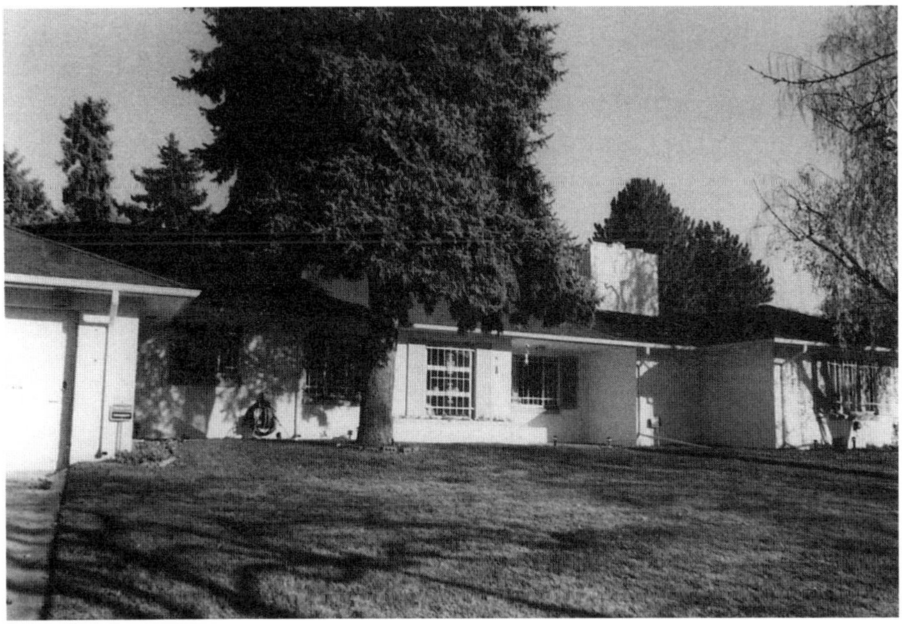

22
2300-2320 EAST 3RD AVENUE
Built: 1910
Architect: unknown

In contrast to the elegant Mediterranean and Tudor homes of the Country Club Historic District, a six-plex of unassuming small red brick apartments lines 3rd Avenue between Gaylord and its eastern alley. One might think they changed hands often, occupied briefly by young couples before they moved on. Perhaps they would be turned into offices or shops. But no, these houses, zoned R-O, are grandfathered, or

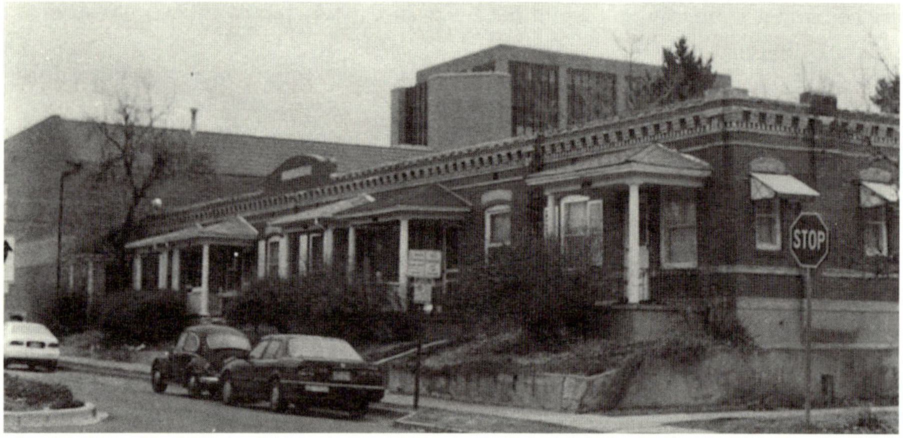

These townhouses, built in 1910 on 3rd Avenue, have remained in the same families for three and four generations.

maybe great-grandfathered, into the historic district, becoming among the oldest, most historic homes in the neighborhood with long-term owners who have lovingly cared for them for three or four generations.

Clara L. Bebout has lived at the house nearest the alley since 1948. She and her husband bought the 825-square-foot residence for $5,000. "The property is worth $113,000 now," she said in 1999. She raised three children in the five-room house. "We put the girls in the dining room and the boy in the other bedroom. Later we made one of the bedrooms into the kitchen because it was such a sunny room," she said. Laundry and storage were in the half basement. The remainder of the 1,600-square-foot lot was used for a garden and a small one-car garage, accessed only by small cars, as the alley is only 16 feet wide.

At the end of the eighties, a median was installed in front of the row of houses to slow traffic from dashing down 3rd from University Boulevard. However, the median also limits space for the residents' cars that must park on 3rd because the garages and access alley are so small. "We had a nice wide street before," Bebout said.

The house farthest west, on the corner of Gaylord, has been in the Hilderbrand-McCleery family since 1920. "The house is deceiving," said Geraldine McCleery, who was born there in 1924. "There's a nice-sized living room, a 12-by-12-foot dining room, two bedrooms, a back porch, and a kitchen large enough for a table and chairs. Then there's a pantry we used for flour and potato bins. The basement was cool and so light you could do sewing and ironing there. One wall had shelves for the canning jars."

When Geraldine was three years old, her parents took in a family of five children from an orphanage. They moved to a larger house three years later, but always kept "The Terrace," as they called it. "We never rented it because there was always someone who needed a house," she said. When her father died, she moved back there with her mother. After her brother finished college, he bought the house. Then a friend of his needed a place to live. "The Terrace" has been in the family for three generations.

Three of the middle houses have been owned by the same family for four generations. "Technically we had the first townhouses in Denver. That means we owned the air above and the ground below," explained Deanna L. Purdy. "My grandparents bought the houses when they were brand new, and I inherited them when my father died in 1996."

Three families came out together from Illinois for health reasons and lived in the three adjacent houses. "They were basically owner-occupied before World War II, but now we rent them occasionally," she said. The family has taken great pride in the houses and has repaired and upgraded them regularly. "They have such a personality and ambiance," Purdy said. "If we want to rent them, we never have to put an ad in the paper."

These six houses are raised from the sidewalk, each reached by seven steps leading to a covered porch. The red brick walls are trimmed with a beige bandbelt or coping. The center of the flat roofline is broken by a decorative red brick and beige parapet.

Although Lawrence Phipps bought the western two blocks of Capitol Annex lining 3rd Avenue to add to Country Club Annex, he did not include this row of houses, which remains in Capitol Annex. The proud owners are an integral, active, and vocal component of Country Club Historic Neighborhood, Inc.

23
316 GAYLORD STREET
Built: 1899
Remodeled: 1992
Architect: Steven Newman

Although the year of construction of this house is listed by the Assessor's Office as 1938, it was 1899 when engineer Robert Beattie bought the lot and a half (37 feet frontage) on Green (Gaylord) Street.[19] He built a small, two-story house and lived there with his wife, Adele; his school-aged stepson, Richard Stanley; and a brother-in-law, Fowler Bryant, also an engineer.[20] No servants are listed as living in the tiny little residences of Capitol Annex. Peter Coffey lived at the small house at 316 Gaylord in 1924, and in 1935, Robert A. Anderson added a 6-by-18-foot brick open front porch and stuccoed the house.

During the mid-forties, owners Margaret "Margie" and John C. "Jack" Davis, who had bought another two lots to the south, built two additions for bedrooms and a utility room and removed the second floor for a low, flat-roofed, ranch-style house, so popular in the fifties.

Joan and Horace F. "Jack" Phelps, who bought it in 1953, made further additions. "We made the attached garage into a den, built a new single garage, and added patios to both the east and south," said Joan. In 1977 they added a brick veneer to the existing masonry walls. Jack had grown up at 191 Race Street.

Next door, at 320 Gaylord, was a vintage, two-story house, again built on only one-and-a-half lots. The house was originally made of soft brick and later covered with stucco for insulation. Jack Phelps said, "There was a neat black family there named Clark. One of them was a schoolteacher, I remember." The house (at 320 Gaylord) is a 1,887 square-foot house built on a mere 5,060 square feet of land. A building permit for that property is dated 1892,[21] the earliest in the District.

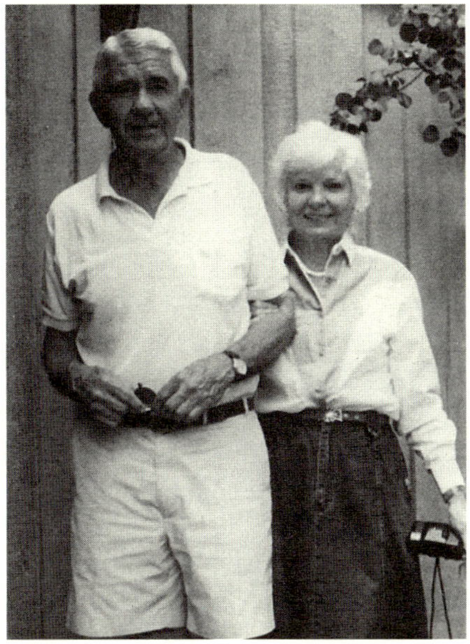

Horace "Jack" and Joan Phelps lived at 319 Gaylord Street for over four decades. They added patios and built a new garage.

Jeannette and Roger S. "Kip" Wotkyns, III, bought the house at 316 Gaylord in 1991. "Originally our house was probably just like the little two-story house next door," Kip said. "With the help of the principal designer of RNL Facilities Corporation, Steven Newman, we changed it drastically. We turned the master bedroom into the kitchen and obtained a variance to build a garage right to the alley property line. The old garage was absorbed into the house, part of it

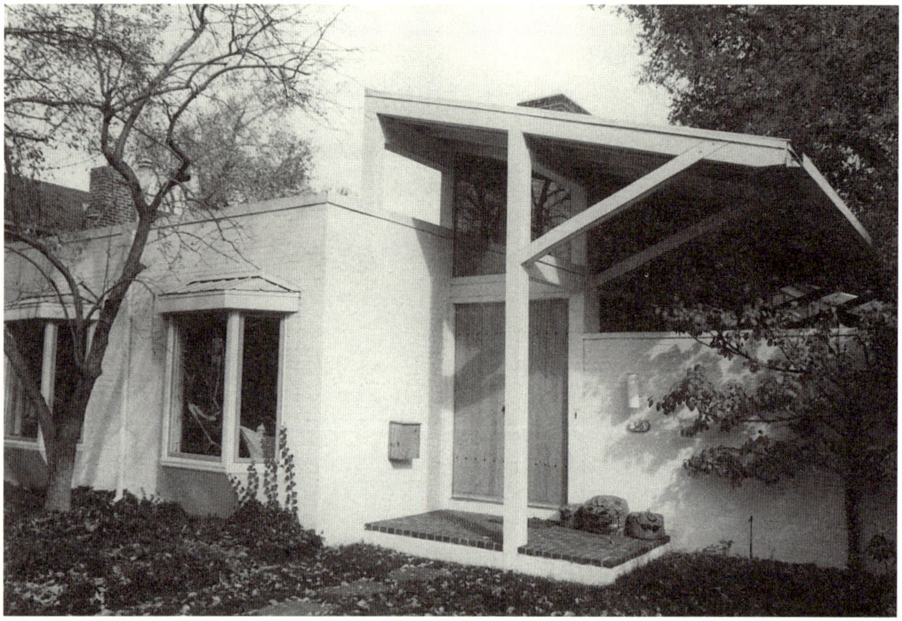

[ABOVE]: *When Roger "Kip" Wotkyns bought the house at 319 Gaylord Street, they added a dramatic tall gallery with clerestory windows*

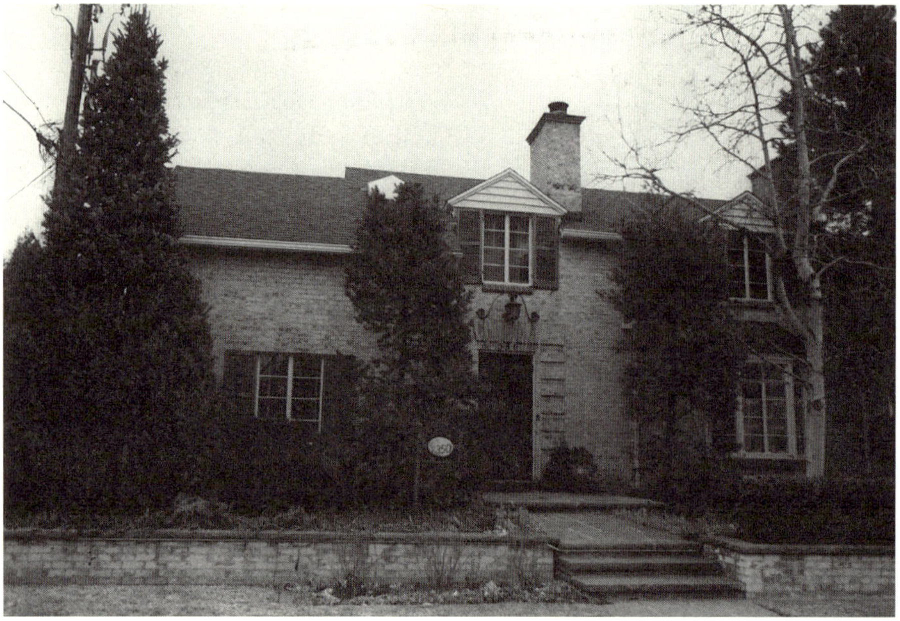

becoming a closet for the new master bedroom. The interior walls were rearranged to form four bedrooms and three baths. Over the south side of the house we built a tall gallery with clerestory windows to add more light and room."

The gallery has a long, dramatic shed roof with wide overhangs, supported by triangular brackets and a small, square wood column. It contrasts with the Modernistic flat roof on the north part of the house, which features two tall bay windows facing west.

24
350 GAYLORD STREET
Built: 1935
Architects: Varian and Varian

This three-lot (75-foot) property is twice the size of others in Capitol Annex, the one-block-wide subdivision that was platted in 1889 as an extension of the farming town of Harman (Cherry Creek North). A 1935 building permit allowed Graland teacher Harold H. Cox to evacuate the property and build a brick, 1,403-square-foot residence with attached garage for $5,000.

[LEFT]
The house at 350 Gaylord Street was owned by two Dines families, both of whom made several additions to the house.

Subsequent owner Dorothy (Mrs. Bruce) Dines said, "The original house had a living room, kitchen, dining room, and tiny powder room downstairs with two bedrooms and a bath upstairs. The garage was by the front door and was made into a family room with a bay window by next owner, Paul MacDowell, in 1948."

The house was then owned by Bruce's brother, David Dines, and his wife, Betty, who added a third bedroom, a bath, and a garage on the side alley during the late fifties. When Dorothy and Bruce bought the house from David, they combined two small bedrooms into a master bedroom and added two more bedrooms for their children, Katherine, Bruce, Jr., and Hildreth. "It's an amazingly quiet neighborhood, although there was a lot of cut-through traffic before the median was built on 3rd Avenue," Dorothy said.

The Dines family has deep roots in the Country Club district. Tyson S. Dines lived at 195 High, where he brought up his sons, Tyson, Courtland, and Eugene. Eugene's widow lived at 1953 East 3rd Avenue. Eugene, Jr., was at 2022 East 4th Avenue; daughter Marcia (Strickland) lived at 360 Gilpin; and both David, a physician, and Bruce, a banker and artist, owned 350 Gaylord.

A branch of the 6th Avenue trolley became the 4th Avenue trolley when it turned south on Downing Street. At Race it turned south to 3rd, then continued through Capitol Annex to Harman. The tracks were removed in 1939 to supply metal for World War II. (Courtesy Colorado Historical Society)

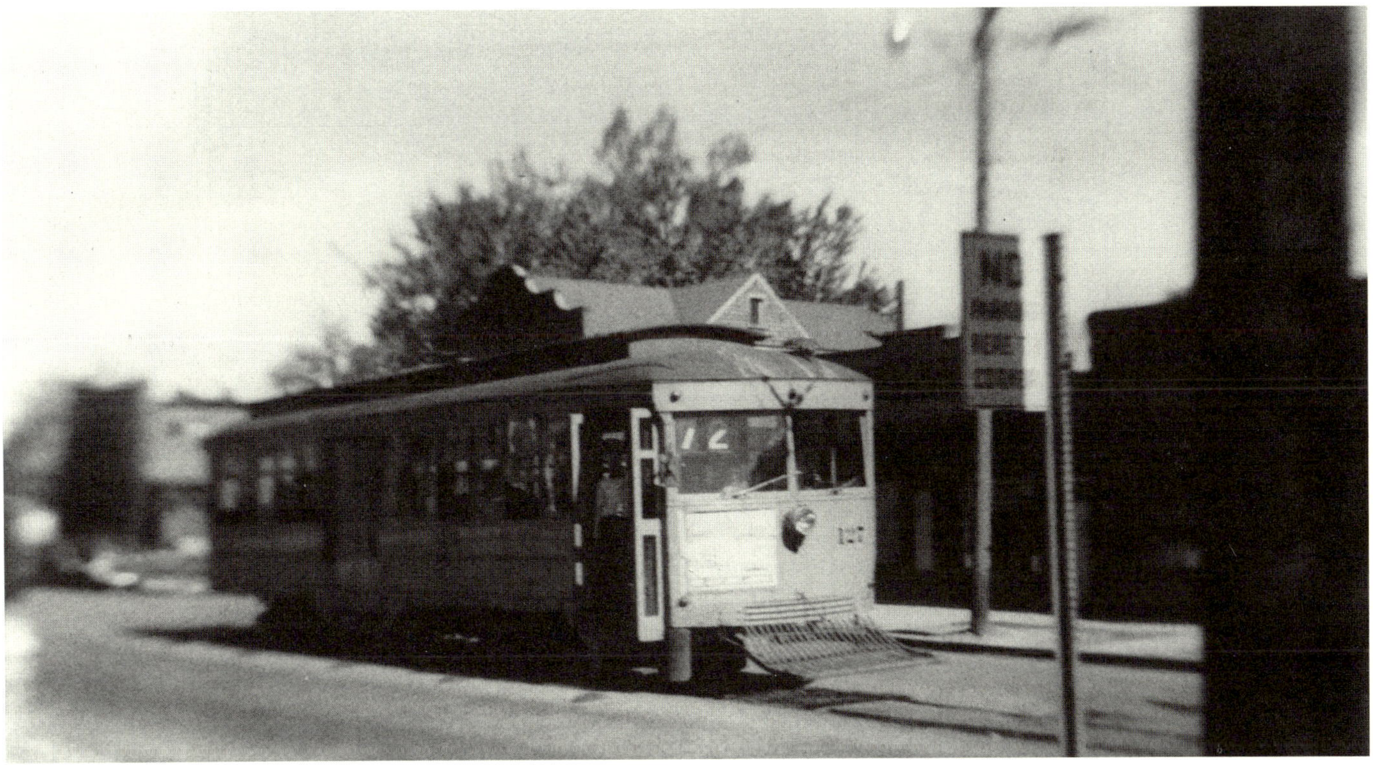

TOUR 4: PARK LANE SQUARE

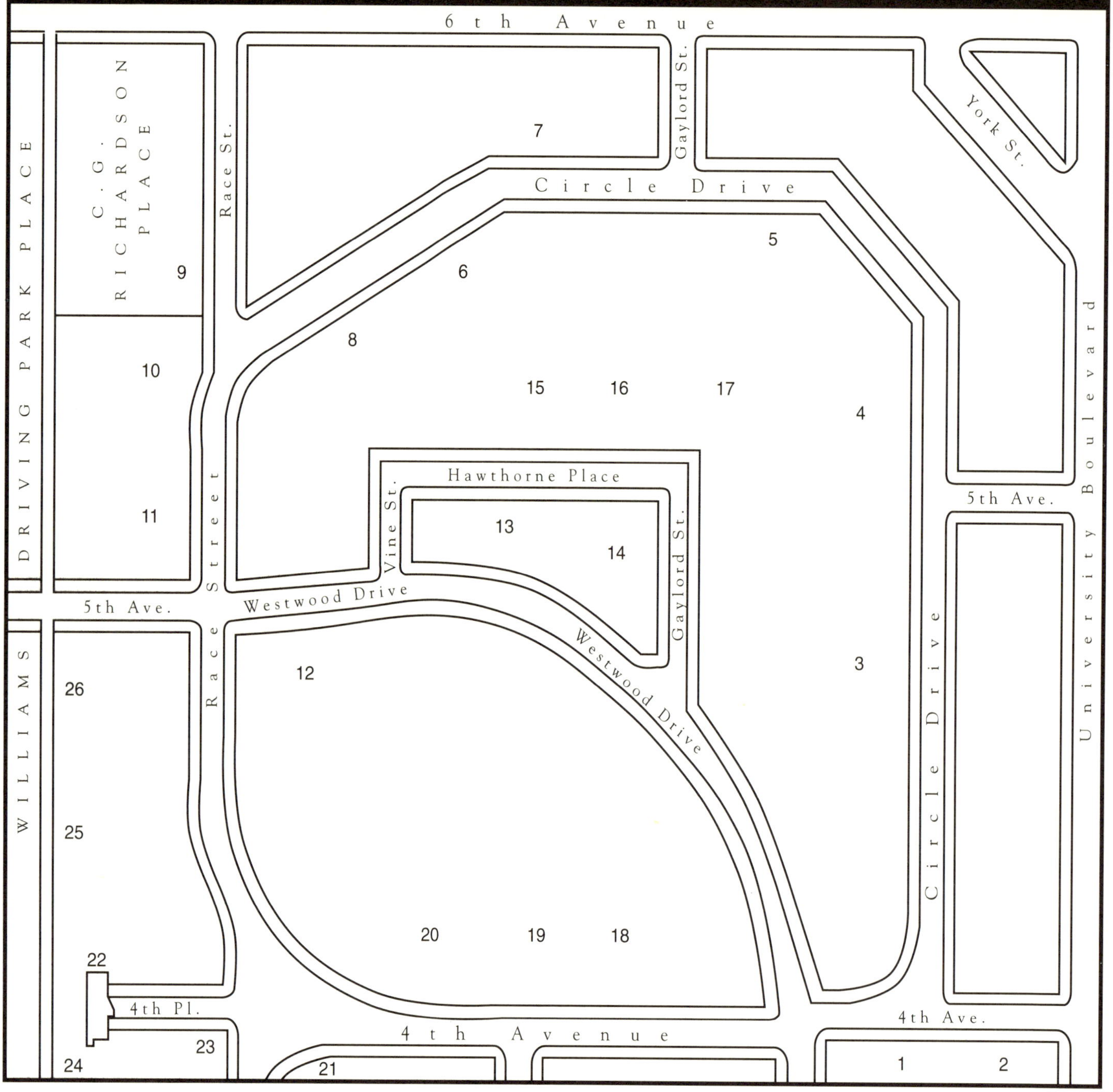

TOUR #4

1 380 Gaylord Street
2 2244 East 4th Avenue
3 475 Circle Drive
4 505 Circle Drive
5 545 Circle Drive
6 575 Circle Drive
7 576 Circle Drive
8 595 Circle Drive
9 C. G. Richardson Place (555 Race Street)
10 545 Race Street
11 515 Race Street
12 490 Race Street
13 460 Westwood Drive
14 450 Westwood Drive
15 2125 Hawthorne Place
16 2151 Hawthorne Place
17 2155 Hawthorne Plate
18 2115 East 4th Avenue
19 2101 East 4th Avenue
20 2025 East 4th Avenue
21 2012 East 4th Avenue
22 1925-7 4th Place
23 401 Race Street
24 1921 East 4th Avenue
25 419 Race Street
26 1920 East 5th Avenue

[OPPOSITE PAGE]
Park Lane Square was designed in the mid-twenties as a country-like suburb within the city. The walking tour winds around the circular streets.

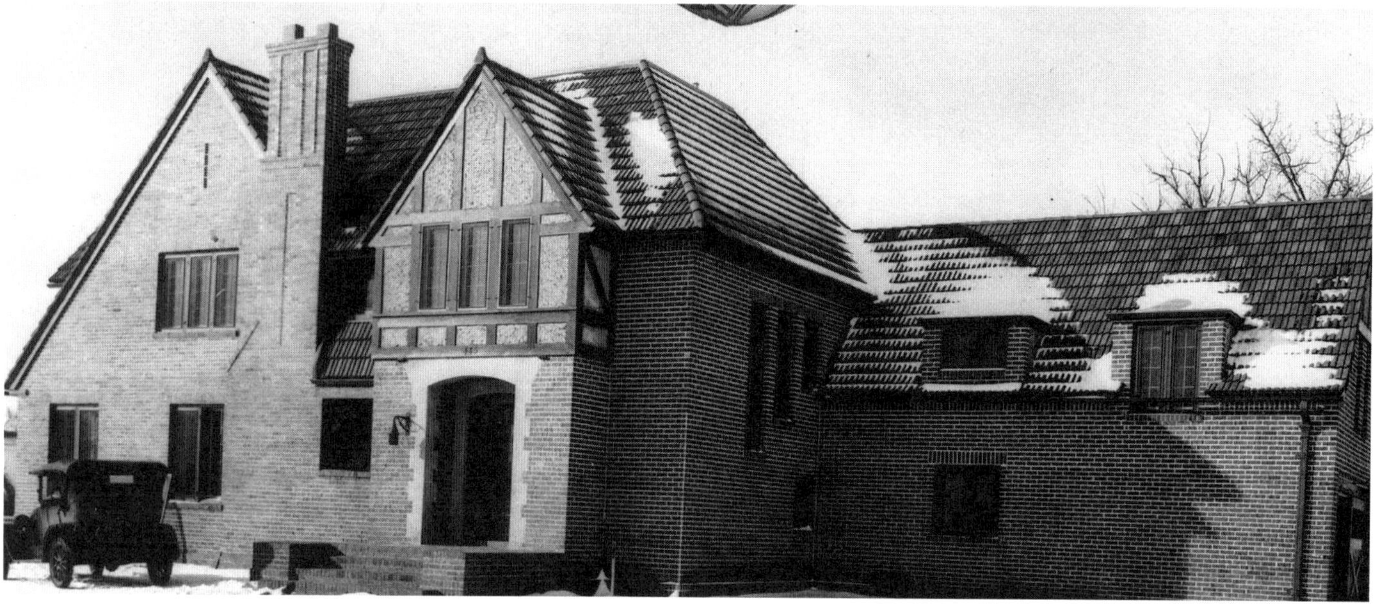

An early Park Lane Square house, built at 485 Race Street, was bought by John A. Ferguson, Jr., whose father purchased the land for the FourthAvenue Realty Company in 1902. (Courtesy Colorado Historical Society)

~ Tour 4 ~

1
380 GAYLORD STREET
Built: 1928
Architect: H. B. Joy

This house, just north of 350 Gaylord, is also north of the alley that divides Capitol Annex from Park Lane Square (Circle Drive), so it is in the latter subdivision. This dividing line is an extension of 4th Avenue, had it not jagged to the north at Race Street.

The building permit for 380 Gaylord was issued in 1928. Mason and Mount Construction Company built a $15,000 masonry residence with full basement and a garage off the alley. Marcus Bogue lived there from 1929 until 1935. Then, for 40 years, this long, extended Georgian house was occupied by Lola and Charles F. Collman, vice-president of H. A. Marr Grocery Company.

Groups of three windows flank the pedimented entry porch, supported by two Doric columns. A fanlight and sidelights surround the paneled door. The symmetrical house and its two wings have side gables with medium-pitched roofs trimmed with dentils.

During the early seventies, neighborhood leaders Christopher "Kit" Dobbins and his wife, Julia "King," lived in the house. Dobbins' father, Cris Dobbins, was president of Ideal Cement Company and managed the several businesses of Claude and Charles Boettcher, which included the American Crystal Sugar Company, Ideal Cement, Denver National Bank, the Potash Corporation of America, Boettcher Realty Company, and the Boettcher Foundation.

2
2244 EAST 4TH AVENUE
Built: 1976 to 1978
Architect: Robert K. Fuller, II

Robert Kenneth Fuller, II, who designed his own house at 2244 East 4th Avenue, is the fourth generation of an eminent family of architects in Colorado. His great-grandfather, Montezuma Fuller, practiced in Fort Collins. He was joined by his son,

On the south side of 4th Avenue, 380 Gaylord Street, the former home of Christopher and Julia Dobbins, is in the Park Lane Square subdivision.

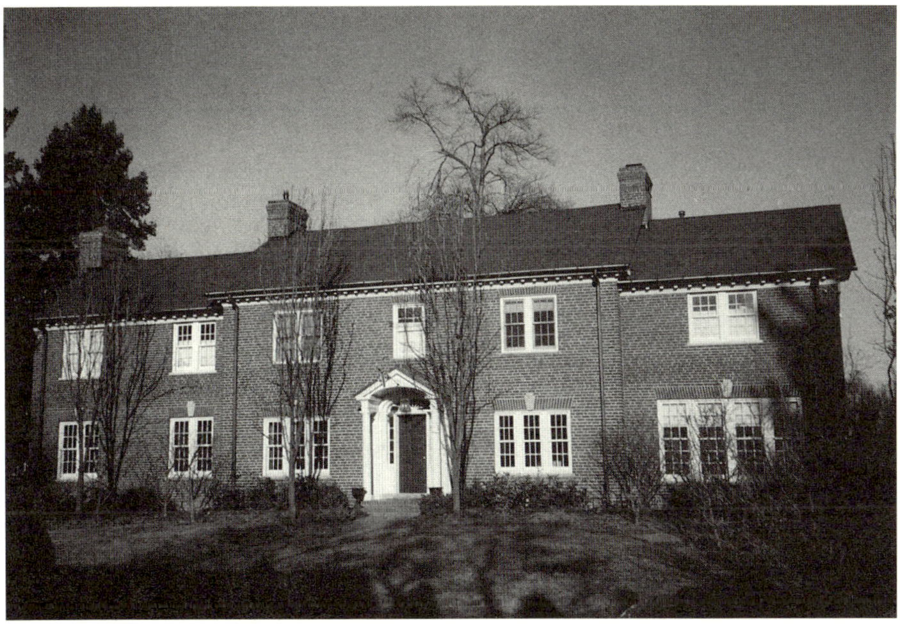

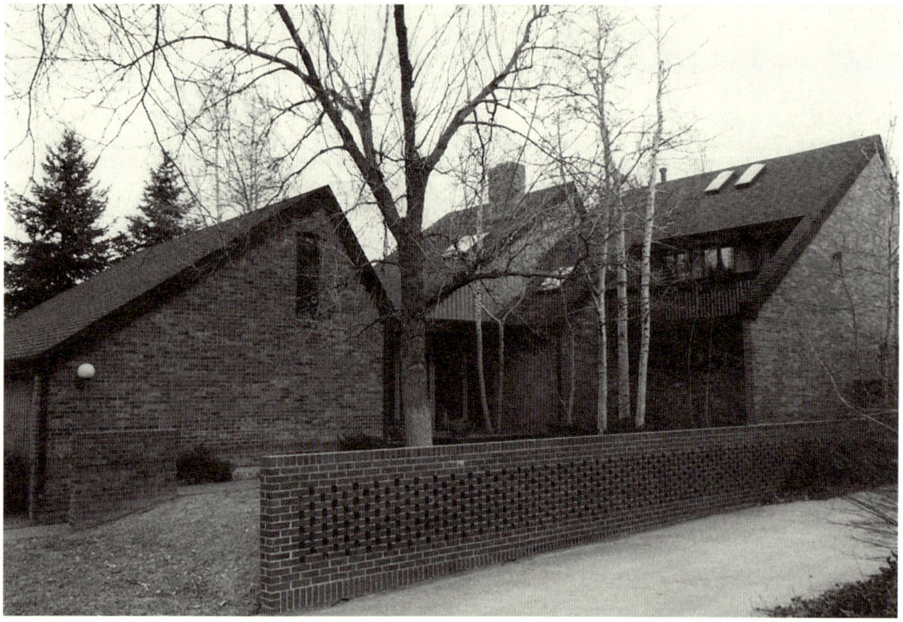

Architect Robert Fuller, II, built this contemporary house on the corner of University Boulevard in the late seventies.

Robert K. Fuller, who later moved to Denver to work with Robert S. Roeschlaub. Roeschlaub, who had brought his family to Denver in 1873, sponsored the Colorado Chapter of the American Institute of Architects (A.I.A.) in 1892, and served as its first president for 20 years. He was named a Fellow of the A.I.A. in 1900 and was instrumental in passing a professional licensing law for Colorado in 1909.

Robert K. Fuller, Sr., who established his own firm in 1917, was joined by his sons, Kenneth R. and Quentin R., and in 1969 by Kenneth's son, Robert K. Fuller, II. Kenneth, who supported the education committee of the A.I.A. in Colorado, donated a beautifully colored collection of Roeschlaub's drawings to the Colorado Historical Society (CHS) while Barbara Sudler (Hornby) was president. "We had a party for him and I had Governor Love and Governor Lamm,"[1] she said. The drawings are exhibited in the CHS museum.

The house Robert K. Fuller, II, built for himself on East 4th Avenue is a contemporary design of three separate gabled buildings: a bedroom wing, public spaces, and a garage, all facing away from busy University Boulevard. The pitch of the gables is asymmetrical because the roofs support solar panels to the south. "We bought one of the few vacant lots left and built a house that opens away from University Boulevard. Between the buildings are open courtyards, accessed by French doors that let in light and air. The garage cuts out the noise and the house works well for us,"[2] Fuller said. The buildings are joined on the west by a common patio. The west edge of the property is defined by a decorative masonry wall.

The property borders both Park Lane Square and Capitol Annex. The commercial properties on the block are zoned as a Planned Unit Development (PUD).

3
475 CIRCLE DRIVE
Built: 1926 to 1931
Architect: Henry James Manning

The castle was built during the late twenties by Mary Dean Reed, whose husband, Verner Z. Reed, had died in 1919.

Reed was a man of many talents and many homes. Born in Ohio in 1864, he traveled with his family to Colorado Springs where he met and married Mary Dean in 1893. His fortune came from opening up the great Cripple Creek Independence mine, and later by investing in the Salt Creek oil fields of Wyoming. His real estate interests necessitated so many trips to London that they lived in England from 1901 to 1912, making frequent trips to the cultural attractions of Italy and France. Back in the United States, his interest in oil irrigation and cattle shuttled him between Wyoming and Denver.

Reed also earned an enviable reputation as a mediator and helped President Woodrow Wilson in settling labor disputes such as telephone workers in California and oil producers and their employees. He was known, too, for his prolific and effective writings and speeches. He published poems; articles on travel, economics, history, and ethnology; and wrote shrewd analyses of business or agricultural problems. Another interest was the Ute and Pueblo Indians, and he also published a volume of essays entitled *Soul of Paris*.[3]

After they settled in the United States, the Reeds considered building a home. Verner wanted to build towards the mountains, but after his death in 1919, Mary turned her attention to 6th Avenue and University Boulevard, incorporating and heading the Dean Realty and Investment Company in 1920. The company accumulated properties from the sparsely populated 1888 C. G. Richardson subdivision during the early twenties. Taking several lots for her own family, Reed then sold the rest of the property to the Park Lane Square Land Company, incorporated in 1926. The subdivision was then replatted in a circular pattern by landscape architect Saco DeBoer, and lots were sold to individuals.[4]

The castle built by Mary (Mrs. Verner Z.) Reed at 475 Circle Drive is the showplace of the Park Lane Square subdiviaion. (Courtesy James D. Simmons)

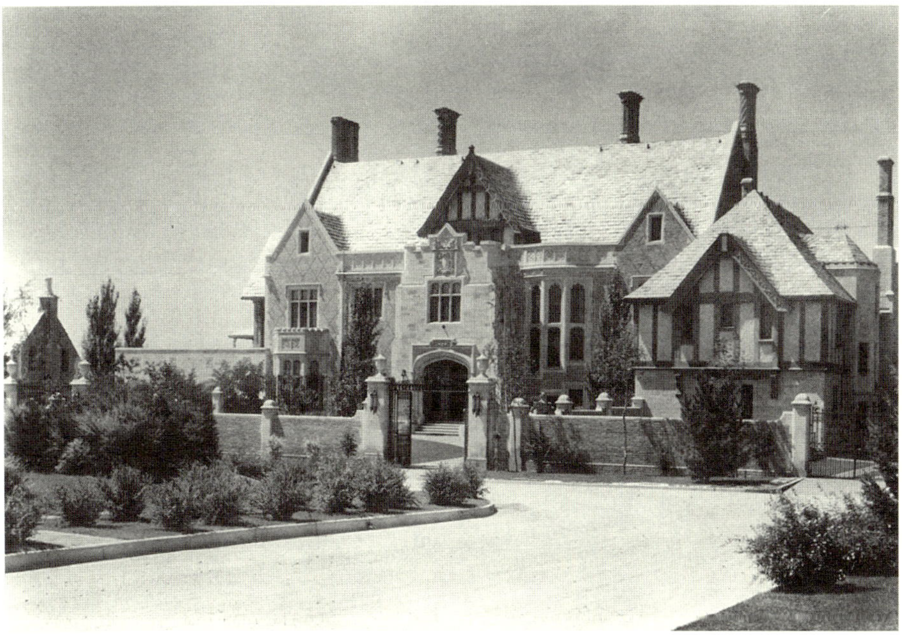

Plans for the house and landscaping of her own two-and-a-quarter acres began in 1926. "The first section completed was the northern timbered servants' quarters, where Mrs. Reed lived for a couple of years while the house was being completed. "We found utility bills from 1929 and plans starting in 1926,"[5] said the current owner (who wishes to remain anonymous).

The Reeds' daughter, Mary Reed (Mayo), had graduated from the University of Denver (DU) in 1919, the year of her father's death, and married Paul Mayo a year later. However, a promising career as a professor of literature was cut short by her untimely death in 1925. After this tragedy, her mother's many gifts to DU in her memory and her own appreciation of the arts led to Reed's membership on the Board of Trustees of the university and an honorary degree bestowed on her in 1945.

In 1959, Italian investment and real estate broker Joseph N. Minissale gave the castle to his wife, Carol, as a surprise gift. They had both come to New York from Sicily and had teamed up to run an upscale bridal shop (Grace Kelly bought her gown there) before coming to Denver in 1940. Minissale was an opera buff, and the castle sparkled with parties.[6]

The mansion, sold in 1977, has been painstakingly preserved by its third owner, who appreciates the detailed workmanship, intricate carving, and quality materials of this home. The stone entrance two-tier portico has an ornate door surround with a Tudor arch. A carved coat of arms above the arched windows crowns the castellated stone parapet. The entrance and doorways are trimmed with elaborate stone and wood carving.

The fireplaces are of Italian and Vermont marble, all carved by Professor Antonio Romanelli of the University of Florence, Italy. Stone door and window surrounds are meticulously sculpted. Animals are carved into the bargeboards of the north wing of the house. Red oak paneling on the library balcony is decorated by dwarfs doing various tasks, carved by architect Manning's co-worker, Edwin Francis. Even the gardener's house to the south features a carved stone plaque of a gardener watering flowers by the front door.

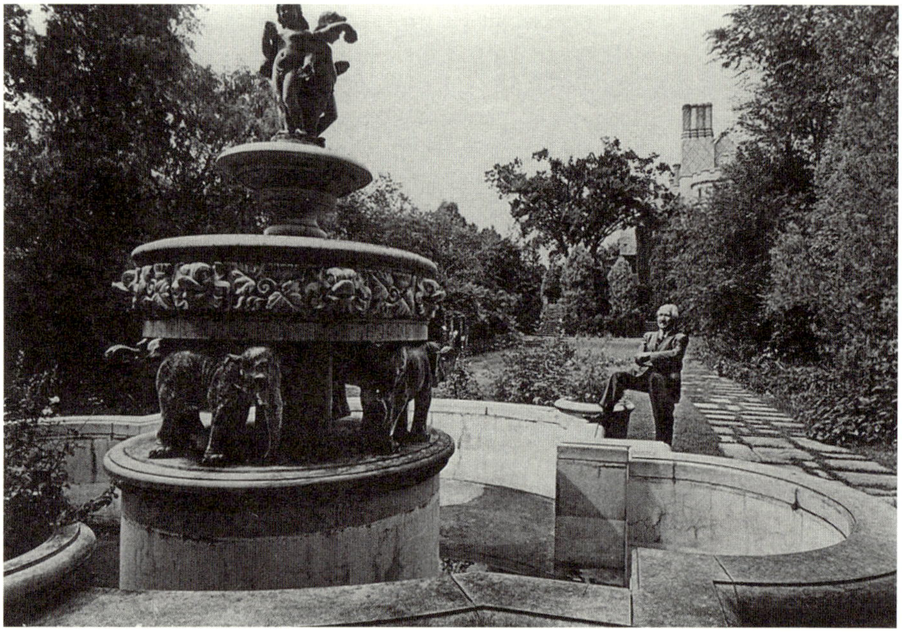

The gardens of the mansion at 475 Circle Drive were proudly maintained by second owner Joseph Minissale. (Courtesy James D. Simmons)

Indiana limestone and custom-made brick of varying sizes are used for the walls, forming a subtle diamond pattern. The floors are of walnut parquet, "like Versailles," said the current owner, who has seen the plans, dated 1928, in Florence. The wide dramatic staircase is of travertine marble with balustrades of carefully twisted iron trimmed with bronze plaques depicting the seasons. Wrought iron is used throughout the house. Polychrome slate covers the roofs.

"Finding screens made of bronze, mottled marble to mend an elephant's chipped foot, Vermont marble from a quarry that has since closed, or a skilled craftsman to spend two-and-a-half years painstakingly painting the house is not easy," the current owner said. Much research and effort is spent preserving the house.

Original features are retained, such as the semicircular paintings of flowers over the dining-room doors, the gold-plated light fixtures, and the canvas stencilled wall covering in the guest bedroom. Also retained are reminders of a bygone era: the men's paneled cloakroom with cupboards under each coat hook for the appropriate hat and the outside steps leading up to the two-foot-square door for the ice man to plunk a cake of ice right into the back of the icebox. The mansion is a combination of many elements, but is largely designed in the style of an English manor house.

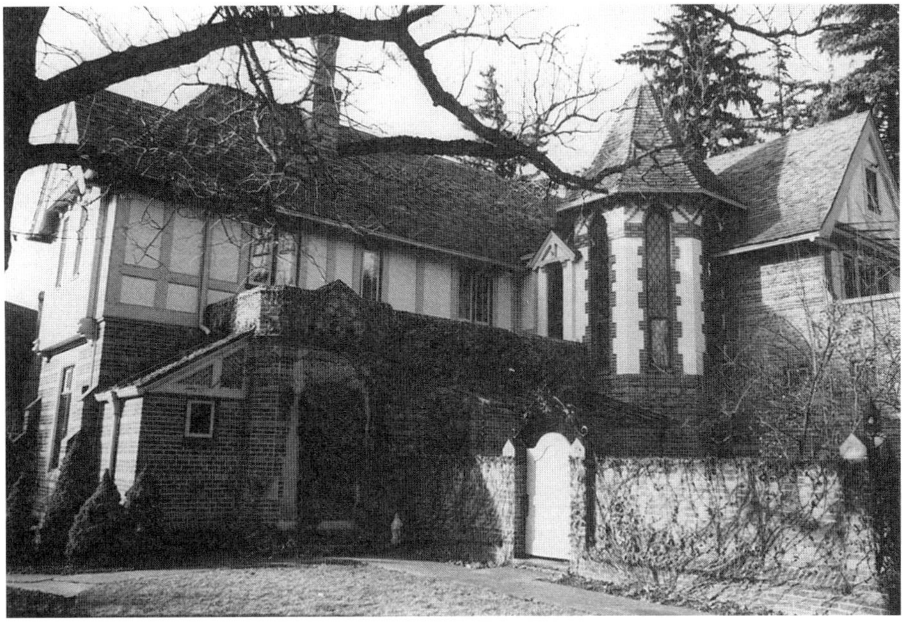

While building her own mansion, Mary Dean retained Henry James Manning to design a house next door for her sister, Florence Titus.

4
505 CIRCLE DRIVE
Built: 1929
Architect: Henry James Manning

While Mary Dean Reed lived in the north wing of 475 Circle Drive, supervising the construction of her castle, she engaged her architect, Henry Manning, to build a smaller but similar house next door for her sister, Florence Dean Titus. This Tudor style house at 505 Circle Drive has a steep front gable and a conical-roofed turret with tall, narrow, leaded windows. Architect Philip Atchison commented, "This house couldn't be built today. The variety of clay tiles rounding the corners of the tower would be impossible to duplicate."[7]

The elaborate patterned brick of the garage contrasts with the beige stucco of the main house. Most of the 17,534 square feet of land are devoted to a large, well-groomed garden. The house was built with garden steps leading from this house to the castle so that Mary could easily go have breakfast with her sister each morning. These steps have become overgrown since Mrs. Titus died, and a wall separates the two properties. The house was sold to *Rocky Mountain News* Associate Editor Robert L. Chase and reporter and Pulitzer Prize-winning playwright Mary Coyle Chase, who lived there until 1986. In 1945, Mary Chase's play, *Harvey*, made her the first Coloradan to win a Pulitzer Prize for drama. She received $1 million for movie rights. The star, Elwood P. Dowd, was played by James Stewart, who came to Denver to attend her reception for the 35th anniversary of the production of the play and later to attend her funeral service in 1981.

Mary Chase wrote other fanciful stories while she lived at 505 Circle Drive. *The Wicked Pigeon Ladies in the Garden* is a delightful children's book about the castle next door. A naughty girl escapes her mother by wiggling through a board in the closed-off "pair of high, wide iron gates across a bricked driveway where once carriages pulled by horses had gone rolling into the grounds." to explore the huge, boarded-up, haunted mansion next door. The house has a "marble fireplace with a

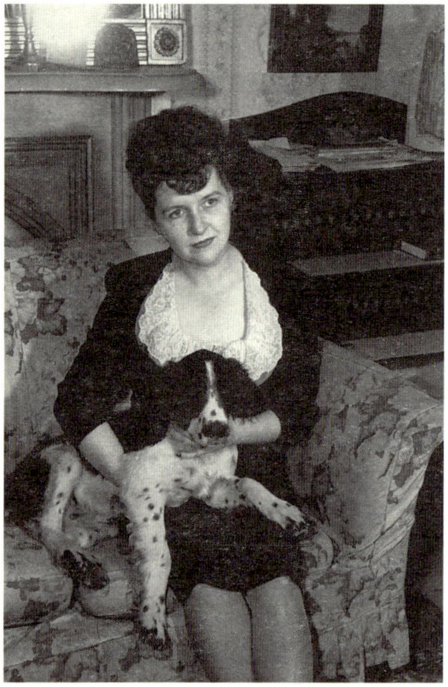

Pulitzer Prize-winning playwright Mary Coyle Chase lived at 505 Circle Drive. (Courtesy DPL Western History Department)

tall mirror above it" and "a summer house, made of wooden strips, criss-crossed," where she met a leprechaun. It had a "big dusty hall with a wide staircase." At the head of the stairs the girl discovers portraits of seven elegantly dressed Victorian ladies who come alive and talk with her.[8]

"Mary Chase was a wonderful neighbor. She used to invite my children over to read them stories,"[9] said Ann Campbell, who lived next door at 525 Circle Drive for 20 years. "She was also one of the most naturally beautiful women I have ever known,"[10] added neighbor Patsy O'Rourke Monaghan of 2012 4th Avenue.

Marilyn Alkire bought this "companion house" from Robert Chase's estate in 1990. This house and the mansion to the south were built at the same time by Manning using many of the same components. "We have lots of the same materials, the same types of wood and fixtures, even some gold door handles," said Alkire. She repainted, redecorated, and re-plumbed the house, redoing the bathrooms, but did few structural changes. "When we bought, you couldn't even see the house because of the overgrown pfitzers, deceased cedars, and a jungle of shrubs. I completely relandscaped."[11] The garden still has the original gazebo and the fountain with a cupid sitting on the front built there in 1929.

5
545 CIRCLE DRIVE
Built: 1941
Architect: Burnham Hoyt

This is one of the few International-style houses in the district. It was designed in 1941 by Burnham Hoyt several years after his brother,

A late International-style house designed by Burnham Hoyt was built at 545 Circle Drive.

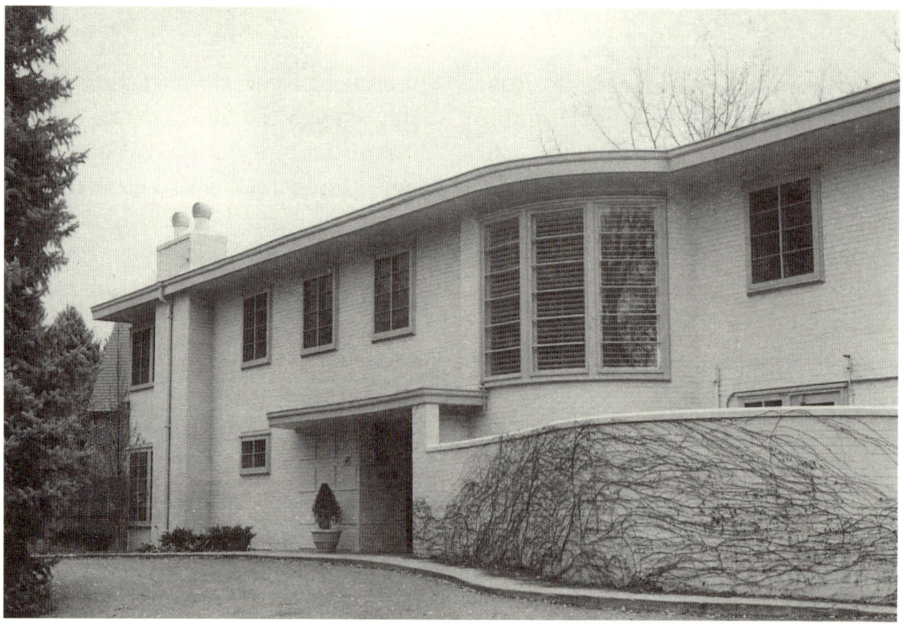

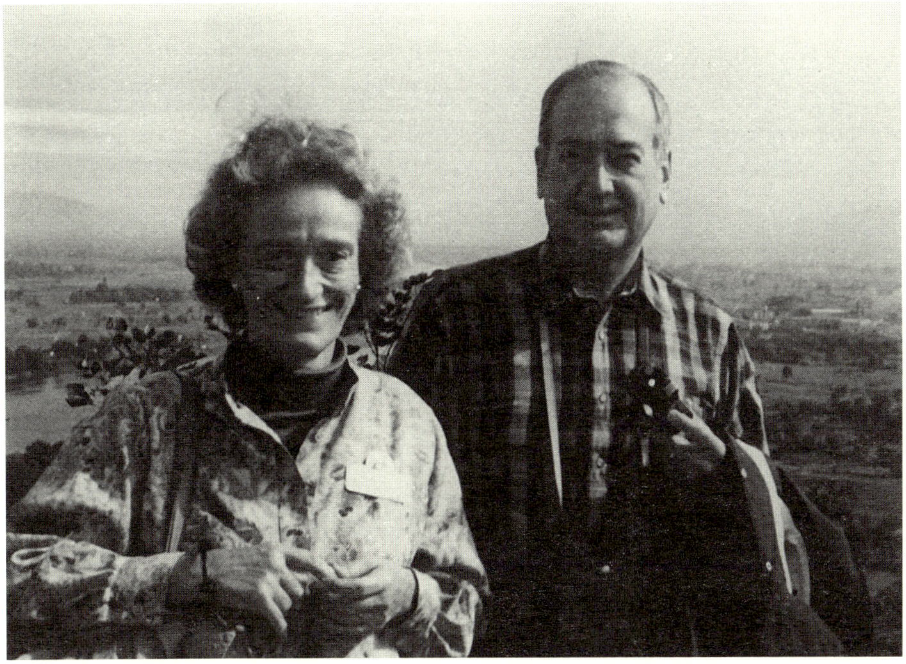

Anne and Claude Maer added a pool room to the house at 545 Circle Drive during the seventies. (Courtesy the Claude Maers)

of Strawn Realty Corporation. The Sullivans put a 26-by-15-foot addition on the rear of the residence in 1950. Sullivan died in 1973, a year after the death of his wife, and the house was sold to Anne and Claude Maer.

For 12 years the Maers lived there with two growing sons, enjoying the large sunken living room and the pool room they had added to the south. Walls of corrugated glass were removed from the entrance hallway and replaced with specially designed shelves to display Anne's collection of pre-Columbian and Japanese art objects. The house had a special attraction for the two teenaged boys, who could escape at night onto the flat garage roof by the alley from one of their bedrooms.[13]

Merrill, had died. This late International style house features simple horizontal lines contrasted with rounded edges. The flush windows, glass bricks, and lack of decoration are typical of the style. A front garage and circular driveway serve the northern entrance.

The home was built for Elizabeth Ferguson Bosworth and Barry Morey Sullivan a year after their marriage in 1940. Elizabeth was the daughter of Arthur H. Bosworth of 301 High Street and granddaughter of John A. Ferguson, purchaser of the Riethmann property for the Fourth Avenue Realty Company, which sold land to the Denver Country Club.

Sullivan's father, Barry Sullivan, was a brother-in-law and business partner of John Morey. Columnist Polly Pry reported on them racing auto cars at Overland Park in 1903: "Johnny had gone out to christen his new machine. . . . Barry took the fence and proceeded to give Johnny plenty of dust to eat."[12] Son Barry was vice-president of the Morey Mercantile Company. When it merged with Continental Foods, he became president of Morey Realty Company as well as vice-president

6
575 CIRCLE DRIVE
Built: 1930
Architect: Henry A. Koch

Referred to as "the other castle" (the first being at 475 Circle Drive) this 6,193-square-foot residence lies on three-fourths of an acre, occupying two 15,000-square-foot lots between Circle Drive and Hawthorne Place. The house was designed by Henry A. Koch, who came to Denver in 1923. He also designed the Centennial Race Track and the Jefferson County Courthouse.[14]

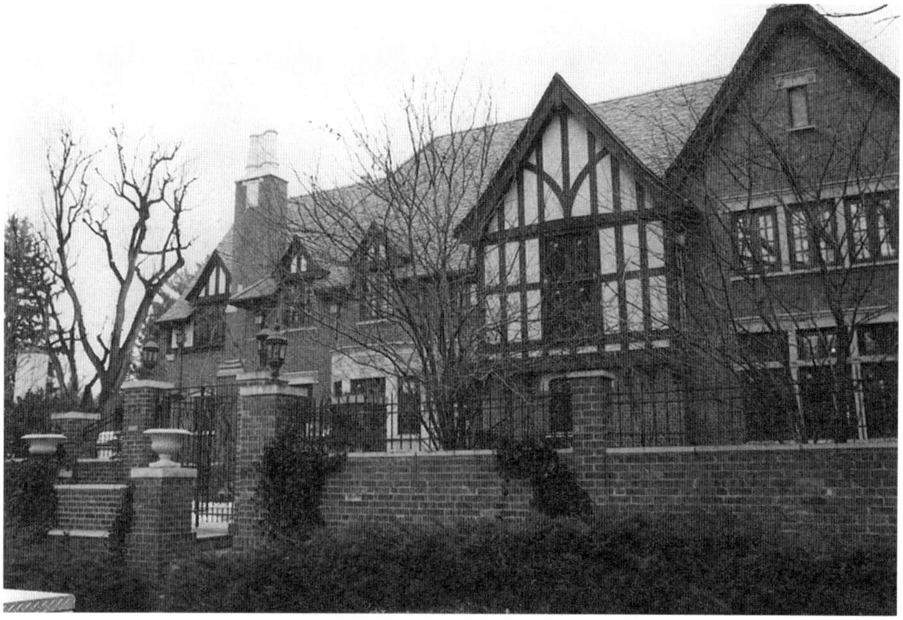

This large Tudor house at 575 Circle Drive includes a garden on a second lot to the south that extends to Hawthorne Place.

The house was built by F. J. Kirchoff Construction Company for $38,000 for Bertha and Albert H. Seep, owner of the Mine and Smelter Company. A fire door was built between the front-drive garage and the rest of the house,[15] and a retaining wall and three-foot, ornamental iron fence were added six months later. "The house was very solidly constructed," said neighbor Charlotte (Mrs. Walter "Bill") Croze of 555 Circle Drive. "You could have set a 20-story building on that basement floor."

Dorothy and Mason Avery Lewis and their two children lived there for three decades. Lewis, a founder of the law firm, Lewis and Grant, was the son of Robert E. Lewis, a judge of the U.S. 10th Circuit Court of Appeals. Mason's two sisters, who often lunched together at the Denver Country Club, were "Weddy" (Mrs. Josiah G.) Holland and Anne (Mrs. Henri) de Compiegne of 140 High Street. His daughter, Sally Lewis (Mrs. David) Keefe, was five years old when she moved there. "It was a wonderful place to grow up, and I remember the milkman clomping down the street in his wagon," she said. "We went downtown on the 6th Avenue streetcar or bus to the movies, or we could walk to the Hiawatha [Esquire Theater]." Dorothy Lewis, active on the Central City Opera and Denver Symphony Society boards, lived there until her death in 1968.

From the entrance on Circle Drive the eclectic Tudor house has a half-timbered front gable and dormers with lead-pane windows. There is fine stone detailing around the entry and terrace windows with terra-cotta ornamentation. The chimneys are notable for their tapered cast pots. The three-car garage is set back and angles toward the garden so the front facade is less massive. From Hawthorne Place a large, serene garden leads to the house. A wide two-story bay is topped by brick battlements with stone coping. The back entrance opens onto a wide glassed terrace overlooking the garden.

The rooms are luxuriously generous. The fireplace surround is of carved stone. "The interior decorator was Havens-Batchelder, and the dining room wallpaper was imported from London," Keefe said. "There were three maids' rooms over the garage with a bath and back stairs. The attic of the house was unfinished. Mother didn't like us up there, but we loved it, as there was a little roof balcony towards the garden."

When Tom Shane, "the Diamond King," lived there he built a high brick wall in the Circle Drive entrance. The wide double entry is centered by a lower brick wall, marked by two large urns.

The house was sold in 1998 for $2.3 million to Kelly and Kevin Gallagher, who have renovated the interior and added rooms over the garage. There are few structural changes. Kevin's father, industrialist and philanthropist Charles Gallagher, is extensively remodeling a historic house at 177 Humboldt for his daughter's family.

7
576 CIRCLE DRIVE
Built: 1929
Architect: Jacques Benedict

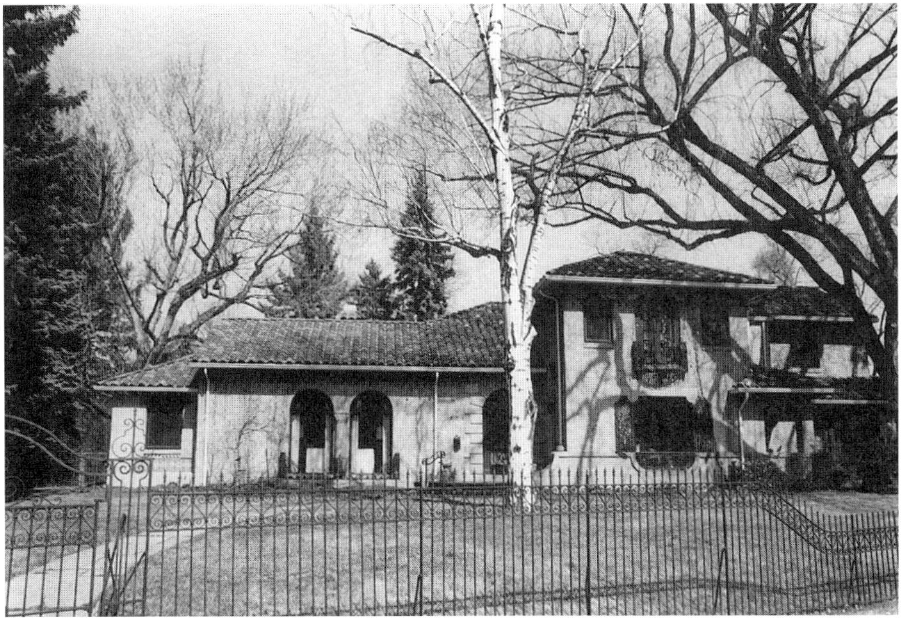

This Benedict- designed, Spanish-style house has been occupied by Lorna Holland Gage Westfeldt since 1964.

This beautifully-crafted Benedict house was built for James W. Douglas, chairman of the board of Whitney Sporting Goods Company.

In 1964 it was bought by F. Wallace "Wally" Gage, president of the Gage Oil and Gas Company, and his wife, Lorna Holland, whom he had married in 1956. Lorna was the daughter of Josiah "Joe" Holland, a founder of the prestigious Holland and Hart law firm. Gage also served on the boards of Denver Country Day School and the Boys Club before his untimely death in 1975 at 51. Lorna, who continued to live there, married attorney Patrick M. Westfeldt 10 years later.

This house is a good example of Benedict's Spanish style. The long tan stucco home has a medium-pitched, red tile roof and rounded arches over the downstairs windows. Wrought-iron balconets are echoed by the front fence and gate.

When the Gages purchased the house from Doribell (the former Mrs. Charles) Hughes, Hughes had remodeled the garage into a bedroom and bath for some of her five children. She then built another garage, but soon moved, finding the three-bedroom house too cramped. "This house has the fine workmanship and generous room dimensions that mark the quality of Benedict houses," Lorna said. "When I wanted to make some changes in the sunroom, the contractor told me, 'Mrs. Gage, you don't want to do that. Those walls are eight bricks thick.'"

After the Gages had moved into the house, 6th Avenue was changed to a one-way street, and the City wanted to take property to widen it. "We were all furious," Lorna said, "but when the Corona Presbyterian Church, the Ascension Episcopal Church, and St. John's [now Good Shepherd] Catholic Church all objected, the City gave up." The street remains at its former width, walled against noise along 6th Avenue.

8
595 CIRCLE DRIVE
Built: 1929
Architect: unknown

This spacious corner between Circle Drive and Race Street has been occupied by the Frank H. Shafroths since 1954. "As a single family, we've probably lived in the same house longer than anybody in the area," Shafroth said.

Shafroth is the son of lawyer Morrison Shafroth and the grandson of John F. Shafroth, Colorado governor from 1909 to 1913 and U.S. senator from 1913 to 1919. Frank, who joined the law firm of Grant, Shafroth and Toll, which his father helped found in 1927, is a hardy outdoorsman and has been active in many community activities, heading the boards of the American Red Cross and Friends of the Denver Public Library.

He and his wife, Sally, raised five children in this symmetrical five-bedroom home. The house is trimmed with block quoins and low-relief window surrounds. A metal canopy protects the front entry. The two-car front garage is attached to the house. In 1975 a one-story, flat-roofed addition extended the library to the southwest. Four years later, the breakfast room was enlarged with an entrance onto a patio. The wide lawn without sidewalks "gives us lots of yard, there's no shoveling, and we have lots of privacy," Shafroth said.

The Frank H. Shafroth family have lived at 595 Circle Drive since 1954.

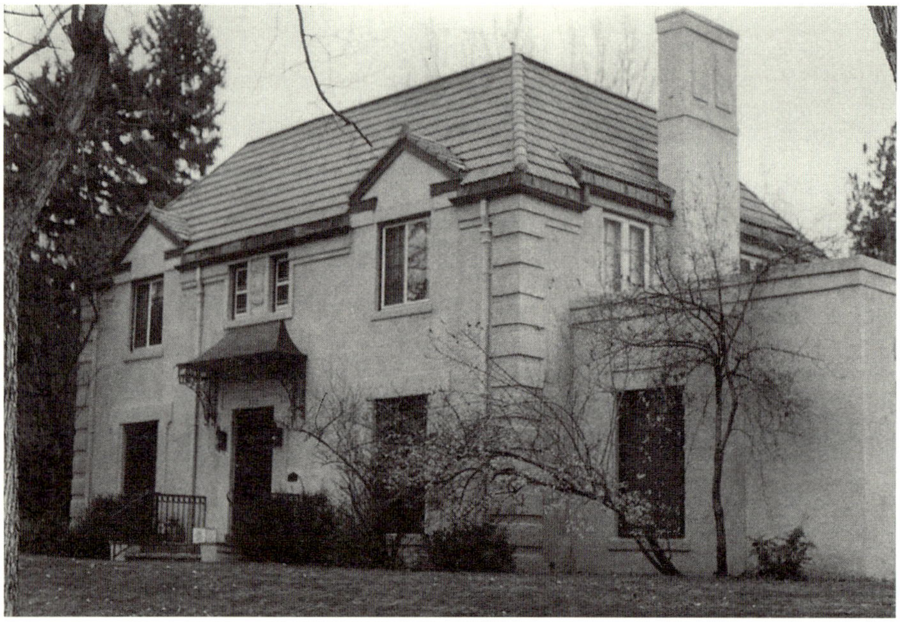

9
C. G. RICHARDSON PLACE
Platted: 1888

Most of the subdivision platted by Cyrus G. Richardson in 1888 was sold to Dean Realty Company (Mary Dean Reed, president) and bought by the Park Lane Square Land Company. In 1925, Saco DeBoer redesigned the property into the circular pattern of Park Lane Square (Circle Drive). However, a strip of 12 lots with turn-of-the-twentieth-century houses along the west side of Race Street is still designated as C. G. Richardson Place.

Since a 10-foot alley to the west was vacated in 1937, most of the properties acquired this adjacent alley land plus the 47.5-foot-wide lots of Williams Driving Park Place to the current alley. A remnant of this alley remains as a driveway east of the little house at 1920 6th Avenue. These houses, then, are on lots 175 feet deep. "Most of those houses didn't have garages. Now, with extended lots, they have garages off the alley," said Rhondda (Mrs. Peter) Grant of 545 Race Street.

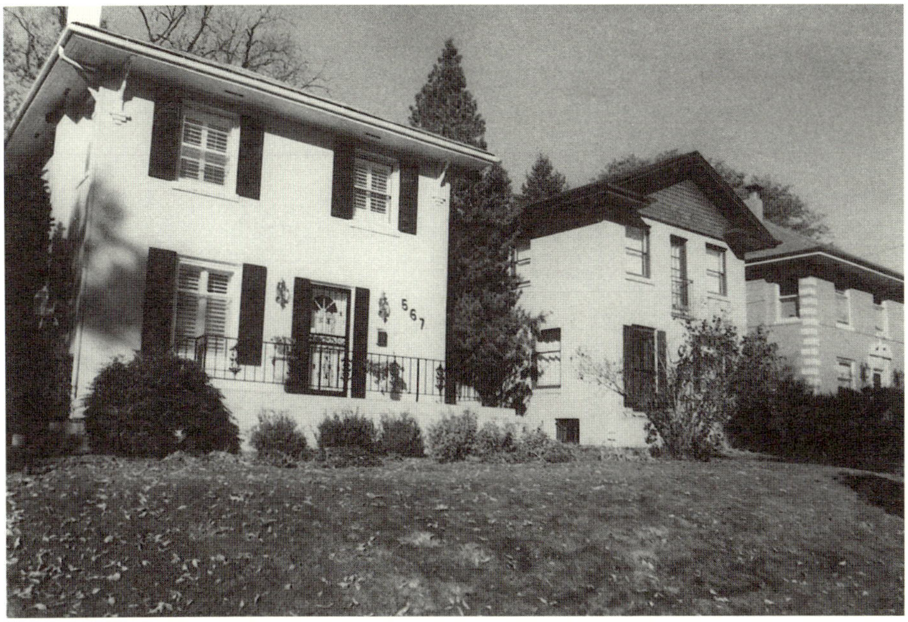

The Foursquare houses on Race Street in C. G. Richardson Place were built between 1900 and 1911, two decades before Park Lane Square was platted.

Five of the seven houses (all but 555 Race Street and 1920 East 6th Avenue) were built when C. G. Richardson Place was developing between 1900 and 1911 on about 7,000 square feet of land and remain in C. G. Richardson Place, complete with sidewalks. "They are good examples of old Foursquares," commented architect Edward D. White, Jr. In 1949 a one-story masonry house with no basement was inserted at 585 Race. The small, 1900 one-story house at 1920 East 6th Avenue was purchased and refurbished by Habitat for Humanity for a 32-year-old single mother of three in 1990. Kathy Stallings had to contribute at least 250 of the total 500 work hours necessary before the house was turned over to her. The renovation vastly improved the neighborhood as well as providing a "dream house" for a needy family.

555 RACE STREET
Built: 1927
Architects: Fisher and Fisher

At the southern end of this row of houses is a Fisher-designed red brick house at 555 Race. It was built in 1927 by lawyer John Pershing, a grandson of General John Joseph Pershing. He practiced with his father, James Hammond Pershing, who moved to Denver in 1892 to join the firm of Pershing, Bosworth, Dick & Dawson. The elder Pershing, a good friend of Mr. and Mrs. Gerald Hughes of 320 High Street, was also a professor of medical jurisprudence at the University of Colorado from 1910 to 1927. He headed the Community Chest and the Public Library Commission. He was internationally known as an authority on the lives of Keats and Milton and served as chancellor of the Colorado Episcopal diocese from 1914 to 1944. His son, John, joined the law firm.

The symmetrical, well-proportioned eclectic Georgian house has a low-pitched hipped roof trimmed with a molded cornice. Double-hung sash windows with divided lights flank the front door, which is capped with a broken scroll pediment. The Denver Public Library publication, *Lookout*, commented that 555 Race, John Pershing's Fisher-designed "small brick colonial house has interesting bond and brick quoins."

The house was later owned by the Gilbert J. Muellers who, in 1935, built a Fisher-designed, two-story brick addition to the rear. This contained a maid's bedroom and bath

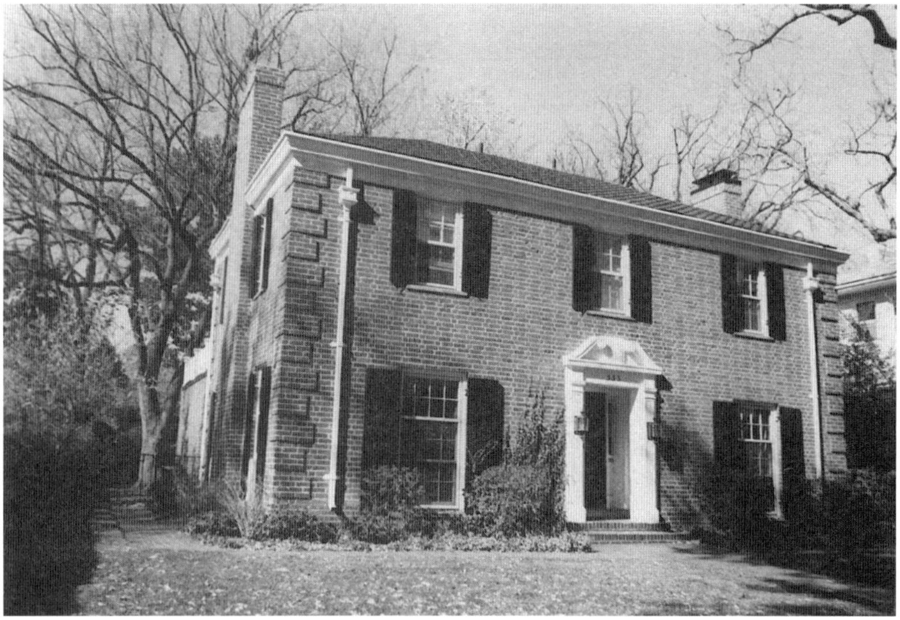

The Fisher-designed home at 555 Race Street was built in 1927 when Park Lane Square was developed.

behind the kitchen with a bedroom and bath over it. A later addition, designed by architect Rodney Davis, consists of a family room under a large balcony with white balustrades. The spacious garden is shielded from the alley by the brick garage.

Jane and Robert O'Donnell bought the house in the early seventies, and Suzanne and realtor James Swanson have lived there since 1984. "An old sewer pipe still runs through the garden on the line of the old vacated alley," Jim Swanson said.

10
545 RACE STREET
Built: 1929
Architect: The Huntington Architectural Company

When Colorado Bank president William W. "Peter" Grant, III, and his wife Rhondda, bought this home in 1964, they were the third owners. The house was built by Myron L. and Eunice Smith, whose only child, Janet, was a good friend of next-door neighbor Barbara Johnson (Hartley). It was one of the early houses in Park Lane Square (Circle Drive). The owners in 1936 were Salisbury E. and Grace Macfarlane Smith and their son, Stuart Salisbury Smith (no relation to the first owners).

The Tudor asymmetrical house has decorative brickwork on the double-stack chimney and half timbering above the arched front entry, featuring herringbone patterned brick. Stone lintels emphasize the windows. The house is bordered on the west by an unused 10-foot-wide alley. Between that and the 20-foot alley now in use is a 47.5-foot-wide strip of land belonging in the next subdivision, Williams Driving Park Place. In 1933 a 12-lot strip of this land was sold by Luther McMahill, Jr., to the Arthur Johnsons, who owned the house to the south, leaving this house only a 17-foot-wide access to the alley. "I had thought of buying that strip for a tennis court, but the Johnsons [to the south] wanted a greenhouse," said Rhondda, whose name is spelled with double ds after her Welsh great-aunt.

The philanthropic Grants are extremely active in the community. Peter is a director of the Denver Museum of Natural History, Channel Six Public Broadcasting, Four-Mile House, and the National Fund for Historic Preservation. Rhondda was on the board of Rocky Mountain Planned Parenthood and is interested in the Women's Foundation

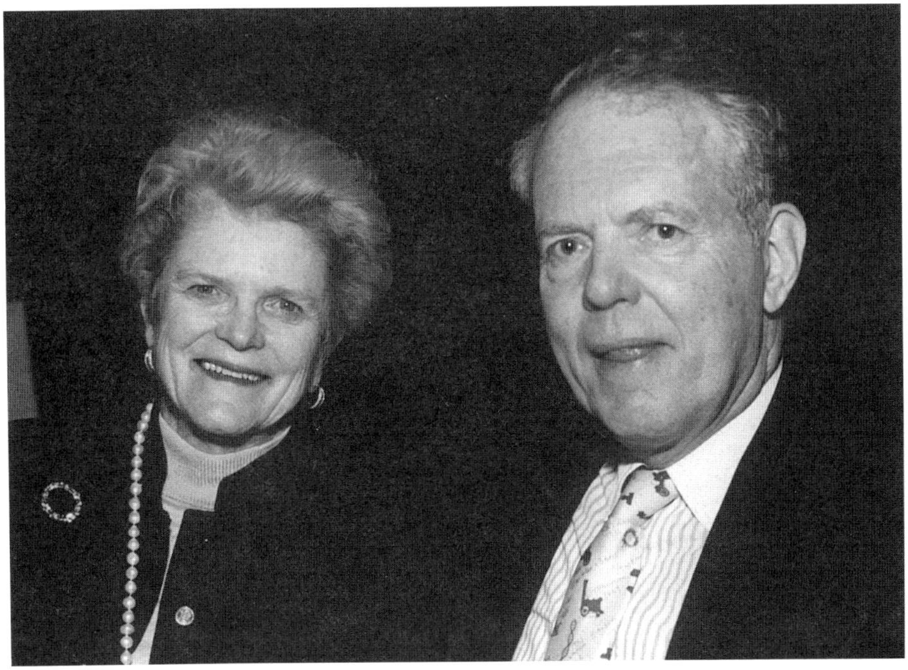

Rhondda and Peter Grant live in the Tudor Revival house at 545 Race Street.

and the Center for Women's Education and Employment. Both are deeply involved with St. Barnabas Episcopal Church and the National Episcopal Church Foundation.

11
515 RACE STREET
Built: 1927 to 1929
Architect: Burnham Hoyt
Contractor: Francis J. Kirchoff

The chancellor of the University of Denver (DU), Dan Ritchie, acquired a new home in 1999. The magnificent 7,237-square-foot three-story house on three quarters of an acre, built for the Arthur E. Johnsons, was recently bought for $1.7 million by the late cable magnate Bill Daniels and donated to DU as a residence for its chancellor.

Although the house was originally built by designer-builder Francis J. Kirchoff,[16] the home was doubled in size two years later as architect Burnham Hoyt designed a circular stairway, a new kitchen, a bedroom to the west, and the large room, variously called the Great Hall and the Music Room. "We called it the Rec Room," said Barbara Johnson Hartley, who grew up in the house. "It was done in bright Swedish colors—blues, greens, and yellows. Vance Kirkland [founder of the Art Department at DU] painted the mural behind the bar, the one thing I insisted be left intact in the house." The Rec Room opens onto a barbecue to the west.

The Tudor mansion has a half-timbered gable over the enclosed front portico. A vine-covered arcade leads to elegant terraced gardens on the south. They are also reached through living-room French doors opening onto a wide stone terrace with a shed roof.

The upstairs guest room doubled as a telephone room. Hartley explained, "My good friend, Janet Smith next door, and I strung up a "telephone" line, a cord with tin cans at either end. It went from my house to a sitting room off her parents' bedroom. Now we use the same system at our house in Evergreen. In a box by the gate is a Calumet Baking Powder can attached to a wire that rings the telephone in the caretaker's house. He then opens the gate."

In 1933 the Johnsons bought land from Luther McMahill behind both their house and the house north of them. The land, actually almost 12 lots of Williams Driving Park Place, was great for baseball practice and

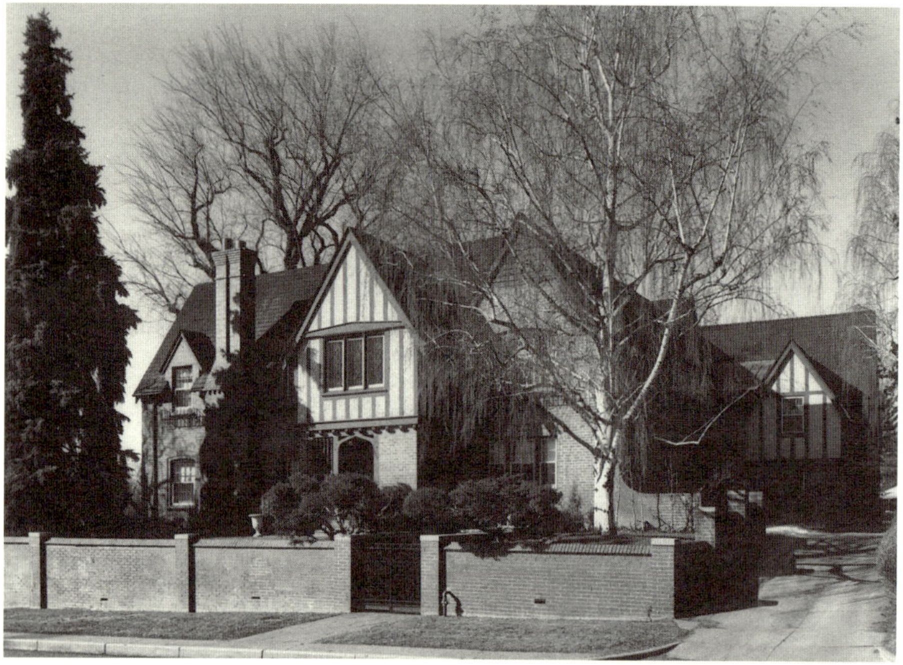

for a large greenhouse where Mrs. Johnson grew orchids, her daughter said. Arthur E. Johnson, president of both Argo and Midwest Oil companies, established the Helen K. and Arthur E. Johnson Foundation, a vehicle for making frequent and generous donations to the Denver Zoo and DU, as well as other nonprofit organizations.

When the Johnsons left, David and Dorothy Murphey bought the house and lived in it during the sixties and seventies.

In 1999, DU completely updated the house. "We renovated with an eye to preservation," explained Stephen Edmonds, director of the Chancellor's Office. "We took out

[ABOVE]
In 1999, cable mogul Bill Daniels donated the house at 515 Race Street to the University of Denver as a home for its chancellor.

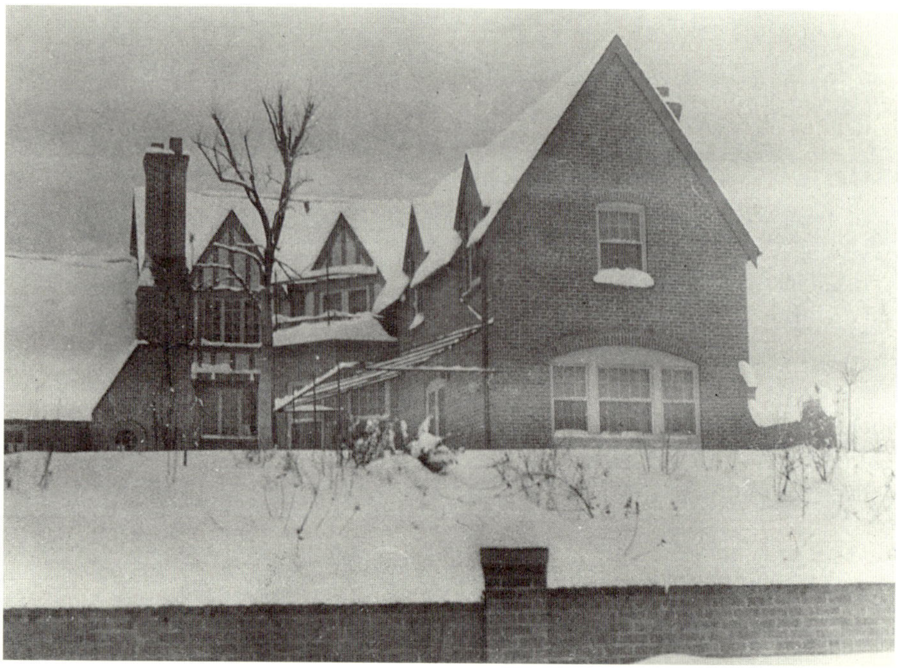

[RIGHT]
When the Arthur E. Johnsons lived at 515 Race Street during the thirties, there were few trees, bushes, or other houses. (Courtesy Barbara Johnson Hartley)

some of the newer things the Murpheys had put in and moved walls back to their original positions to maintain the integrity of the house. It was a collaborative project. We used two architects: Arthur "T." Cowperthwaite, Jr., and Edward D. White, Jr., because of their interest in preservation. Barbara Johnson Hartley helped us, and her husband, Jim Hartley [Hartley House Interiors, Ltd.], did the interior design, integrating pieces from Ritchie's ranch. Major high-tech changes include extensive additions of fiber-optic technology. There are miles and miles of cabling throughout the house. Every room has computer access."

Two other chancellors of DU have lived in the Country Club district. The Mitchell house at 1640 East 3rd Avenue was occupied by Caleb F. Gates, Sr., while he was chancellor. Then, when Lawrence C. Phipps built a mansion in Bel Caro, he gave DU his house at 360 High Street, which was occupied by Chancellor Chester Alter.

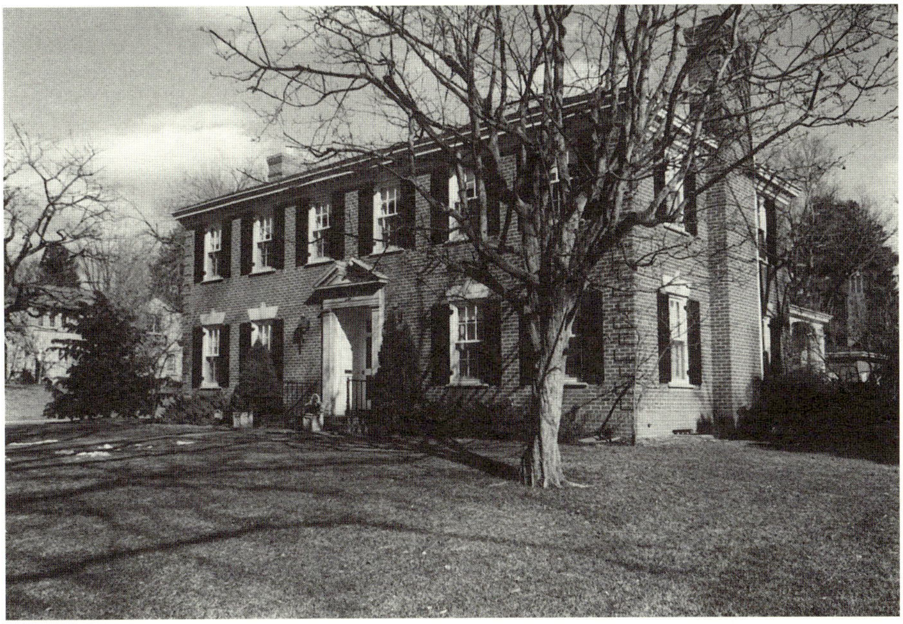

The Richard E. Pate family lived in this 1938 Georgian house at 490 Race Street until 1996.

12
490 RACE STREET
Built: 1938
Architect: Gordon White, with suggestions from the Richard E. Pates, Jr.

This beautifully-proportioned Georgian Revival house "was basically designed by my mother and father," said Richard E. Pate, III. "They had already built a house on Clermont Street, had traveled extensively on the East Coast, and had a pretty good idea of just what they wanted." The house has a low-hipped shingle roof. The paneled front door surround has fluted pilasters and a broken pediment with acorn finial. "As many of their ideas were from Fredericksburg, Virginia, my mother called it a 'Fredericksburg design,'" Pate said. The keystones over the windows were modeled after those in their home state, Pennsylvania, the "Keystone State." The hardware was obtained from Fann Hardware Company in Pennsylvania, the company Richard E. Pate, Sr., represented when he came to Denver in 1897 to recover from chronic catarrh. Later, the senior Pate founded the successful Davis and Shaw Furniture Company, which was maintained by three generations of Richard E. Pates. Richard Pate, Jr., remained active in the company for 76 years, until his death in 1995 at 97.

He lived on this corner of Westwood Drive and Race Street until 1974 when he married Dorothy (Mrs. John C.) Moore and moved into her Georgian Revival house at

369 Humboldt Street. His son, Richard Pate, III, then moved into the Race Street house with his wife and five children. "The children were pretty much grown at that point, but we have lots of grandchildren who loved running all over the house," Pate said.

The second owners of the house were Brian and Mary Minturn, who bought it in 1996. "We moved from Boston and were looking for an older traditional house," Brian Minturn said. They had lived in an apartment for a year and a half looking for the perfect house. They expanded the typical 1930s small kitchen and added a family room and upstairs master bedroom and bath, using brick from the demolished garage for a perfect match. The other large bedroom connects to a smaller bedroom with a "Jack and Jill" bathroom. They then built a detached three-car garage. "We talked with Dick Pate," he said. "The last thing we wanted to do was detract from the original lines of the house."

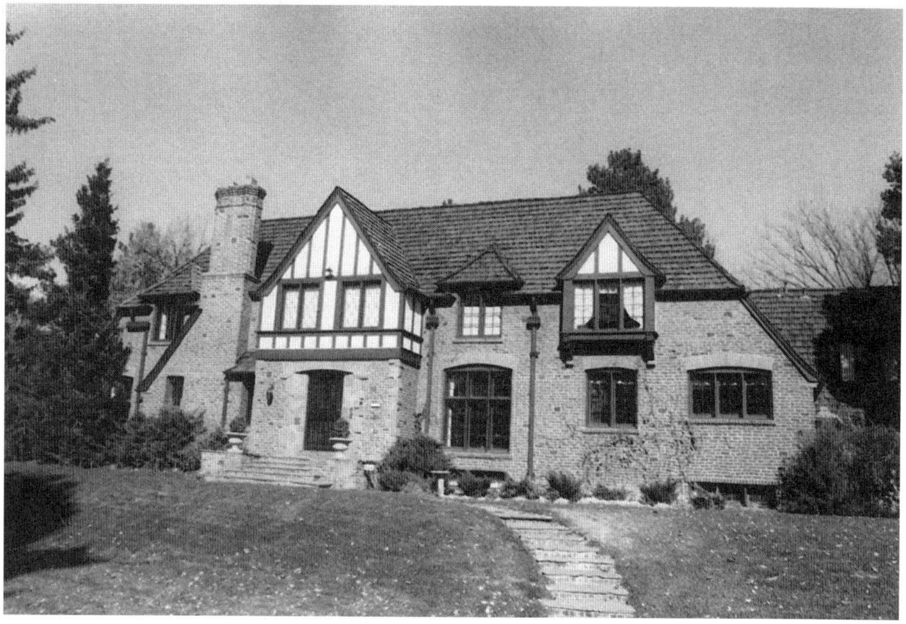

The Tudor Revival house at 460 Westwood Drive was one of the earliest homes built in Park Lane Square.

13
460 WESTWOOD DRIVE
Built: 1928
Architect: unknown

James M. Patterson bought this property when it was first platted by the Park Lane Square Land Company and engaged their contractor, Morton Herres, to build a 96-by-30-foot Tudor residence with a partial basement and attached garage.[17] The house, one of the first in Park Lane Square, was soon purchased by president of the Shirley-Savoy Hotel J. Edgar Smith, who lived there for 25 years.

Smith was the son of James B. Smith, who came to Denver in 1919, merged the Shirley and the Savoy Hotels, and managed the joint operation until his death in 1930. Convenient to the capitol, the hotel was a second headquarters for the legislature when it was in session. In 1952, Smith passed on the management position and the residence to his son, 32-year-old Britton Smith.[18]

Mildred and Stanley Russell moved in during the sixties. "Madcap Mildred," as she was dubbed by a journalist, was married to a successful, quiet, and long-suffering cement tycoon. She was a savage gossip, loved attention and publicity, liked to garden, and was never seen without a hat and five orchids draped over her shoulder, reported the *Rocky Mountain News*.[19] "Teenagers used to tease her, and she would call the police. On one occasion she had the cops chasing

150 of them. One night she saw a young neighbor girl get in the car with her boyfriend. Mildred quickly jumped in her car and followed them," said neighbor Mary Alice Krill. "But Mildred had another side. She always had beautiful flowers, and once, when we were away, she took it upon herself to tend our garden. When we came back, it was blooming better than it ever had been," Krill added.

The red brick Tudor Revival house has two half-timbered front gables and a double-stack chimney. Large window spaces facing south let in sunlight. In 1977 the house was bought by Judith and realtor P. Baxter Lanius.

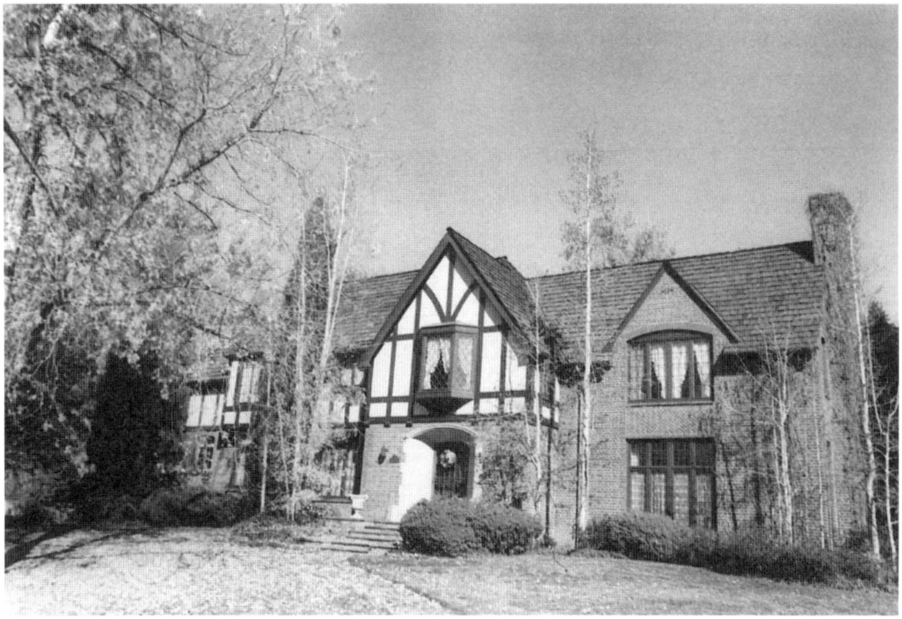

A similar eclectic Tudor house was built at 450 Westwood Drive in 1941.

14
450 WESTWOOD DRIVE
Built: 1941
Architect: Henry A. Koch

This Tudor Revival house is much like the one to the west at 460 Westwood Drive, built 13 years earlier. Both have half-timbered front gables over the entrance, and dormers with multipane windows topped by Jack arches. Both houses are raised and stand together on an island bounded on either side by Hawthorne Place, which circles north from Westwood Drive.

Although the lot was first sold to W. Oscar Temple,[20] this 4,607-square-foot house was built for Katherine and civil engineer Frank Freeman. Their son, Frank, Jr., opened a studio there in the sixties.

After 27 years, Mary Alice and Arthur Krill moved in. Mary Alice was director of research and associate executive director of the Medical Group Management Association, a national organization headquartered in Denver. Art, a mechanical engineer, became president of the Ken R. White Company, an engineering, architectural, and planning firm with worldwide operations. One engineering feat occurred after the crippling accident of a friend. The company developed and built a wheelchair for quadriplegics that could be guided by slight finger gestures, or even by eye movements. The wheelchair was appropriately named the "Independence."[21]

For several years Krill was a president of the Cherry Creek Improvement Association that was the foundation of Country Club Historic Neighborhood, Inc. Marie Vest, vice-president and "fireball" of the association said, "Krill was a good president, too."

From Hawthorne Place there is an excellent view of the south side of the mansion and garden at 575 Circle Drive.

15
2125 HAWTHORNE PLACE
Built: 1953
Architect: Burnham Hoyt

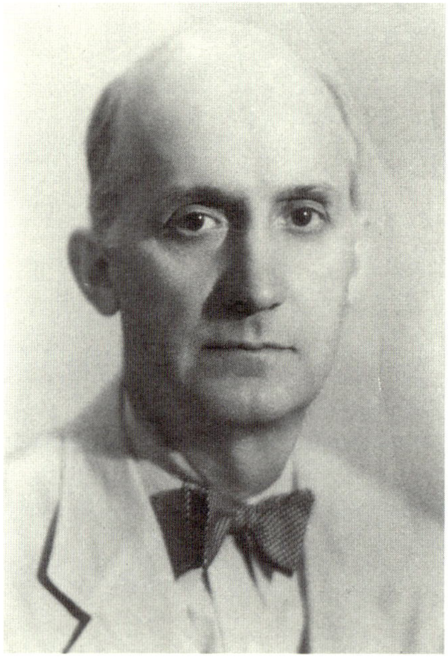

[LEFT]
Dr. James Johnston Waring, a founder of the Webb-Waring Institute for Biomedical Research, built the house at 2125 Hawthorne Drive. (Courtesy Webb-Waring Institute)

James Johnston Waring came first to Colorado Springs, then to Denver in 1908, ill with tuberculosis he had contracted during his third year at Johns Hopkins Medical School. After finishing his M.D. at the University of Colorado, he joined the teaching staff and became the school's first chairman of the Department of Medicine. Though cured of his pulmonary disease in Denver's healing clime, he pursued an interest in lung diseases, working with his physician and colleague, Dr. Gerald Webb of Colorado Springs. The resulting Webb-Waring Lung Institute, located on the southwest corner of the medical school campus, was built, through Waring's perseverance, five years after Webb had died.

"Waring's great love of knowledge—be it in the form of books, clinical research, or student papers—never faltered. He maintained it even in the final chapters of his life," wrote Patricia Paton in her biography,[22] *A Medical Gentleman*.

Ruth Porter Waring, the daughter of prominent businessman Henry M. Porter, raised champion orchids, helped found the Botanic Gardens, and, as an accomplished musician, was a staunch supporter of the Denver Symphony Orchestra.

The 1953 house at 2125 Hawthorne Drive was one of the last designed by architect Burnham Hoyt.

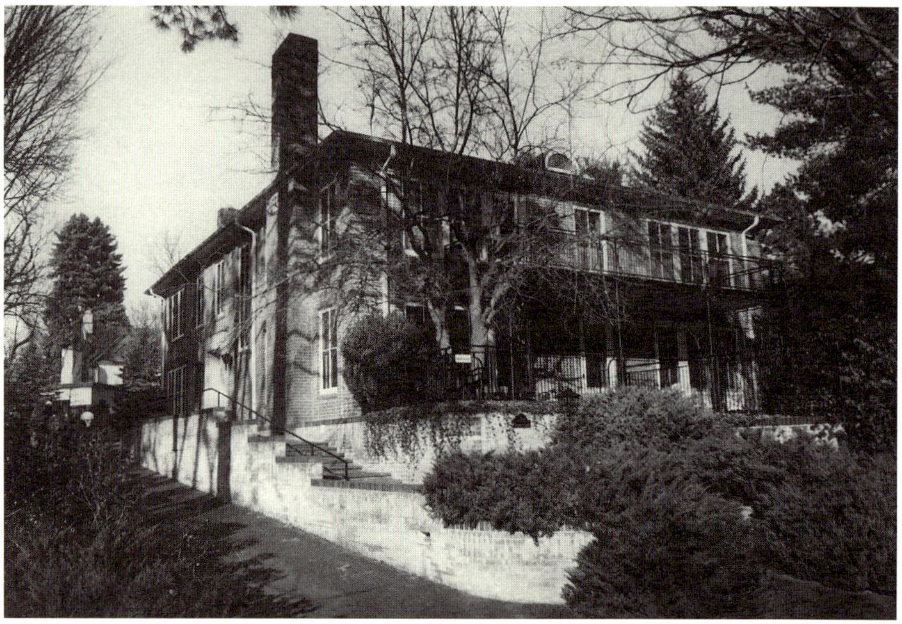

After their two daughters left their home on Gaylord Street, the Warings asked Burnham Hoyt to design this "smaller," 6,318-square-foot, contemporary home with a small garden. The house has large, double-hung, glass areas; generous interior spaces; a library; an extensive master suite; a guest suite; and servants' quarters. The low-pitched roof has wide overhangs. The property lies at the top of a hill, and the side entry is up several steps beside the driveway. A covered terrace on the south overlooks the garden, the quiet street, and, at one time, the mountains. The house has a simple elegance with minimal ornamental elements.

As Edward D. White, Jr., wrote in *City Beautiful*, "Hoyt's later work is characterized by the abandonment of applied decoration and the adoption of proportion and rhythm to create vitality of architectural design, by the use of large, glass areas to welcome light and views and by the natural and open expression of materials—brick as brick, wood as wood, stone as stone—unadorned by superficial finishes and ornamentation."

16
2151 HAWTHORNE PLACE
Built: 1931
Architect: Palmer Sabin
Local Architects: Fisher and Fisher

Probably no one knows more about the houses in the Country Club Historic District than realtor Kennard P. "Ken" Perry. His childhood, from the age of nine until he went to Dartmouth College, was spent in the house he now lives in. The home was designed for his father, Robert M. Perry, by Pasadena, California, architect Palmer Sabin, a cousin of his mother's.

Ken's adulthood was spent as a real estate broker, first at (Arthur) Bishop-(Gordon) Brown Company, then at Bishop-Perry. Co. In 1971 he started his own firm, Perry & Company. "I did lots of business in the Country Club district because I live there, I know the people, and I like the houses," Perry said. "Back in the fifties, insurance companies were the primary source for financing homes, and ranch style was all the rage. Travelers refused to give loans on two-story houses. They said they were out of style and old-fashioned. They missed the market completely."

Perry's father, Robert Perry, was not only president of the Moffat Coal Company but also held the prestigious position of president of a railroad company. "It was a farce, really," Ken said. Because the Rock Island, Burlington, and Union Pacific companies refused to allow

The house at 2151 Hawthorne Drive is owned by realtor Kennard P. Perry, whose family built the home in 1931.

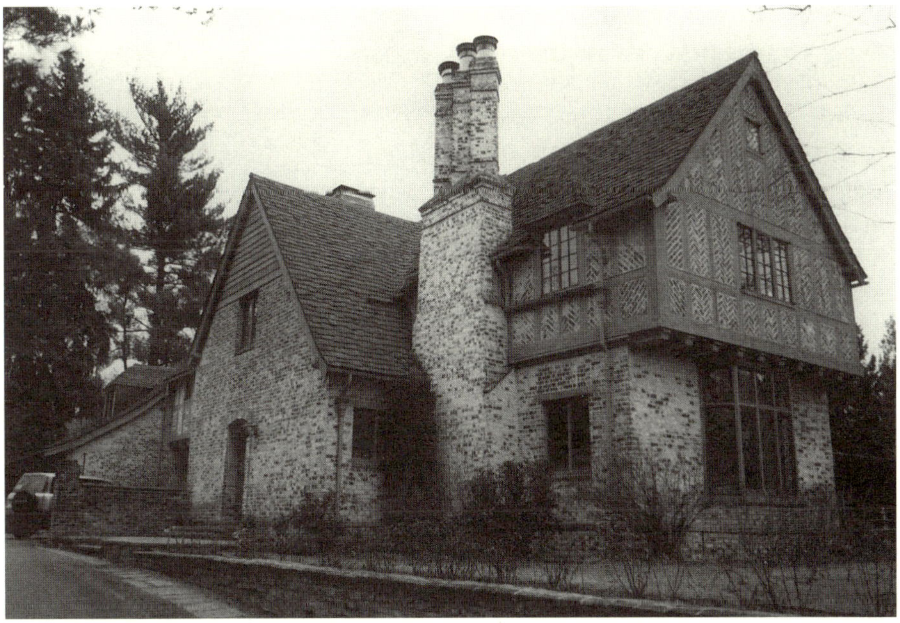

the Moffat Railroad into Union Station, another arrangement was necessary. Perry's grandfather, Samuel M. Perry, built seven miles of track from 15th Street to the main railway line and dubbed this stretch the Denver Northwestern Pacific Railway. Upon his father's death, Robert Perry became president. "It was great because we all got railroad passes because he had the title of president of a railway company," Ken said. In 1934, Robert Perry succumbed at the age of 50 to complications after an operation.

In 1956 Ken's widowed mother, Rosamund, married a family friend, rancher-lawyer Ferrington Carpenter, and moved to Hayden, Colorado. Years earlier, after her graduation from Smith College, she had come to this rural part of Colorado to teach school and help Carpenter start a school district. At that time Ken and his wife, the former Martha Brodhead, moved into the Hawthorne Place house. Their three children are Barbara, a real estate broker with Perry and Company; Anne, a proofreader of court records; and Kennard, Jr., a realtor in California.

The setting for the house, Hawthorne Place, runs along a natural strip of high land. "A lot of the land below us on Westwood Drive is fill. I was told it was once an old dump," Perry said. "We had a great view of the mountains, and people said, 'Why don't you have bigger windows?' However, with the rapid growth, the view didn't last. We can still see Pikes Peak from the attic, but I doubt if many houses still have a good view."

The rusticated brick of this Tudor eclectic house is similar to that of the Fisher-designed house at 100 Franklin Street. The second story is cantilevered with a steep timbered gable filled with brick in a herringbone design. The bay off the living room has leaded windows. Three pots top the diagonal brick stacks of the large chimney on the west. The side driveway leads to a timbered two-car garage.

Only four houses lie on the secluded circular Hawthorne Place. "We don't have many trick-or-treaters," Perry said, as he passed around leftover lollipops and bite-size Butterfingers.

17
2155 HAWTHORNE PLACE
Built: 1927
Architect: Jacques Benedict

The Geddes (previously spelled Geddis) family played a key role in the development of the eastern subdivisions of the Country Club Historic

William John Geddes, whose father platted the Capitol Annex subdivision in 1889, built the house at 2155 Hawthorne Place in 1927.

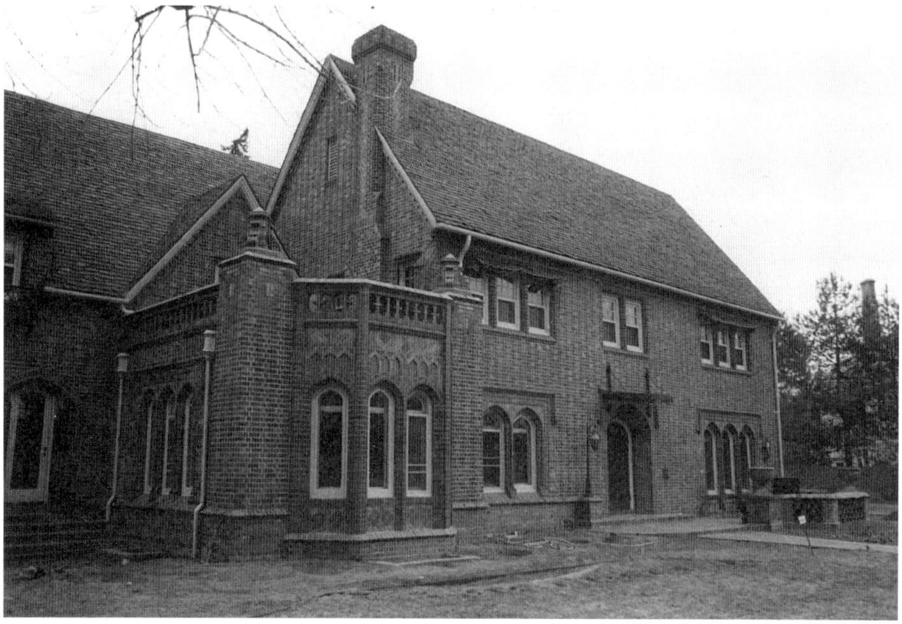

District. When William Geddis, a contractor from Northern Ireland, came to Denver during the 1880s, he and his partner built the foundations for the Brown Palace Hotel and the capitol, among other buildings. He bought the Denver Sewer Pipe and Clay Company in 1892 and expanded it into a large and highly reputable company. "The productions of the company are constantly specified by architects and engineers having found especial favor with their price and quality," reported the *Times* in 1902.[23]

Geddis also invested in real estate. In 1889 he bought and platted the Capitol Annex subdivision bounded by Bridger (3rd) and Vasquez (4th) Avenues and York (University Boulevard) and Vine Streets. This open farmland was, at that time, merely an expansion of the newly incorporated town of Harman (Cherry Creek North).

He became known as William F. Geddes, married, and in 1890, William John Geddes was born. Later they had two girls, Jean (Mrs. W. Oscar Temple) and Ethel (Mrs. George Simson, Jr.).

When the major eastern subdivisions were developed in about 1925, William John Geddes, who was now married to Vivian Hoffman, and president of Denver Sewer Pipe and Clay, used the firebricks to build this house on Hawthorne Place for himself. He also built a house for his widowed mother and persuaded his two brothers-in-law to build adjacent houses on Vine Street. His widow, Vivian, continued to live on Hawthorne Place until 1995.

The second owner of the house, Laurie G. Nichols, moved in with her real estate developer husband and three sons in 1995 and did an excellent and extensive job of remodeling the house. "We had rehabilitated an old house in Chicago and wanted a historic home with charm," she said.

The large Tudor mansion is well hidden in the middle of Park Lane Square on 30,218 square feet behind the Reed castle and the access road, Hawthorne Place. "Even Pizza Hut can't find it, and I was attracted to the privacy here. The boys can go out roller blading and I don't worry," Nichols said. She describes the house as Deco Gothic. Tudor or flattened Gothic arches top the front door and windows. The gable is echoed by the small front gable over the one-story, three-sided bay, which has a stone balustrade above. The molded patterned brickwork is unusual. The house is eclectic. Even the architect, Jacques Benedict, said it was "tough to categorize."

"The new owner did a nice job of restoring this house," said Landmark Commissioner, architect Edward D. White, Jr.

Nichols plans to plant an English herb garden near the kitchen and build a gazebo. Her gardener told her a story about the hospitality of the Geddes family. "They used to have a white globe on top of their chimney. When it was lit they were having a party, and the whole neighborhood was invited."

18
2115 EAST 4TH AVENUE
Built: 1936
Architect: Paul Atchison

This 2,754-square-foot, Georgian-style house was built by surgeon William W. Haggart during the depressed thirties. Business was then as slow for home construction as it was for everyone else. Subsequent owner Edward D. White, Jr., was told by the architect, "Business was so slow during the Depression that I couldn't afford an office. I had the plans for this house spread all over the dining-room table."

The house has a side gable with end chimneys. The white door surround has sidelights and a decorative broken pediment centered with a pineapple design. Symmetrically placed sash windows are flanked by green shutters.

The home was bought by Anne and Edward D. White, Jr., during the sixties, where they raised two

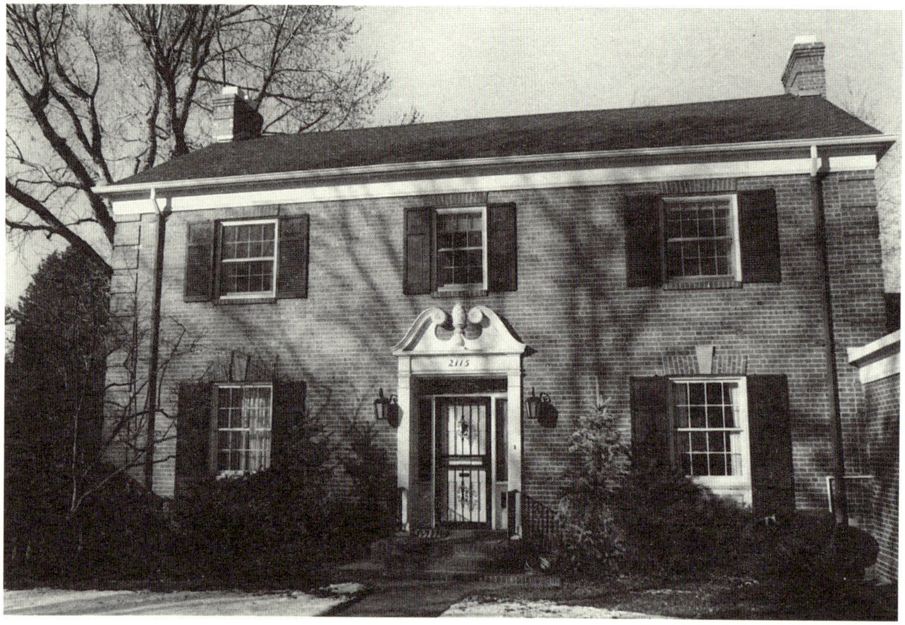

[ABOVE]
The Georgian-style house at 2115 4th Avenue was built during the Depression in 1936.

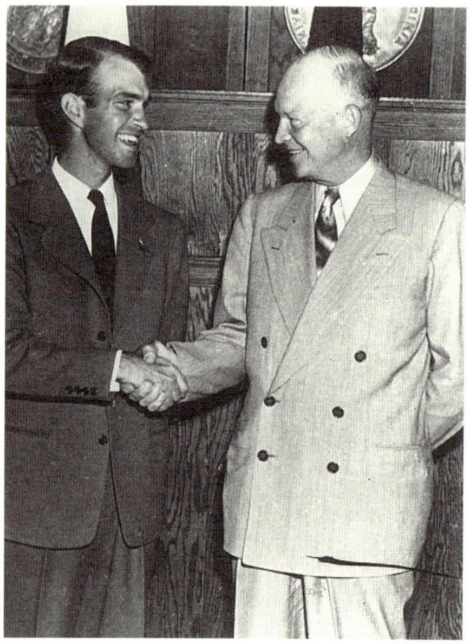

[LEFT]
During the 1960s the house was occupied by Landmark Commissioner, architect Edward D. White, Jr., shown greeting Dwight David Eisenhower. (Courtesy E. D. White, Jr.)

sons, Edward D. White, III, and James Waring White. After East High School and Columbia University, where he earned a degree in architecture, White returned to his native Denver to practice. White practiced with Victor Hornbein, who designed many Denver buildings, including the Humphreys, Gates Science, and Foundation buildings at Graland School plus additions; the Bethesda Hospital buildings; the Children's Day Care Center and Kennedy Center for Retarded Children at the University of Colorado Health Sciences Center; and the dramatic Denver Botanic Gardens. White specializes in remodeling, preservation, and restoration, and restored the Governor's Mansion during the 1980s. He was a pioneer on the Denver Landmark Commission, where he has served for 30 years.

Alice and Dr. Robert G. Bosworth, Jr., purchased the house in 1982.

19
2101 EAST 4TH AVENUE
Built: 1950
Designer: Sewell Thomas

After the war, mining construction engineer Sewell Thomas designed and built two houses simultaneously, one for the family of his daughter, Lenore (Mrs. John Stoddart), at 280

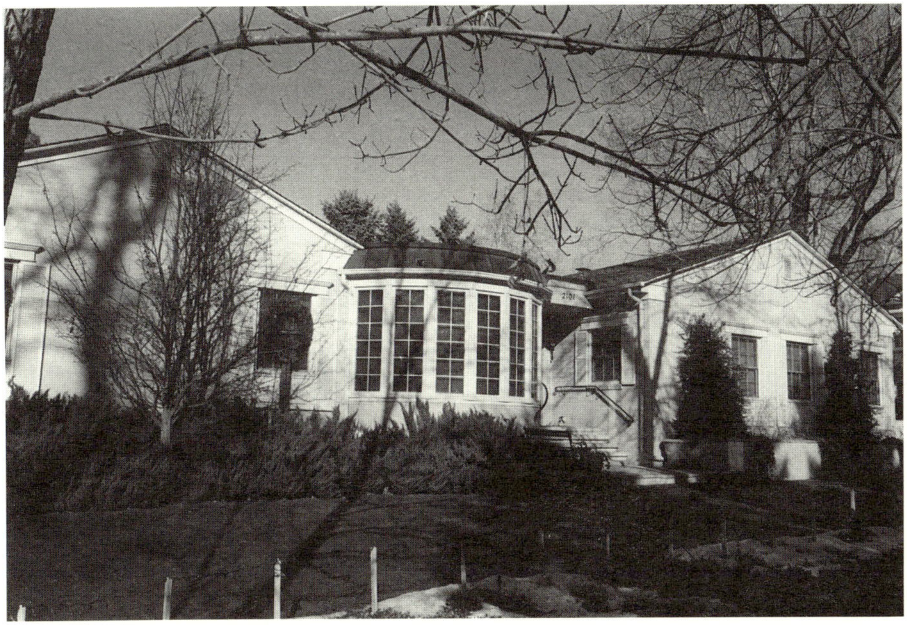

Sewell Thomas built his fourth house in the Country Club area at 2101 East 4th Avenue in 1950.

Race and one for himself at 2101 East 4th Avenue. "These were the last vacant lots available in the late 1950s," Lenore said.

The one-story house has two low-pitched gabled wings and a balustrade over the prominent curved library bay. Double glass doors on either side of the fireplace lead to a rear flagstone terrace and flower gardens. "The house has a definite California feeling," said architect Philip Atchison.

During the fifties, Thomas turned to writing. His book, *Silhouettes of Charles S. Thomas* gives insight into his father's, Charley Thomas, acquaintance with Woodrow Wilson. An anecdote describes the senator's habit of wearing a toupee over his balding head, but only in winter to keep warm: "In the first warm days of April when he removed the covering and climbed the Hill to attend a session of the Senate, the Sergeant-at-Arms barred him at the door of the Chamber."[24] A subsequent book, *Yaqui Gold*, is a novel about mining in an isolated Mexican mining village based upon Thomas's extensive experience in that country.

"When Mother died, she left us 2101 East 4th," said Lenore. The Stoddarts raised the living-room ceiling and put in a huge skylight. They added lights over the doors and a bay window in the dining room.

After the Charles L. Warrens moved there in 1983, they noticed a leak in the ceiling of the library—the curved center section of the house. The solution was to line the roof with copper, but the metal was so shiny that it detracted from the house. "E.J." Warren explained how to rectify the situation: "Charles, who was then chairman of the board of the Zoo, returned from a meeting with a possible solution: spray elephant's urine on the copper to give it an aged patina appearance." The technique has yet to be tried.

20
2025 EAST 4TH AVENUE
Built: 1928
Architect: Fisher and Fisher

Early in the history of Circle Drive, cofounder of Neusteter's women's clothing store Meyer Neusteter and his wife, Bernita, built this Fisher-designed home. The large, 63-by-36-foot, beige stucco Mediterranean house has a low-pitched hipped roof. The entrance is flanked by Doric pilasters under an ornate, painted metal balconet.

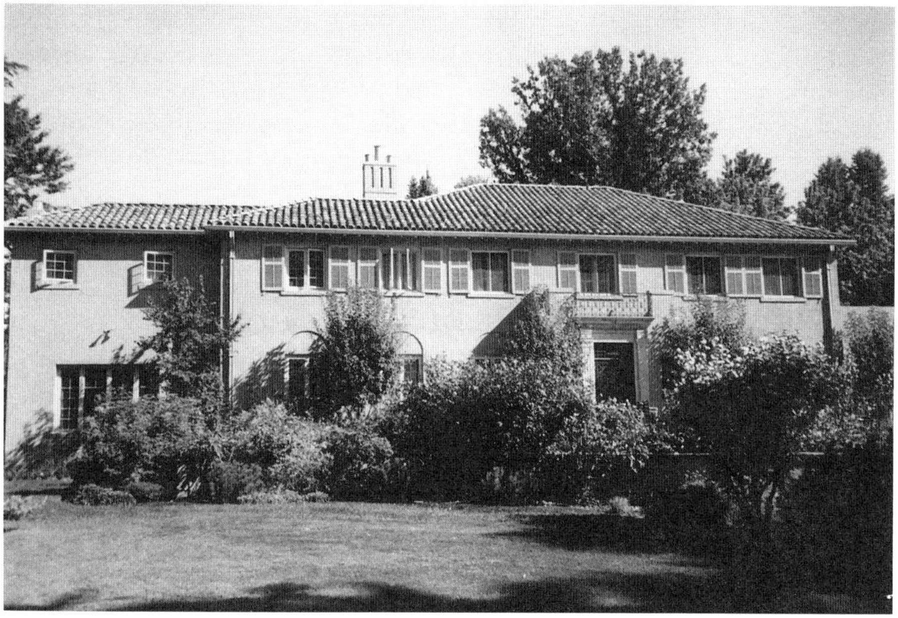

One of the first houses in Park Lane Square was built by Meyer Neusteter at 2025 4th Avenue in 1928.

Simple round arches and similar balconets trim the lower windows, flanked by accordion-type shutters. The house, built for $22,000 with a half basement and front-drive garage, occupies a spacious 36,200 square feet of beautifully landscaped property.

In 1934 a two-story, 18-by-27-foot sitting room with bedrooms above was added to the west. About that time William F. "Bill" Wilbur was busily carving out caves with "leftover" boards from the surrounding construction in the then-vacant lot at 450 Circle Drive. "The Neusteters loved gambling. On the west they had a big room with a roulette table. We used to watch from the lot, now [George] Hopfenbeck's house, and see these nice-looking people, all in evening dress, having a grand old time," Wilbur said.

During the sixties, dashing aviation pioneer Harry Combs and his wife, Virginia, moved into the house. Combs, who founded Combs Aircraft, was the first to introduce jet aircraft for private ownership. Besides running the Bijou Springs Ranch near Colorado Springs, he was a historian and novelist. His 1992 book, *Brules*, tells of an old mountain man recounting his Wild West life of horses, cattle, and Indians to an 11-year-old admirer.

Stockbroker Thomas P. Owen, and his wife, Mary Ellen Kelly Owen, lived in the house during the seventies and eighties.

21
2012 EAST 4TH AVENUE
Built 1927
Architect: unknown

Part-owner and chief contractor for Park Lane Square Herres Construction Company built this house on the east half of the lot for president of Sechrist Manufacturing Company Kenneth L. Francis and his wife, Della.[25]

Two years later the house was sold to ophthalmologist Donald H. O'Rourke and his wife, Elease "Mickey," who lived there for several decades. "There were only two other houses on the block, the Neusteter mansion at 2025 4th Avenue and next door at 2022," said Patsy O'Rourke Monaghan, who grew up in the house. "There were lots of vacant lots to look for horny toads from our house to the Perrys' [2151 Hawthorne Place]," she added.

The red brick house has a medium-pitched roof with dentils. Four steps lead to the protruding, brick, gabled portico that frames the entrance. The door surround includes sidelights with a fanlight above.

In 1936, Dr. O'Rourke bought the west half of the pie-shaped lot and put on an 18-by-20-foot, brick, two-story addition.[26] A white wooden picket fence divides this section of the garden. To the south of the house, at 390 Race Street, was a little shack used as a guard house. "Whenever a burglary occurred, a big bright light on a 50-foot pole alerted the neighborhood," said William F. "Bill" Wilbur. The proprietors of Guardian Signal, Victor and Ziska Simer, lived nearby at 1921 East 4th Avenue. According to Tom O'Rourke, Victor spent his time stealing from the neighborhood while hiring a guard to sit on an old wooden chair inside a tiny green metal shack, turning on the light every month or so. "As a boy I used to go down and visit with Fred while he stuffed Prince Albert tobacco into his pipe," he said. Barbara Johnson Hartley added, "The guard used to date one of our maids."

The Robert M. Perrys didn't use the guard house. "My father had been kidnapped when he was younger and was concerned about adequate protection. We had our own security system, but I heard the Guardian Signal people were in cahoots with crooks," said Kennard Perry of 2151 Hawthorne Place. "You'd call up to tell them you would be out of town, and that was their signal to rob your house."

Richard Weil, III, and his wife bought the house in the early seventies and sold it to Jocelyn and Douglas K. Childs in 1988.

The red brick house at 2012 4th Avenue was built on a pie-shaped lot in 1927.

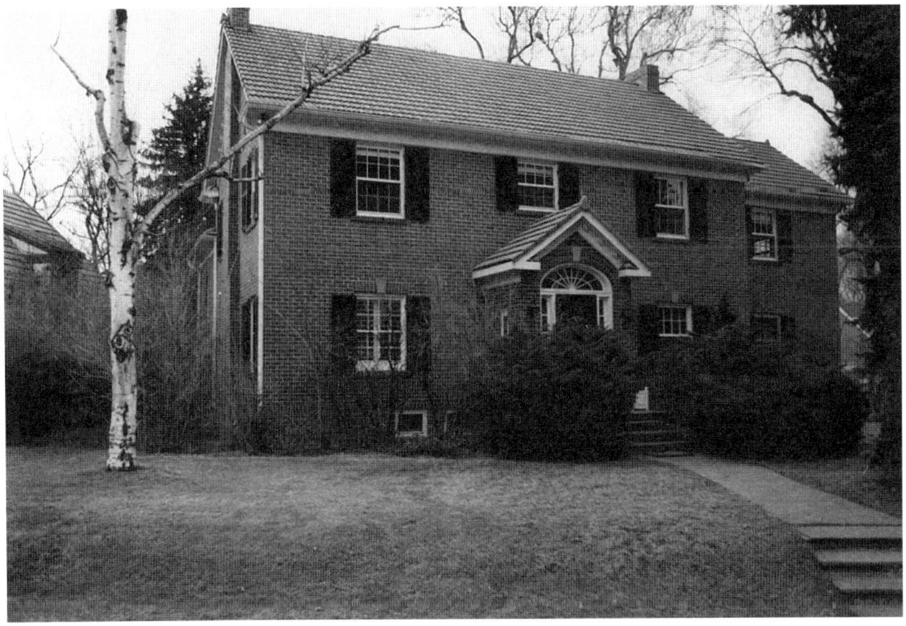

22
1925-1927 EAST 4TH PLACE
Built: 1901
Architect: unknown

This house was built in 1901 near the City Ditch by teamster Luther McMahill and his wife, May. It is located on 12 narrow lots in the southeast corner of Williams Driving Park Place, near the corner of Race Street and 4th Avenue, at that time south of the city limits at 6th Avenue. To the east between 4th and 6th Avenues was nothing but barren prairie and a half dozen scattered farmhouses in the subdivision C. G. Richardson Place (Circle Drive), which was platted in 1888. The lots are located on a narrow, 47.5-foot strip between two alleys. The eastern one was vacated in 1963[27] and incorporated into the property. Access is gained through 4th Place, a 20-foot-wide driveway leading from Race Street. "The history of this property is unique and

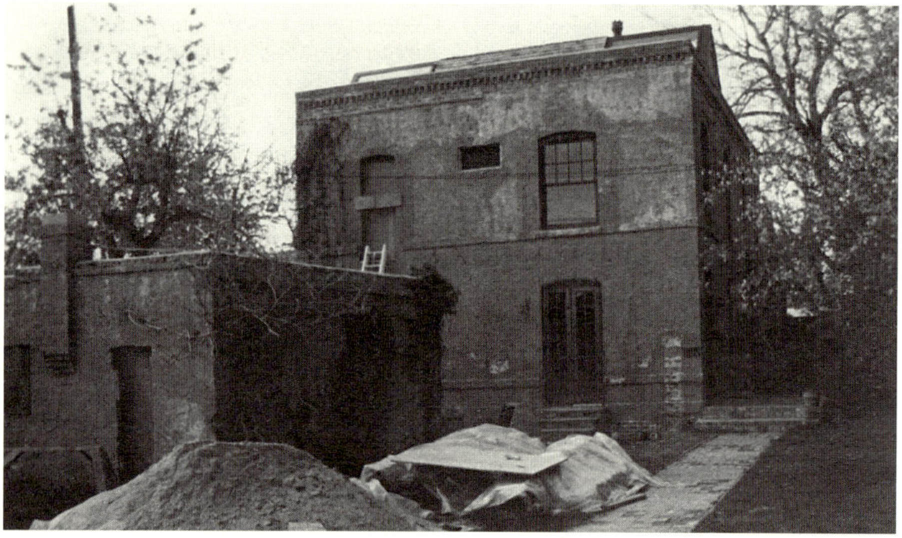

[ABOVE]
This 1901 house on 4th Place became part of the Country Club neighborhood when the alley to the east was vacated in 1957.(Courtesy Sandra Klinger)

really intrigues me," wrote historian Rhonda Beck, who researched this house extensively in 1998.

Although the assessor lists 1896 as the year of construction for the house, the property wasn't transferred to the McMahills until 1900[28], and a building permit was issued in 1901.[29]

The flat-roofed, two-story house is made of old soft brick covered with stucco for insulation. The 24-by-40-foot residence cost $1,800 and fronted east toward Race Street, but was bordered on the east by the

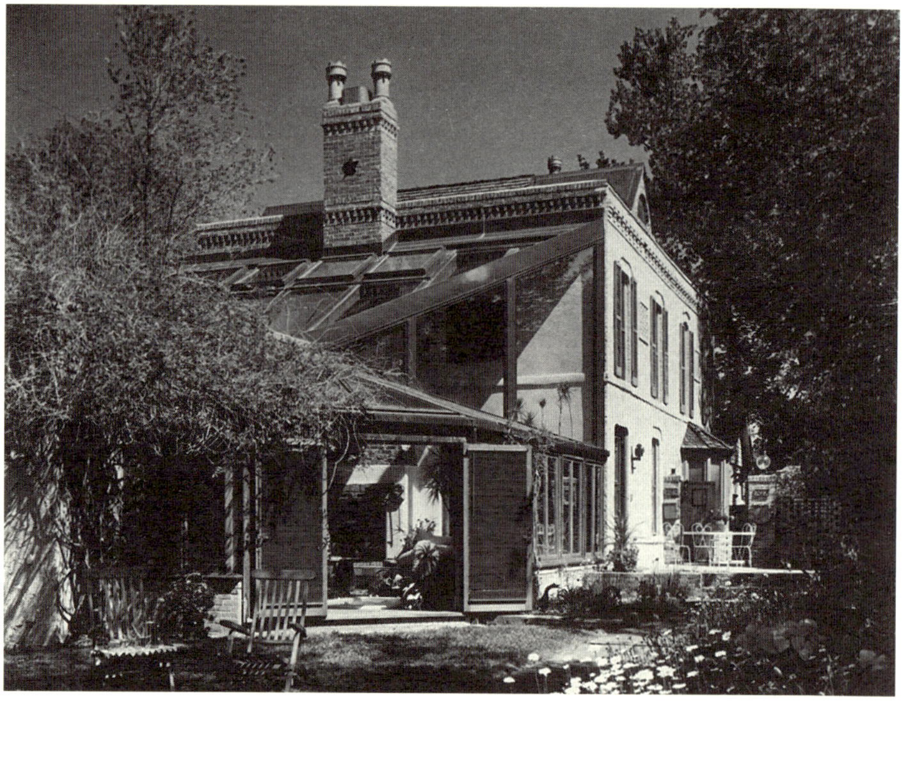

[RIGHT]
The historic house was renovated during the 1980s by interior designer Sandra Klinger. (Courtesy Sandra Klinger)

vacated alley. McMahill, later a carpenter, lived there with his wife, May. Their son, bricklayer Luther, Jr., lived in a small house to the south at 1921 4th Avenue.

The McMahill house was built as a dual residence. "The rounded window corners, the flat arch, and the original front doors are strictly Italianate," said current owner, Sandra A. Clinger, an award-winning interior designer who bought the house in 1981 and has renovated it to preserve its nineteenth century character. "The two front doors, the checkerboard designs on the front wall, and the decorative parapet on the front of the house were original," she said. Clinger added a coach lantern from Austria by the front door, a wooden beam from a Summit County mine shaft over the south opening of the fireplace, and duplicated the masonry front parapet on the south wall and garage. She also installed skylights and designed a master suite on the second floor. Later she added a large, sunny conservatory and patio to the south. The old 18-by-20-foot original garage off the alley, built by May McMahill in 1923, is remodeled into her office and tastefully decorated. A four-stall carport with guest quarters above was built inside the graceful, brick serpentine wall on the alley.

The address of this house, listed as 1921 East 4th Avenue in 1900, was changed to 405/409 Race Street by 1910, then changed again to 1925/1927 4th Place after the alley was officially vacated in 1963. In 1982 these seven lots were zoned PUD (Planned Unit Development #800) to allow for a residential duplex.

McMahill died in the early twenties, and his widow, May, lived there until 1941. After May died, the house reverted to the Colorado National Bank, who removed rubbish, made repairs, reroofed, and rented through an agent in Idaho Springs. By 1946 the new owner was Col. James Hoffman.

From 1891 to 1900, before building this house, McMahill had lived nearby in Capitol Annex at 313 York Street. This property was later a Texaco station, then Homer Reed, Ltd. clothing store. By 1892 a streetcar was rolling up 4th Avenue from Corona Street, turning south at Race Street and continuing east through the town of Harman (Cherry Creek North).

According to local folklore, the home on 4th Place was once a brothel. Anne Waring (Mrs. Claude) Maer said, "I used to go to see a seamstress, Rose Edgerton [who lived at 1927 4th Place during the sixties]. She told me that teenaged boys would come and knock at her door and say, 'Where are the girls?' Finally I asked them, 'How would you like it if boys came knocking on your grandmother's door asking for girls?' She was the dearest woman and used to tell me stories about the brothel."

Privacy is ensured as the house is neatly hidden behind large Race Street houses lined with 70-year-old trees. The joined houses were owned by Gerald H. and Peggy Stokes from 1970 to 1981.

23
401 RACE STREET
Built: 1932
Architect: unknown

The two-story house at 401 Race Street was built by Dr. Harry H. Wear in 1932. "Wear was a shining light as a surgeon. He was a protegee of my grandfather, Dr. Francis H. McNaught, who thought very highly of his professional skills," said William F. "Bill" Wilbur.

In 1940, movie mogul Frank H. Ricketson, Jr., called "Mr. Showman" by *Denver Post* journalist Joanne Ditmer,[30] moved into the house and installed a complete theater with projection booth on the third floor. He could then show movies to friends every Sunday evening. Ricketson, who built his first theater in Montrose in 1925, soon owned 30 Fox-Intermountain theaters. During the Depression he stimulated attendance by creating "Bank Night," a Tuesday night

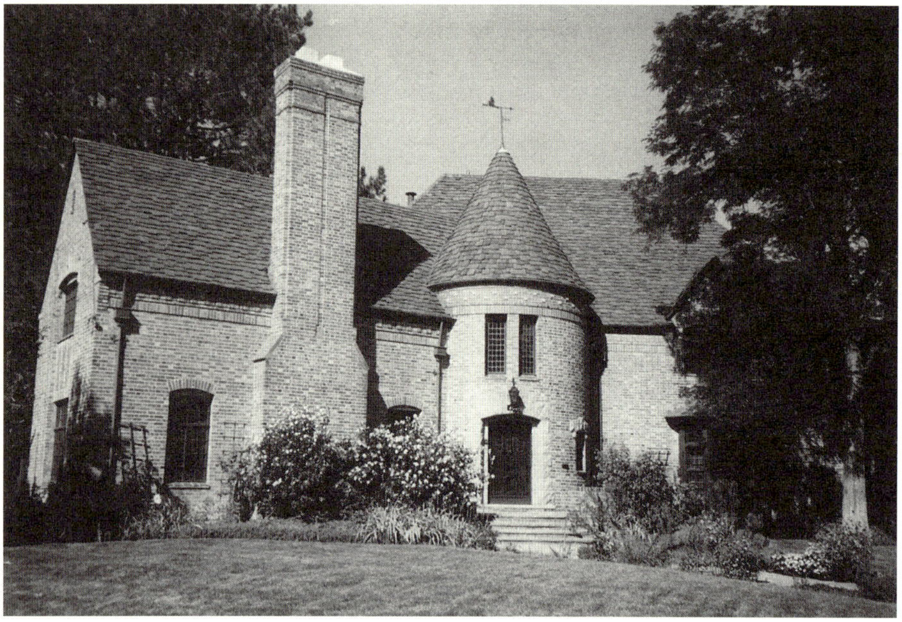

When movie mogul Frank H. Ricketson, Jr., lived at 401 Race Street, he installed a movie theater on the third floor.

drawing for cash prizes awarded only if the winner were in the audience.

Subsequent owners of the house were the Richard Hugo Olsons, who lived there from 1960 to 1985. At Purdue University, Olson met his wife, Virginia, an Indianapolis native. He came to Denver to set up a branch of Sundstand, a firm his father had started in Rockford, Illinois, where he grew up. After the Denver firm was established, he resigned, bought Gerry Mountaineering, and expanded the business into Colorado Outdoor Sports.

"We used the third-floor theater for a playroom for the kids," Virginia said. During the nineties, while David and Catherine Dorn lived there, Catherine promoted and nurtured the landscaped islands that deter traffic from racing through the Race and 4th Avenue intersection.

The red brick house is perched on the pie-shaped lot between 4th Avenue and Race Street. The segmented stone door surround is in the round tower, topped by a pinnacle, which dominates the front facade. The door is topped by two long narrow windows. A wide chimney rises over the moderately steep, tile gable roof south of the tower.

24
1921 EAST 4TH AVENUE
Original house built: 1923
New house built: 1996
Architect: unknown

For several decades this address was given to the strip of Williams Driving Park Place along the alley owned by May and Luther McMahill at the turn of the twentieth century.

In 1923 they built a 28-by-40-foot brick Bungalow with full basement for $3,000 for their son, Luther, Jr., on five narrow lots facing 4th Avenue.[31] The tiny one-story house, bought by Ralph Grabell, was sold to Victor Simer, who lived there with his wife, Ziska, managing the Guardian Signal System and maintaining a small guard house at 390 Race Street. After Victor died, Ziska remained in the house until the nineties, operating the business from the rear of their property.

Those five narrow lots, which are directly behind 401 Race Street, would be a desirable addition to that land. "We vacated the alley behind us in 1957 for a play yard and tried to buy that property to the west when we moved in,"[32] said Virginia Olson who, with her husband, Richard, bought the house at 401 Race Street during the fifties. "A rather reclusive lady lived alone behind us," Ginny said. "I almost never saw her."[33]

After Ziska Simer died, the little house was torn down and a beige stucco "spec" house was built in 1996. Some residents refer to it as a "typical Highlands Ranch-style" house. Neighbor Charlotte (Mrs. Walter "Bill") Croze said, "They managed to build a darling house on this narrow lot with a magnificent master bath with skylights."[34]

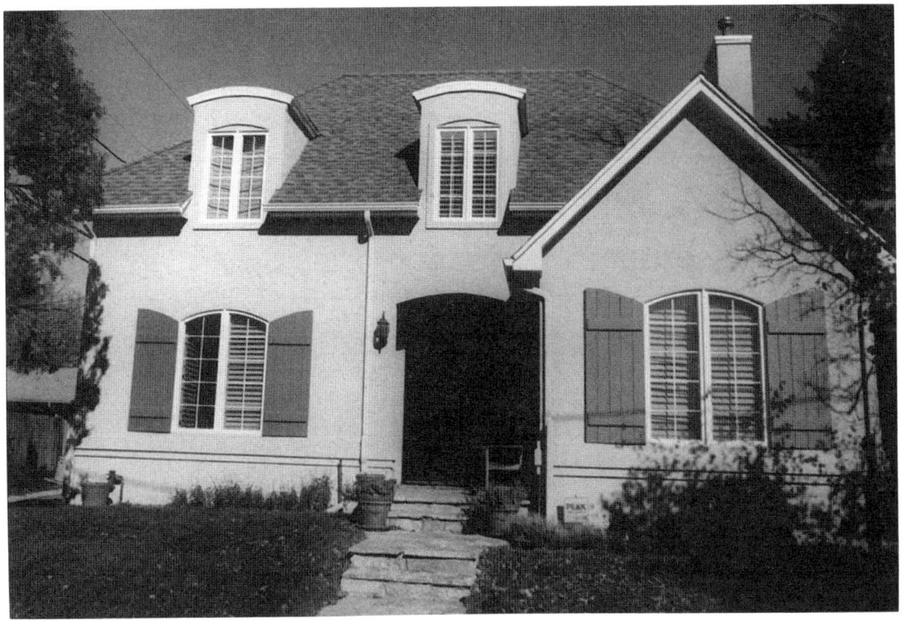

[ABOVE]: A tiny house built on the alley in 1923 was demolished and replaced with a beige stucco home at 1921 4th Avenue in 1996.

25
419 RACE STREET
Built: 1900
Architect: unknown

This tiny, 490-square-foot house was one of the early homes built on the east edge of the Williams Driving Park Place subdivision facing Race Street. Now stuccoed, like the main house to the east at 461 Race Street, the front-gabled home has a frame entrance portico that projects toward the alley and a second-floor dormer to the south.

"When we bought 461 Race Street in the fifties, a little old lady lived in that house. We bought the property after she left, fixed up the house, and acquired the ten-foot unused alley in between our houses,"

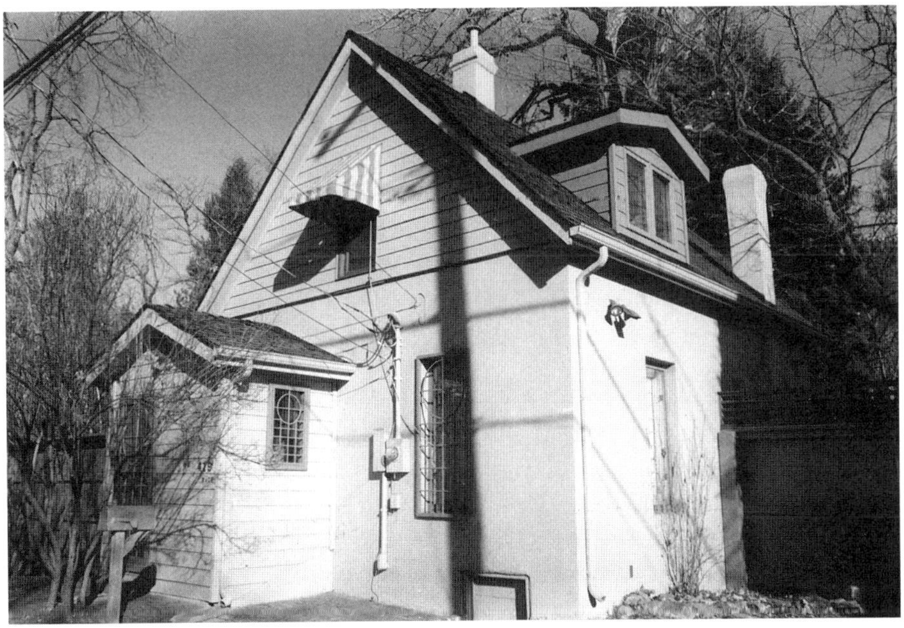

[RIGHT] The entrance to the 490-square-foot house at 419 Race Street is on the alley.

said John F. Sweeney who, with his wife, Vivian, lived at 461 Race Street for 33 years. "A friend helped me take down the fence and the old vacated alley became part of our property. During the sixties we let Joe [Jerome] Strickland rent it and live there with his children."

The only access to this residence is on the alley, where a mailbox with a flag identifies the entrance to this historic little home. It is now owned by Tim Gill of 461 Race Street.

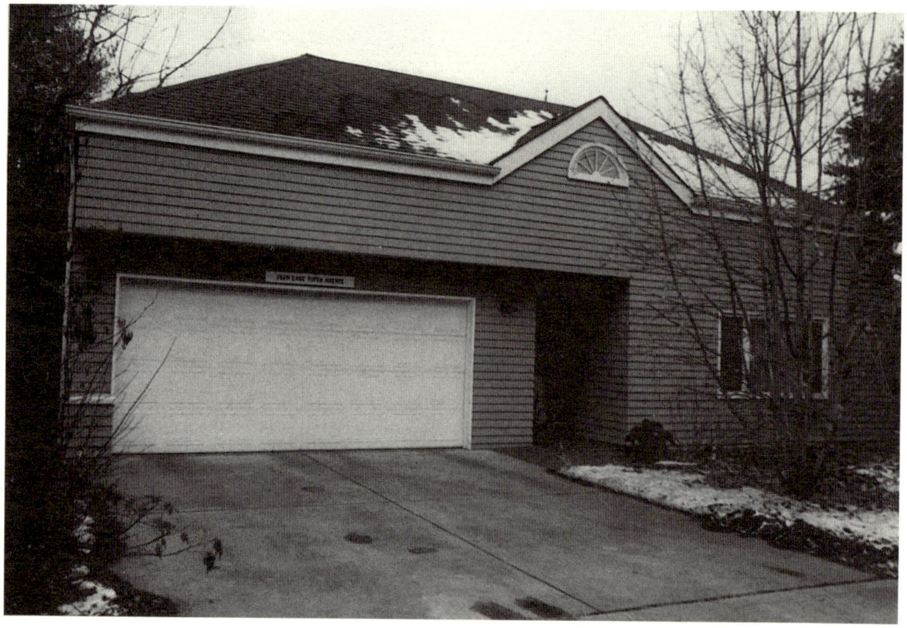

On the alley at 1920 East 5th Avenue is a narrow house that is 88 feet long.

26
1920 EAST 5TH AVENUE
Built: 1954
Architect: unknown
Designer for 1989 additions: Robert Caudle

In 1954 financier William Merriam Bart "Bill" Berger squeezed a tiny one-story red brick house into the 47.5-foot space between the alley and a 10-foot unused alley vacated in 1963 west of 485 Race Street. The property extends for 165 feet, occupying lots 42 through 48 of block 25 of Williams Driving Park Place.

During the mid-eighties, the garage, the front bedroom, and the laundry room were added, resulting in a house 88 feet long. Robert Caudle was the designer of the additions, which included moving the kitchen to the east and making a dining room out of the original kitchen. He put a bay window in the dining room where the original front door was. A further change was a second floor added over the garage, now a bedroom and a combined study darkroom workshop with a bath for current owner Dr. William Cable "Buzz" Jackson.

"The City doesn't have the word yet that this alley has been vacated. We see men with long tools going up and down our side of the fence, looking for the old sewer pipes," Jackson said.

The bedrooms of this house are accessed through a long hallway. The living room and terrace face the south, with a side garden in back. A wide overhang on the terrace keeps the living room cool in summer and lets the winter sun in. "If it's too hot, we use the terrace with a fountain that we put in between the garage and the dining room," Jackson said.

Berger built the house to take advantage of the sun. "We were advised not to buy the land south of us but we bought it anyway,"[35] he said. Berger was the chief Colorado

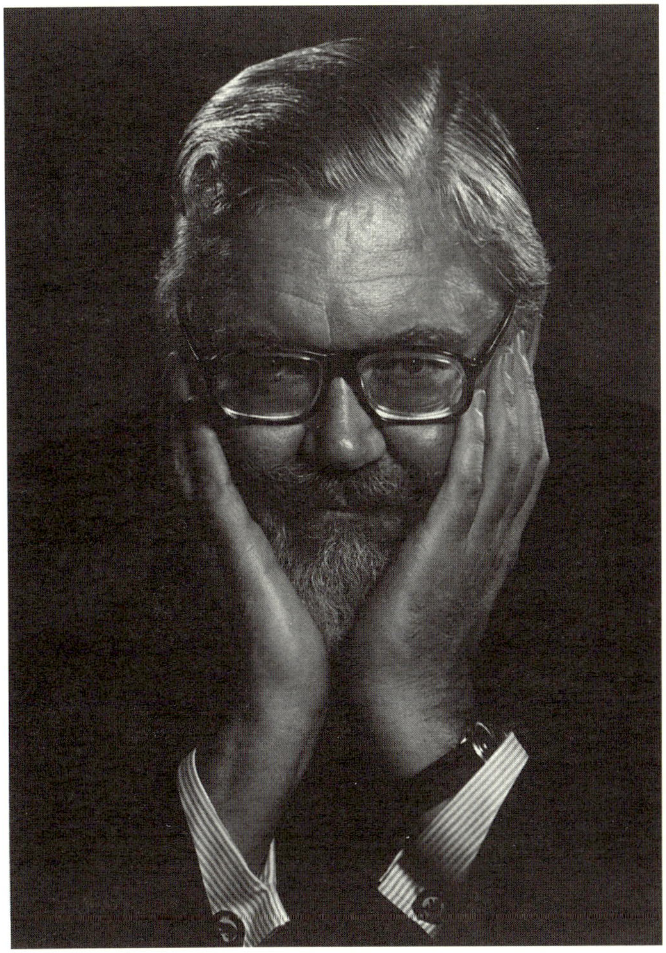

[Left]
The small house on the 47.5-foot-wide lot of Williams Driving Park Place at 1920 5th Avenue was built by William M. B. Berger, founder of Berger Funds. (Courtesy Susan Berger Tweedy)

National Bank investment manager at the age of 25. "It so happened that Uncle George [B. Berger, president of the bank] had been buying stocks for the trust department, and he [suddenly] died. There I was behind his desk with $100 to learn on," reported the *Rocky Mountain News* on December 6, 1970. Berger launched Berger Funds, an aggressive and highly successful investment business. It was so successful that Bill was asked to appear on the Louis Rukeyser program on National Public Television in 1994 or 1995. Close friend James S. Holme said, "Just before his appearance, he slipped on the ice and fell flat on his face. For his screen debut he appeared so battered and bandaged that Rukeyser commented on what a good sport he was to join the program."

Berger and his wife, Bernadette, lived at the Polo Club, land, as Bill pointed out, that was owned by his great grandfather, William Bart Berger, during the late 1800s. The two collected countless magnificent British paintings and, in 1998, displayed them at the Denver Art Museum "for the express purpose of introducing new friends to the joys of art and to the Denver Art Museum."[36]

The Jacksons bought the house in 1987. "It's very private," Jackson said. "We put up an eight-foot cedar fence between us and 485 Race, and on the alley we put a six-foot fence on top of a three-foot retaining wall."

Dr. William Jackson was a dentist before his retirement. His wife, Elaine "Lainey" Wallbank Jackson, is a professional gardener who volunteers much time at the Botanic Gardens. "Lainey is also a Master Gardener. She's indispensable to the organization." said Botanic Garden's board chairman Charles "Cal" Cleworth. Architect Edward D. White, Jr., echoed the sentiment: "She has two green thumbs," he said.

~ Appendix I ~

Country Club's Most Prolific Architectural Firms

The Country Club Historic District is a showplace of elegant, well-preserved homes, custom-designed by many of Denver's outstanding twentieth century architectural firms. Like their prestigious owners, they have contributed much to the shaping of Denver.

JULES JACQUES BENOIS BENEDICT

Jacques Benedict (1879-1948), born in Chicago, studied for four years at the l'Ecole des Beaux-Arts in Paris, then practiced in New York City before moving to Denver in 1909. Opinionated, dapper, witty, and eccentric, Benedict was popular socially and was Denver's prime Beaux-Arts architect, incorporating detailed European features into his designs. Stone lintels, carved stone doorways, ornate plaster ceilings, stairways of hand-carved wood, and travertine marble are common in his structures.

Benedict designed Woodbury branch library, the Waring house used as the Botanic Gardens office building, Graland School, the George E. Cranmer home on Cranmer Park, the Chapel at St. Thomas' Seminary, the Divine Science Church, the Holy Ghost Catholic Church, the Central Savings Bank, and the Washington Park pavilion

In the Country Club neighborhood he designed:

330 Gilpin Street	1912
1700 East 3rd Avenue	1912
120 Humboldt Street	1912
161 Race Street	1919
360 High Street	1920
476 Westwood Drive	1927
576 Circle Drive	1929
355 Gilpin Street	1932

MAURICE BISCOE

Maurice Biscoe (18?? to 1953) came to Denver in 1905 to supervise the construction of St. John's Episcopal Cathedral for the New York firm of Gordon, Tracy and Swarthwout. During the fifteen years he spent in Denver he designed many residences plus the Dickinson Branch Library and the Clayton School for Boys. Two of his projects in Colorado Springs were the Myron Stratton Home and several buildings for Colorado College. Although he moved back to Boston in 1920, he collaborated with Arthur and William Fisher to design Colorado General Hospital (at 8th Avenue and Colorado Boulevard) in 1925. Biscoe died in Massachusetts in 1953.

Biscoe designed several houses in the Country Club neighborhood:

320 Humboldt Street (his own house)	1908
100 Humboldt Street with Henry Harwood Hewitt	1910
121 Lafayette Street	1913
140 High Street	1914
1640 East 3rd Avenue	1916
190 High Street	1917

WILLIAM E. FISHER AND ARTHUR A. FISHER

William Ellsworth Fisher (1874-1937) came from Ontario, Canada, to Denver with his family in 1885 and opened his own architectural office in 1895. He formed a partnership with Daniel R. Huntington in 1901, the year before incorporation of the Fourth Avenue Realty Company that developed the Denver Country Club and the adjacent residential area. The realty company hired Fisher as the chief designer of their residential area, Country Club Place. He laid out three streets with wide parkways, each introduced by elaborate Mediterranean gates on Fourth Avenue. After Huntington moved away, Fisher's brother Arthur moved to Denver to join the firm. The office became a prestigious training ground for young architects and received many commissions, including the Denver Tramway Building and the Railway Exchange Building. Banks include the Colorado National Bank, the International Trust Company, the United States National Bank, and the Midland Savings Building. The firm designed the Neusteter Department Store and the Davis and Shaw furniture store. They planned Morey Junior High and South High School. During the 1920s the firm designed several hospitals including Presbyterian and National Jewish Hospitals. Colorado General Hospital was designed in collaboration with Maurice Biscoe.

The firm won numerous awards in both national and local competitions. Fisher was elected president of the Colorado American Institute of Architects (A.I.A.) in 1915 and Regional A.I.A. Director in 1922. He also founded a local division of the Architects' Small House Bureau to design low-cost housing. When William Fisher's suicide occurred in 1937, the vacancy was filled by his son, Alan Birney Fisher, a founder of the Denver Landmark Preservation Commission.

Arthur Addison Fisher (1878-1965) graduated from Denver schools, then settled in New York after studying at the Beaux-Arts Atelier Barber. Before he returned to Denver in 1905 to practice with his brother, he traveled extensively in Europe and brought his Mediterranean influence to Denver. He was especially interested in church architecture, served on the Church Art Commission of the Episcopal Diocese of Colorado and designed the Church of the Ascension at 6th Avenue and Gilpin Street. Arthur died in 1965, six years after his retirement.

William E. Fisher and Arthur A. Fisher, Architects, was the most influential and prolific firm in the Country Club area. Their designs include:

Gates and parkways of Country Club Place	1903
100 Franklin Street	1906
370 Humboldt Street	1907
135 and 145 Humboldt Street	1908
120 Franklin Street	1909
128 Gilpin Street	1909
110 Franklin Street	1910
345 Gilpin Street	1911
140 Humboldt Street	1912
320 High Street	1912
140 Humboldt Street	1912
314 Lafayette Street	1912
300 High Street	1913
160 Downing Street	1915
350 Gilpin Street	1916
323 High Street	1916
149 Gilpin Street	1921
380 High Street	1924
1625 Third	1926
555 Race Street	1927
2025 East 4th Avenue	1928
2151 Hawthorne Place	1931

FREDERICK LOUIS HARNOIS

Frederick Harnois (1872-1921) moved to Denver from New York about 1896 and formed a partnership with Theodore Davis Boal in 1901. The firm received many commissions because of Boal's social connections, although Harnois did most of the designing. Two of the firm's projects were the Grant-Humphreys mansion in 1902 and a Shingle-style clubhouse for the Denver Country Club in 1904. By 1907, Harnois decided to form his own firm and built several residences, including the Crawford Hill mansion on Sherman Street and the Wolhurst estate near Littleton. He died in 1921.

Harnois had opened his own firm by the time he built some of the earliest houses in the Country Club district:

164 Lafayette Street (his own home)	1907
170 Lafayette Street	1907
142 Marion Street	1911
140 Gilpin Street	1912
195 High Street	1912
149 High Street	1912
336 Marion Strcct	1914
160 Downing Street	1915

MERRILL AND BURNHAM HOYT

Merrill Hoyt (1881-1933) worked in the office of Fisher and Fisher before opening an architectural office in his native Denver. The Hoyt partnership began in 1919 when his gifted brother, Burnham (1887-1960), returned to Denver from New York City to join the firm. Burnham had studied at the Beaux-Arts Institute in New York City where he won six design competitions. In 1926, when he was chosen as chief designer of Riverside Church, he was often in New York, but, after his brother's fatal heart attack in 1933, he settled in Denver to fulfill his brother's commitments.

Among their projects were the Park Hill Library, the Nurses' Home (Tammen Hall) at Children's Hospital, Cherry Hills Country Club, Lake Junior High School, St. Martin's Chapel and the Parish House of St. John's Cathedral, the Educational Building at Montview Boulevard Presbyterian Church, Lake Junior High School, and Valverde School. After Merrill's death, Burnham's most noted designs were the Red Rocks Amphitheater and the Boettcher School for Crippled Children. Burnham retired in ill health in 1955, after designing the Denver Public Library, incorporated into the main library in 1995.

In the Country Club neighborhood, the Hoyts designed:

101 High Street	1920
177 Race Street	1922
369 Humboldt Street	1922
375 Humboldt Street	1922
101 High Street	1923
385 Gilpin Street	1925
380 Gilpin Street	1925
210 Vine Street	1926
101 Gaylord Street	1928
130 Gaylord Street	1928
515 Race Street	1929

After Merrill died, Burnham designed

127 Gaylord Street	1935
100 Gaylord Street	1937
545 Circle Drive	1941
2125 Hawthorne Drive	1953

HENRY JAMES MANNING

Harry James Manning (1877-1933) had come to Denver from Illinois in 1904 and practiced with Franz C. Wagner. Specializing in sanitaria, the firm was awarded the Roosevelt Medal of the International Congress on Tuberculosis for a design for a sanitorium. When Wagner died in 1912, Manning practiced by himself and designed Bethesda Sanatorium, the Fairmont Elementary School, Cathedral High School, and St. Thomas Episcopal Church. He designed the Capital Life Insurance Building and was an associate architect for the City and County Building. He met Mary (Mrs. Verner Z.) Reed and designed the Marjorie Reed Mayo Nursery and Reed Memorial Library at the University of Denver in memory of her daughter, Margery Reed Mayo, who had died in 1920. During the late twenties he designed Mrs. Reed's mansion at 475 Circle Drive and the house beside it at 505 Circle Drive for her sister. While working on these projects Manning traveled to Europe with Mrs. Reed to view architectural details and choose ornamental artifacts for the homes. Manning died in 1933 at St. Luke's Hospital in Denver.

Homes he designed in the Country Club Historic District are:

165 High Street	1923
300 Gilpin Street	1910
475 Circle Drive	1926-1931
150 Vine Street	1928
177 Humboldt Street	1929
505 Circle Drive	1929

MAREAN AND NORTON

Willis Adams Marean (1853-1939) came to Denver from New York in 1880 and practiced with Frank E. Edbrooke until 1895, designing the Brown Palace Hotel, the Interstate Trust Building, Central Presbyterian Church, the Ernest and Cranmer Building, and the Cooper Building.

In 1895 he formed a partnership with Albert Julius Norton (1867-1944), a draftsman at Edbrooke and Co. Marean died in 1939, three years after his retirement. Norton, also a New Yorker, had traveled and studied art in Europe, and, like Marean, served as a long-term member of the Denver Art Commission. Norton was active in Denver art circles and a trustee of the Denver Art Museum. He died in 1944.

The firm designed the Chamber of Commerce building, the Y.M.C.A. Building, the Shirley-Savoy Hotel, the Sara Platt Decker branch library, the Governor's Mansion, and the Washington Park Community Church. Both men promoted and added to Denver's City Beautiful plans by designing the Open Air Theater at Civic Center and the Greek Pavilion in Cheesman Park

During the early teens the partners designed several houses in the Country Club area:

1601 E. 3rd Avenue	1909
300 Humboldt Street	1910
165 Franklin Street	1911
111 Gilpin Street	1913
301 High Street	1914
300 Lafayette Street	1916

STERNER AND WILLIAMSON

Frederick Junius Sterner (1862-1931), who came to Denver during the late 1880s, formed a partnership with Ernest Philip Varian until 1910. They designed the University Club, and the Antler's Hotel in Colorado Springs.

In 1910, Sterner opened an office with their chief draftsman, George Hebard Williamson (1872-1936). However, Sterner shortly started practicing in New York City, so spent less time in Denver. Williamson carried on the business under the same name. In 1923 Sterner retired to his native England where he died in 1931.

Together they designed the Daniels and Fisher Tower, the Denver Athletic Club, and Smiley Junior High School. Williamson is especially remembered for his award-winning design of his alma mater, East High School, completed in 1924. During the thirties Williamson served as the Federal Housing Administrations' chief architectural supervisor for Colorado, vice-president of the Denver City and Country Zoning Board, and was honored as a fellow in the Colorado Chapter of the American Institute of Architects. He died in 1936.

In the Country Club Historic Neighborhood the firm designed some of the earliest homes:

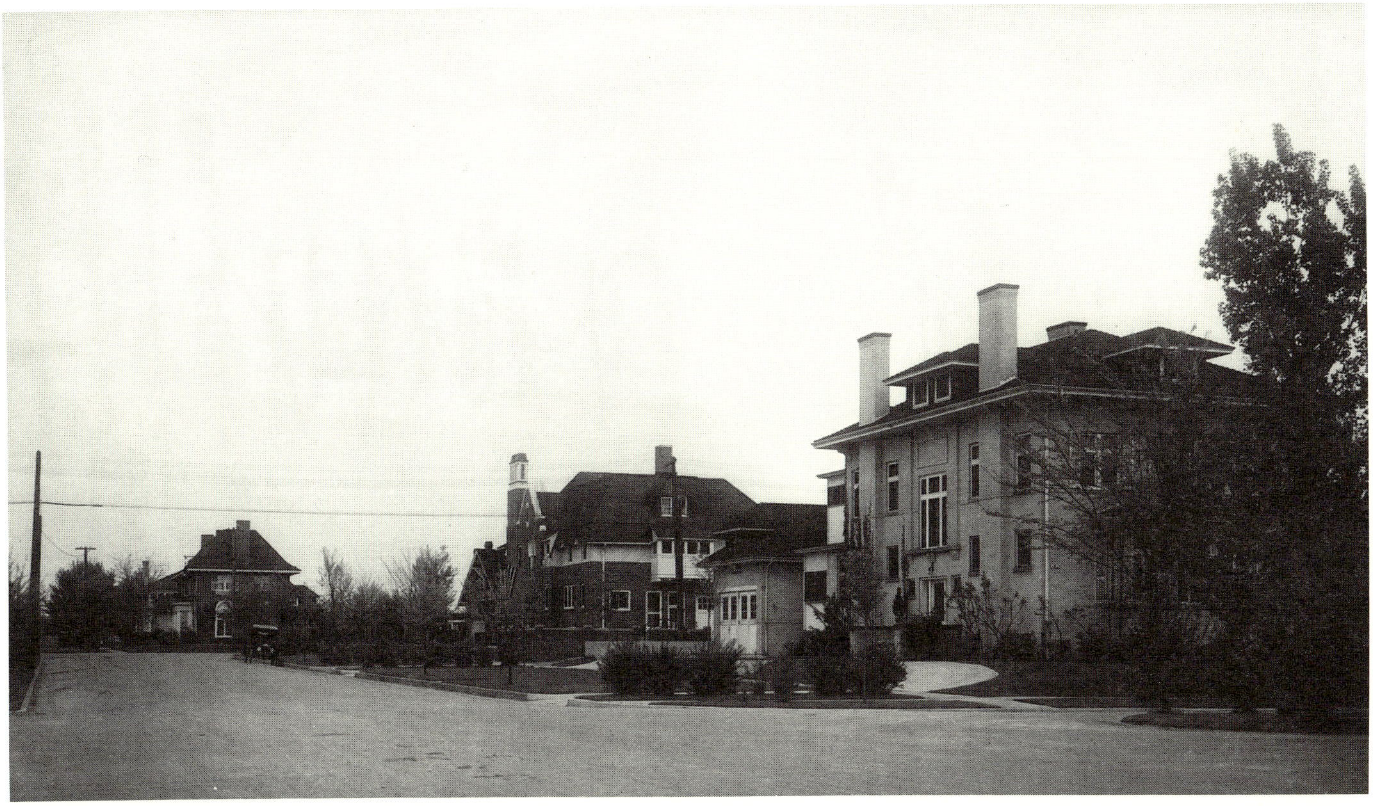

Early homes in Country Club Place were 180 Franklin Street, designed by Glen W. Huntington and remodeled by Fisher and Fisher; 1640 East 3rd Avenue, designed by Maurice Biscoe; and 1700 East 3rd Avenue designed by Jacques Benedict, all built before 1917. (Courtesy DPL Western History Department).

379 Marion Street	1905
350 Humboldt Street	1905
330 Humboldt Street	1910
301 Humboldt Street	1908
140 Gilpin Street	1912
165 Gilpin Street	1910
141 Gilpin Street	1912

SOURCES

1. Withey, Henry F. and Elsie Rathburn. *Biographical Dictionary of American Architects*. Los Angeles: New Age Publishing Co., 1956.
2. Noel, Thomas J. and Barbara Norgren, *Denver: The City Beautiful.* Denver: Historic Denver, Inc., 1987. "The Architects: Biographical Sketches," with articles by Artha Pacha Frickell, Rutherford W. Witthus, Carol J. Callahan, Edward D. White, Jr., Sharon Elfenbein, Ellen T. Ittelson, Bette D. Peters, and Tyson Dines, III.

~ Appendix II ~

Architectural Styles in the Country Club Historic District

Most Denver homes do not fit neatly into a pure architectural stylistic category, but have characteristics of one or more styles. Most are "eclectic" or "Revival." Elements of the styles most prevalent in the Country Club Historic District are described below

BUNGALOW

Following the tradition of the Craftsman movement which stressed utility, simplicity, and heavy exposed woodwork, the Bungalow style became a symbol of the movement with its low, overhanging roof, broad porches, and simple horizontal lines. Identified as the most common example of Craftsman architecture, the Bungalow Style spread quickly across the country during the early twentieth century. In Colorado, this style was popular from 1900 to around 1930.

The typical early Bungalow is a one or one-and-a-half story, wood or masonry structure with a gently pitched front or side gable roof. An additional gable occasionally covers an open porch, and the overhang is usually supported by battered or "elephantine" porch piers or thick columns. Some bungalows have clipped gables, shed dormers, or exposed rafters. Later Bungalows may be enlarged, but all have a wide front porch. Examples in the District are:

145 Lafayette Street, page 57
167 Lafayette Street, page 57
330 Humboldt Street, page 75
160 Franklin Street, page 96

An example of Craftsman Style is 171 Franklin Street, page 95.

ENGLISH/NORMAN COTTAGE

The English or Norman Cottage is generally composed of brick, stucco, or occasionally stone. The most distinguishing feature is the steeply pitched roof and steeply pitched projecting front entrance. The eaves sometimes flare upward at the roof-wall junction. Many have arched or straight-headed picture windows on the front facade, but otherwise fenestration is limited. Windows are occasionally casements divided by heavy metal mullions. Decorative brickwork, arched entrances, and small-paned windows are characteristic. Examples in the District are:

128 Gilpin Street, page 106
330 Gilpin Street, page 114
130 Gaylord Street, page 165

FOURSQUARE

One style found after 1900, the Foursquare, is so common in Colorado as to be a vernacular building and is also called the Denver Square. It is recognized by its square plan and its simplicity. The majority of these homes were built during the first three decades of the twentieth century. The typical Foursquare has a hipped roof with central formal decoration, broad overhanging brackets or modillions, classical dentils, and a porch with hipped roof, supported by simple Doric columns or square posts. Occasionally, a Foursquare will feature a gable.

Some will be considerably larger, with elaborate ornamentation. But, in general, a basic square plan is predominant. Examples in the District are:

330 Lafayette Street, page 49
181 Franklin Street, page 94
C. Richardson Place, page 185

GEORGIAN

Georgian houses are formal, symmetrical two-story, wooden or red brick boxes. The paneled front door is often capped by a decorative crown supported by fluted columns or pilasters. The roof is usually a side gable with a cornice decorated with dentils. Aligned vertically and horizontally, the double-hung sash windows have small panes separated by wooden muntins. Examples in the District are:

144 Downing Street, page 50
369 Humboldt Street, page 78-79
160 Race Street, page 144
490 Race Street, page 189
2115 East 4th Avenue, page 196

GREEK REVIVAL

The most striking feature of Greek Revival architecture is the one or two-story columns supporting a front portico or full-length porch. The hipped or gabled roof is low pitched. The cornice lines are emphasized with a wide band, usually divided into two parts. The front door surround has long, narrow sidelights with transom lights above. Examples in the District are:

Former 140 Humboldt Street, page 61
180 Humboldt Street, page 66
350 Humboldt Street, page 76

INTERNATIONAL STYLE

The chief characteristics of the International Style are smooth surfaces, flat roofs, a large expanse of windows, asymmetrical composition, and occasionally rounded corners. Ornamentation is generally absent, thus distinguishing the International Style from the usually highly-decorated Art Deco. Horizontal lines are a characteristic, particularly on commercial buildings where alternating bands of windows and solid planes created a horizontal effect. Wood or metal casement windows were common. The style, which dates from the 1930s through the 1950s, also emphasized a lack of color, contrasting black and white. Examples in the District are:

450 Race Street
545 Circle Drive, page 180

MEDITERRANEAN

The key to distinguishing the Mediterranean Style is the tile roof and restrained ornamentation (as opposed to the elaborate details on a Spanish Colonial structure). Built in Colorado during the 1920s, these structures are generally stucco or brick, often painted white to contrast the brightly colored roof tiles. Roofs are low-pitched gable or flat on smaller homes and are low-pitched hipped on some larger homes. Another characteristic feature is the extension of a side or front wall to form an arcaded entrance or porch. Windows are sometimes casements, framed by wooden or wrought-iron grills or small second-story balconies, called balconets.

In comparing a Mediterranean Style home to a Spanish Colonial home, the Mediterranean example will have a flat or planer surface, few projections, and limited ornamentation. The heavy tile roof is generally the dominant characteristic.

Mediterranean is the predominant style of architecture in the older (western) Country Club subdivisions, heralded by the entrance gates to Country Club Place on East 4th Avenue. Examples in the District are:

135 Humboldt Street, page 63
381 Franklin Street, page 87
190 High Street, page 129
101 High Street, page 138

SPANISH COLONIAL

The Spanish Colonial Revival Style, popular during the 1920s and 1930s, is characterized by elaborately carved decorations surrounding windows, entrances, and cornices. In contrast to the plainer, flat surfaces of the Mission and Mediterranean styles, the Spanish Colonial Revival building has more complex, deeply sculptured surfaces. Curvilinear shaped gables, parapets, arcaded entrances and porches, wrought-iron detailing around openings, round-arched or straight-headed windows and heavy tile roofs are also characteristic elements of this style. Stucco is the most common building material used and is generally painted white or a light color. Examples in the District are:

320 Humboldt Street, page 74
385 Gilpin Street, page 116
380 High Street, page 118
576 Circle Drive, page 183

TUDOR REVIVAL

The most dominant features of the Tudor Revival style are the half-timbering, which covers the upper story, and the very steeply pitched roof. The exterior uses textures: brick, stone, or stucco, and together with the timbering, give the house a picturesque composition. Constructed in Colorado during the late teens and twenties, these homes also feature gabled or hipped roofs covered with tile, slate, or shake shingles, and decorative chimney detailing. Windows are generally mullioned casements, with an occasional bay window. Examples in the District are:

120 Humboldt Street, page 60
1625 East 3rd Avenue, page 110
210 Vine Street, page 159
100 Gaylord Street, page 163
515 Race Street, page 188

SOURCES

Material for this section is largely from *A Colorado Guide to Architecture*, published by the Colorado Historical Society in 1983. Other sources are *A Field Guide to American Houses*, by Virginia and Lee McAlester. This section was reviewed by Edward D. White, Jr., A.I.A.

~ Endnotes ~

South of the City Limits

1. Bethuel M. Webster, Jr., "A Letter to Eleanor," July 11, 1967.
2. Louisa Arps, *Denver In Slices*, p. 145.
3. *Rocky Mountain News*, January 10, 1882.
4. *Encyclopedia of World Sport*, Vol II, David Levinaon and Karen Christensen, Editors.
5. *Daily News*, July 12, 1895.
6. Abstract of 446 Lafayette Street
7. *Denver Tribune*, January 22, 1882.
8. *Denver Municipal Facts*, Vol 1, August 14, 1898, p.7.
9. Advertisement Driving Park Land Company, DPL Western History clippings file.
10. Carla Swan Coleman, "Driving Park Place 9-12," a paper presented to the Denver Fortnightly Club in 1959, based on the abstract of her property.
11. *Denver Post*, November 19, 1931.
12. Condemnation Permit, Lots 23-24, Driving Park Place, October 22, 1931.
13. Louisa Ward Arps, *Ibid*, p. 22
14. *Denver Times*, January 22, 1901.
15. Abstract of 100 Franklin Street.
16. *Ibid*.
17. Sanford, Albert B., *The Trail*, April 1925.

The Western Subdivisions

18. *Denver Times*, December 6, 1901.
19. Abstract of 100 Franklin Street.
20. Barbara Sudler [Hornby], National Register for Historic Places Nomination Form, 1986.
21. *Republican*, January 1, 1905.
22. Building Permit, #2420, 1914.
23. *The Denver Republican*, November 7, 1909.
24. Abstract 100 Franklin Street.
25. "Ahead of the Crowd," Vol. I, Robert D. McPhee, 1993.
26. Interviews with Barry and Rich Oliver in 1999.
27. Building Permit, October 22, 1931.
28. Abstract of 301 Marion.
29. Building Permit #1130, 1905.
30. Denver Country Club Minutes of the Board of Directors.
31. *Ibid*.
32. *Ibid*.

Speer Boulevard

33. *Denver Municipal Facts*, 1912, p.11.
34. *Denver's Speer Blvd: Revitalization*, Urban Design Committee of the Denver Chapter of the American Institute of Architects.
35. "Bob Speer's Challenge to Denver," *Denver Post Magazine*, November 21, 1965.
36. *Denver Municipal Facts*, 1912, p.11.
37. Minutes of the Denver Country Club board of directors.
38. *Denver Municipal Facts*, 1912, p.11.
39. *Denver Post*, June 15, 1912.

40 Louisa Arps, *Denver In Slices*, p.83.

41. Saco DeBoer papers filed at the DPL Western History Department.

Eastern Subdivisions

42. Map of Capitol Annex.

43 Hall, Frank, *History of the State of Colorado*, Volume V, 1895, p. 454.

44. *Denver Times*, November 17,1902, Sec. 2;, p.6, c2.

45 *Rocky Mountain News*, January 1, 1901, Sec. 3, p.2, c.4.

46. *The Town of Harman and the Harman-Bromwell School*, Citizens Advisory Planning Organization of Denver, Colorado, 1976.
47. Denver Building permit, 1892, #305 to H.L. Moore.
48. 1900 Census report.
49. *Ibid*.
50. Baist map, 1905.
51. Refer to the Baist map to define the boundaries of Capitol Annex, which stretch from York Street (University Boulevard since 1907) to the Race-Vine alley (Blocks 1, 2, and 3).

The northern boundary lies 12 lots (300 feet) south of 4th (Vasquez) Avenue on a line that would continue 4th Avenue east if it did not make a jag at Race Street. Half alleys now exist on this dividing line.

The southern boundary included three lots (75 feet) lining the south side of 3rd Avenue between Race and York Streets, including the Lawrence C. Phipps to form Country Club Annex in 1925.

52. Map of Capitol Annex
53. Interview with Alberta Iliff Shattuck in 1999.
54. Denver Assessor's Office
55. Abstract of 361 Race Street.
56. Denver City Ordinance #36, 1920.
57. Denver City Ordinance #116, 1909.
58. Denver City Ordinance #25, 1984.
59. Interviews with Mary Lee Anderson in 1998 and 1999.
60. Denver Assessor's Office.
61. National Register of Historic Places Inventory Nomination Form, Barbara Sudler (Hornby), 1986).
62. Interview with Jane Bromfield Foster in 1999.
63. Interview with Diana Warren in 1999.
64. Baist Map, 1905
65. Abstracts of 545 Race Street and 460 Westwood Drive.
66. Denver City Ordinance #37, 1926.
67. Abstracts of 545 Race Street and 460 Westwood Drive.
68. Baist map 1905.

Cherry Creek Historic Neighborhood, Inc.

69. *Rocky Mountain News*, March 10, 1946.
70. *Rocky Mountain News*, January 26, 1947.
71. *Rocky Mountain News*, March 10, 1946.
72. *Denver Post*, November 9, 1950.
73. *Denver Post*, October 14, 1962.
74. *DenverPost*, December 22, 1968.
75. *Rocky Mountain News*, August 10, 1981.
76. *Ibid.*
77. Minutes of the Country Club Historic Neighborhood, Inc. board meetings.

Introduction to Walking Tours

1. *Design Guidelines* of the Country Club Historic Neighborhood.
2. Interview with Lenora Thomas (Mrs. John) Stoddart.
3. Interview with Helen (Mrs. Gary) Christy in 1999..
4. Denver City Ordinance #116, 1909.
5. Denver City Ordinance #36, 1920.
6. Denver City Ordinance #59, 1933.

Park Club Place

301 Marion Street

1. *Denver Post*, February 18, 1937, p.10.

379 Marion Street

2. Abstract of 379 Marion Street.

1333 East 3rd Avenue

3. Building Permit #144, 1914.
4. Interviews with Philip Atchison and Edward D. White, Jr, in 1999.

300 Lafayette Street

5. *Real Pioneers of Colorado*, Volume 2, p. 266.
6. *Rocky Mountain News*, "Have Faith," an interview with Edwin S. Kassler, April 19, 1959.
7. Philip K. "Pete" Alexander, Jr., Diary of G. W. Kassler, from, *George W. Kassler, Colorado Pioneer, Vol. II*.
8 Stephen Leonard and Thomas J. Noel, *Denver: Mining Camp to Metropolis*, p. 28.
9 *Rocky Mountain News*, "Have Faith," an interview with Edwin S. Kassler, April 19, 1959.
10 Alexander papers, 1930, from Denver Public Library Western History Department.
11. Louisa W. Arps, *Denver In Slices*.

199 Lafayette Street

12. Philip K. "Pete" Alexander, Jr., family history, p. 86. (Courtesy Gladys Barkalow Alexander)
13. *Ibid.*, p.104.

140 Humboldt

14. Alexander, Philip K. "Pete", Jr., family history, p.78.
15 Brochure for Dora Moore School House Tour, 1989.

135 Humboldt Street

16. Dayle Friedman, *The Saga of Leopold Henry Guldman: An American Jewish Success Story*, Brandeis University, 1978, p. 9.

17. *Ibid.*, p.10.
18. *Rocky Mountain News*, May 6, 1937, p.14.

145 Humboldt Street
19. Brochure for Dora Moore School House Tour, 1987.

180 Humboldt Street
20. Building permit #341, 1908.
21. *Sketches of Colorado*, 1911, p. 291.

300 Humboldt Street
22. Land transfer, (number not given), March 11, 1904.
23. Building permit #536, 1911.
24. Charles A. Johnson, *Denver's Mayor Speer*, p. 224.

320 Humboldt Street
25. *Denver Post*, December 29, 1953, p.3.

330 Humboldt Street
26. Land transfer #263, March 1, 1904.
27 Building permit. 1910.
28. Interview by Helen Christy on July 12, 1959. Stephen Hart Library, Colorado Historical Society.

350 Humboldt Street
29. 1920 Census report.

335 Humboldt Street
30. *Rocky Mountain Herald*, Jan. 15, 1972, DPL Western History clipping file.
31. Interviews with Charles A. Moore and W. Bart Berger in 1999.

370 Humboldt Street
32. "A Letter to Eleanor," from Bethuel M. Webster to his daughter, July 11, 1967.

Country Club Place

381 Franklin Street
1. Building permit #3687, 1922.
2 *Rocky Mountain News*, January 30, 1953, p. 12.

350 Franklin Street
3. *Denver Post*, November 18, 1962.

314 Franklin Street
4. Building permit #460, 1911.
5 Building permit #152, 1913.
6. *Rocky Mountain News*, February 22, 1953.

180 Franklin Street
7. Fisher and Fisher plans, Denver Public Library Western History epartment.
8. *Rocky Mountain News*, April 3, 1974, p.37.

171 Franklin Street
9. Lorna Grindley Moore, "The Denver Crafstman Era." Paper presented to the Denver Fortnightly Club on February 6, 1990.
10. 1910 Census.

160 Franklin Street
11. *Denver Times*, February 16, 1912, p. 7.
12. *Colorado Magazine*, October 1959, p. 289.
13. *Ibid.*
14. *Sons of Colorado*, June 1906.
15. *On and Off the Wall*, May/June 1992. Published by the Denver Art Museum.

120 Franklin Street
16. 1910 Census.
17. Building permit #2645, 1909.
18. *Rocky Mountain News*, February 25, 1962, 6A.
19. *Rocky Mountain News*, December 6, 1991, p. 215.

100 Franklin Street
20. Building permit #1890, 1906.

103 Franklin Street
21. Building permit #2159, 1906.
22. Building permit #1288, 1906
23. *Denver Times*, undated article in clipping file, Denver Public Library Western History Department.
24. Ralph Ball, *The Colorado Lawyer*, July 1999.

111 Gilpin Street
25. *Denver Post*, August 11, 1913.
26 Robert D. McPhee, "Ahead of the Crowd," Volume II.

141 Gilpin Street
27. Building permit #550, 1912.
28. 1920 Census
29. *Rocky Mountain News*, July 1, 1984, p. 14M.

128 Gilpin Street
30. *Denver Post*, March 25, 1965, p. 31.

31. *Ibid.*
32. Building permit #1288, 1909.
33. Building permit #764, 1923.

170 Gilpin Street
34. *Rocky Mountain News*, December 5, 1955.
35. Building permit #1168, 1919.
36. Noel and Norgren, *City Beautiful*, p. 216.

1640 East Third Avenue
37. *The Denver Kiwaian*, Denver Public Library Western History clippings file.
38. Building permit #851, 1919.

1625 East 3rd Avenue and 323 Gilpin Street
39. *Sketches of Colorado*, 1911, p. 137.
40. DPL Western History clipping file.
41. *Rocky Mountain News*, September 26, 1919.
42. *Rocky Mountain News*, August 16, 1994.
43. *Denver Post*, February 25, 1951, p. 9AA.
44. *Cervi's Rocky Mountain Journal*, May 20, 1970.
45. Pat Hanna, *Rocky Mountain News*, Festival, June 25, 1967, p. 9.

300 Gilpin Street
46. *Sharp Scrapbook*, Volume 1, p. 63.
47. Denver Museum of Natural History collections, Catalogue #1476.
48. *Denver Post*, January 4, 1918, p.11.
49. *Denver Post*, May 28, 1930, p. 3.

330 Gilpin Street
50. *Rocky Mountain News*, September 23, 1946.
51. *Denver Post*, September 23, 1946.
52. *Rocky Mountain News*, March 24, 1963, p. 22A.

380 Gilpin Street
53. Building permit #7987, 1925.
54. Junior Symphony Guild Showhouse brocure, 1996.

399 High Street
55. *Denver Post*, March 9, 1999.

380 High Street
56. Assessor's Office.

360 High Street
57. *Denver Post*, Empire section, July 25, 1965.

320 High Street
58. Wilbur Stone, *History of Colorado*, 1918.
59. *Denver Post*, January 12, 1945.
60. Polly Pry, Volume 1, #5, October 5, 1905, p. 4.
61. Brett Halliday, "Murder at the Brown Palace," from *Denver Murders*, New York: Duell, Sloan and Pearce, 1946.
62. *Cervi's Rocky Mountain Journal*, September 14, 1950.
63. Leonard and Noel, *Denver: Mining Camp to Metropolis*, p. 241.
64. *Cervi's Rocky Mountain Journal*, July 7, 1955.
65. *Denver Post*, April 9, 1969, p. 45.

300 High Street
66. Building permit #617, 1919.
67. Building permit #909, 1920.
68. Fisher and Fisher plans at DPL Western History Department.
69. *Rocky Mountain News*, May 28, 1939.

310 High Street
70. *Rocky Mountain News* Sunday Magazine, March 10, 1985, p. 2M.

200 High Street
71. *Denver Post*, October 20, 1970.
72. *Ibid.*
73. *Denver Post*, January 8, 1971.
74. *Denver Post*, January 22, 1971.
75. *Denver Post*, February 24, 1971.

301 High Street
76. *Denver Commercial*, August 6, 1925.

190 High Street
77. *Denver Post*, October 4, 1933, p. 3.
78. *Denver Post*, July 26, 1959.
79. *Pueblo Star Journal*, October 23, 1955.
80. *Denver Post*, August 13, 1943.
81. Interview with Julius Wassenaar.

149 High Street
82. Tom Gavin, *Denver Post*, May 8, 1970, p. 17.

170 and 180 High Street
83. James Sudler, interview taped on February 18, 1975. Stephen Hart Library, Colorado Historical Society.

84. *Ibid.*
85. Joanne Ditmer, *Denver Post,* March 27, 1982.
86. Leonard and Noel, *Denver: Mining Camp to Metropilis*, 1990.

140 High Street
87. *Rocky Mountain News*, March 9, 1954, p.8.
88. Noel and Norgren, *Denver: The City Beautiful*, p. 75.
89. Robert D. McPhee, "Ahead of he Crowd: Growing Up in the Twenties and Thirties," Volume II, p.4.

Country Club Annex

161 Race Street
1. *Rocky Mountain News*, May 17, 1978.
2. *Denver Post*, March 13, 1989.

300 Race Street
3. *Rocky Mountain News*, January 15, 1978.

338 Race Street
4. *Rocky Mountain News*, July 26, 1980.

300 Vine Street
5. Building permit #1471, 1911.
6. *Historic Denver News*, June 1999.
7. Building permit, March 13, 1988.

265 Vine Street
8. Building permit #3, 1936.
9. *Denver Post*, June 29, 1957, p.6B.

230 Vine Street
10. Charles A. Johnson letter to Denver Public Library Western History Department.
11. *Denver Post,* Empire Magazine, DPL Western History clipping file.
12. *Denver Post Roundup*, September 15, 1957.
13. *Denver Post*, February 22, 1970, p.40.

210 Vine Street
14. Building permit #5218, 1926 by Mrs. W. Oscar Temple.

127 Vine Street
15. Alexander family papers at the Stephen Hart Library of the Colorado Historical Society.

100 Gaylord Street
16. *Green Thumb*, April 1950, p. 112. Published by the Denver Botanic Gardens.

140 Gaylord Street
17. *Men and Women of Colorado, Past and Present,* Denver: Pioneer Publishing Co., 1944, p. 31.
18. *Denver Post*, December 30, 1944.

316 Gaylord Street
19. Abstract of 316 Gaylord Street.
20. 1900 Census.
21. Building permit #305, 1892.

Park Lane Square

2244 East 4th Avenue
1. Interview with Barbara Sudler Hornby, 1999.
2. Interviews with Robert K. Fuller,II , 1998 and 1999.

475 Circle Drive
3. *Men and Women of Colorado*, p. 65.
4. Abstracts of 460 Westwood Drive and 465 Race Street.
5. Interview with current owner in 1999.
6. *Rocky Mountain News*, October 6, 1990.

505 Circle Drive
7. Interview with Philip Atchison, 1999.
8. Mary Coyle Chase, *The Wicked Pigeon Ladies*, pp. 4-6.
9. Interview with Ann Campbell.
10. Interview with Patsy O'Rourke Monaghan, 1999.
11. Interview with Marilyn Alkire, 1999.

545 Circle Drive
12. Polly Pry, vol. 1, #3, Sept. 13, 1903.
13. Interview with Anne Waring Maer in 1999.

575 Circle Drive
14. *Rocky Mountain News*, March 7, 1959, p.56.
15. Building permit #1021, 1930.

515 Race Street

16. Building permit #2562, 1927 (for the address of 509 Race)

460 Westwood Drive

17. Building permit #2774, 1928.
18. *Denver Post,* June 1, 1953, p.17A.
19. *Rocky Mountain News,* December 8, 1965.

450 Westwood Drive

20. Original map of Park Lane Square showing owners.
21. Interview with Arthur Krill.

2125 Hawthorne Place

22. Pat Paton, A *Medical Gentleman,* Denver: Colorado Historical Society, 1993, p. 149.

2155 Hawthorne Place

23. *Denver Times,* November 17, 1902, p.6, c2.

2101 East 4th Avenue

24. Sewell Thomas, *Silhouettes of Charles Sewell Thomas.* The Caxton Printers, Ltd., Caldwell, Idaho, 1959, p. 176-7.

2012 East 4th Avenue

25. Building permit #2489, 1927.
26. Building permit #2622, 1936.

1925-1927 East 4th Place

27. Denver City Ordinance #38, 1963.
28. Land transfer Block 25 Lots 25-36 to May McMahill #1378 on February 11, 1900.
29. Building permit #1270, 1901.

401 Race Street

30. Joanne Ditmer, *Denver Post,* June 19, 1967, p. 1B.

1921 East 4th Avenue

31. Building permit #6210, 1923.
32. Interviews with Virginia Olson in 1998 and 1999.
33. Interviews with Virginia Olson in 1998 and 1999.
34. Interview with Charlotte Croze in January 2000.

1920 East 5th Avenue

35. Interview with W. M. B. Berger, 1999.
36. *600 Years of British Painting: A Preview of the Berger Collection,* Metaphor Publishing, 1998.

~ Sources ~

BOOKS

Arps, Louisa Ward, *Denver In Slices*. Athens, Ohio: Swallow Press, 1959.

Davis, Sally and Betty Baldwin, *Denver Dwellings and Descendants*, Denver, Sage Books, 1963.

Dodds, John W., *Everyday Life in the Twentieth Century*. New York: G.P. Putnam's Sons, 1965.

Ferril, William Columbus, *Sketches of Colorado, Volume 1*. Denver: The Western Press Bureau Company, 1911.

Johnson, Charles A., *Denver's Mayor Speer*. Denver: Green Mountain Press, 1969.

Levinson, David and Karen Christensen, Editors. *Encyclopedia of World Sport: From Ancient Times to the Present*, ABC-CLIO, Denver. 1996.

Kohl, Edith Eudora, *Denver's Historic Mansions*. Denver: Sage Books, 1957

Hall, Frank, *History of the State of Colorado*: The Blackely Printing Company, 1895.

Leonard, Stephen J. and Thomas J. Noel, *Denver: Mining Camp to Metropolis*. Niwot, Colorado: University Press of Colorado, 1990.

McAllester, Virginia and Lee, *A Field Guide to American Houses*, New York: Alfred A. Knopf, 1989.

Noel, Thomas J., *Denver Landmark's Historic Districts*. Niwot, Colorado: University Press of Colorado, 1996.

Noel, Thomas J. and Barbara S. Norgren, *Denver: The City Beautiful*. Denver: Historic Denver, Inc., 1993.

Press Biographies, Representative Men of America. Compiled by the Press Syndicate of America. Denver, 1906.

Vickers, William B., *History of the City of Denver*, 1996.

White, B. S., *Representative Men of the West in Caricature*, Denver: Press of Carson-Harper, 1904.

Wilk, Diane, *A Guide to Denver's Architectural Styles and Terms*, Denver: Historic Denver, Inc., 1995.

Williams, Henry Lionel and Ottalie K., *The Treasury of Great American Houses*. New York: G.P. Putnam's Sons.

PERIODICALS

On and Off the Wall, Denver Art Museum. September/October 1998 and May/June, 1990.

The Lookout,. "Art In Denver," Denver Public Library, April 1928.

Sanford, Albert B., "Early-Day Experiences of John J. Riethmann," in *The Trail*, April 1925.

UNPUBLISHED MANUSCRIPTS

Alexander, Philip K., Jr., *Hugh John Alexander ,1975; and George W. Kassler, Colorado Pioneer, Volume* II, 1977. Privately printed.

Coleman, Carla Swan, "Driving Club Place 9-12." Paper presented to the Denver Fortnightly Club, 1959.

Denver's Speer Boulevard: A Revitalization Urban Design Committee. Denver Chapter AIA, (no year given)

Design Guidelines for the Country Club Historic District, Denver Landmark Preservation Commission & Planning and Development Office, May 1995.

Elfenbein, Sharon, National Registry of Historic Places Inventory, Nomination Form, 1979.

Hornby, Barbara Sudler, Nomination form of the Country Club Historic District, Expanded, for the National Registry of Historic Places, 1985.

McPhee, Robert, "Growing Up in the Twenties and Thirties," Volumes I and II, 1993.

Minutes of Cherry Creek Improvement Association 1982-1995.

Minutes of the Board of Directors of the Denver Country Club.

Moore, Lorna Grindlay, "The Denver Craftsman Era." Paper presented to the Denver Fortnightly Club, 1990.

Norgren, Barbara, "Nomination of the Denver Country Club for the National Registry of Historic Places," 1985.

ABSTRACTS OF PROPERTIES

100 Franklin Street
316 Gaylord Street
180 Humboldt Street
466 Lafayette Street
301 Marion Street
379 Marion Street
361 Race Street
545 Race Street
460 Westwood Drive

PEOPLE WHO HAVE CONTRIBUTED TIME, PHOTOGRAPHS, OR INFORMATION TO THIS PROJECT:

Albi, Charles
Alexander, Bruce and Phyllis
Alkire, Marilyn
Anderson, Margaret
Anderson, Mary Lee
Arkell, James
Arndt, Karl
Atchison, Philip
Atchison, Robert
Ball, Ralph W.
Bebout, Clara L.
Beck, Rhonda
Benton, Barbara and Field
Berger, W. Bart
Berger, William M. B.
Black, Regina and Robert C., III
Blanchet, Loraine
Boswell, Rhonda
Bosworth, Robert and Alice
Brooker, Kathleen
Brooks, Laurene "Baba" Berger
Campbell, Ann
Catherwood, Jean
Caughey, Judith Stearns
Christy, Helen (Mrs. Gary)
Clanahan, Virginia
Clinger, Sandra E.
Close, Anne Merryweather
Cochran, Elizabeth Millett
Coleman, Thomas H. and Lorraine
Coss, Gerald and Jaculine Harrier
Cowperthwaite, Arthur T., Jr.
Cowperthwaite-Davis, Blanche
Crotty, Brenda
Croze, Charlotte
Dabney, William C., Jr.
Dalton, Gigi and Matthew
Dean, Robert and Virginia
Dines, Allen
Dines, Dorothy Hildreth
Dines, Tyson, Jr.
Dohse, Jeff
Douden, Medora Wilson
Ebrahami, Patricia
Edmonds, Steve
Elfenbein, Sharon and William
Ellett, Elizabeth
Falkenburg, Janis and William S.
Ferrugia, Mona
Filley, Giles, Jr. "Josh"
Filley, Mary (Mrs. Giles)
Flobeck, Polly Sargeant
Foster, Jane Argall
Freeman, Joe
Freeman, Nancy Widmer
Fuller, Robert K.
Gates, Caleb and Sidney
Grant, Helen Prindle
Grant, Hugh
Grant, Rhondda and Peter
Grier, William M., Jr.
Hanson, Bruce
Hartley, Barbara Johnson
Heitler, Dorothy

Henry, Richard A.
Higbie, Lorraine
Hodges, Jean (Mrs. Joseph, Jr.
Holme, James S. and Alice
Holyoke, Polly
Hoover, Betsy and George
Ivy, Logan
Jackson, Betty Lynn (Mrs. Dennis)
Johnson, Charles A.
Jones, Jill Cowperthwaite
Jorst, Mike
Keefe, Sally Lewis and David
Kemp, Polly
Kennedy, Kelly and Michael
Koether, Sally
Krill, Arthur and Mary Alice
Lanius, Paul Baxter, Jr.
Leuthold, Tony and Merrilyn
Macdonald, Jedeane
Maer, Claude and Anne Waring
Mason, Margurite "Peggy" Simson
McKenna, Joan
Mead, Judy
Millett, Katherine
Millett, William D., Jr. "Pete"
Minturn, Brian
Mitchell, John C.
Monaghan, Patsy O'Rourke
Moore, Charles M.
Moore, Dorsey
Moore, Gerald
Neidecker, Dora Shaw
Newton, Virginia Shafroth
Nichols, Laurie G.
McCleery, Geraldine
Medina, Dan
Olson, Virginia
O'Brien, Anne
O'Donnell, Jane Garnsey
Oliver, Barry
Oliver, Christopher
Oliver James
Oliver, Richard
O'Rourke, Thomas
Pate, Dorothy Moore
Pate, Richard A., III
Perry, Kennard
Phelps, Dorothy Thomas
Philipp, Zina Spore Moore
Ridgeway, Elizabeth Lynn
Ross, Mary and Jeffrey
Purdy, Deanna L.
Shattuck. Alberta Iliff (Mrs. Robert)
Sheldon, Barbara
Shroads, Jim and Merrillyn
Simmons, James D.
Smith, Constance Whiteley
Smith, Dudley, Jr.
Smith, Ruth Hollister (Mrs. Dudley)
Sneed, Eunice (Mrs. John L.)
Steele, Patsy White
Stockmar, Suzanne
Stocks, Alison
Stoddart, Lenore Thomas
Strickland, Marcia Dines and Joe
Swanson, James
Sweeney, John F.
Talmage, E.T.H., Jr.
Tanner, Patsy Prey
Temple, Marjorie (Mrs. William G.)
Toll, Giles
Toll, Lydia and Henry Wolcott
Trevor, Libby
Tweedy, Marjorie Stovall Sargent
Tweedy, Susan Berger
Van Gilder, Dell
Vest, Marie (Mrs. Walter)
Warner, Daniel
Warren, Emma J. and Charles
White, Edward D., Jr.
Widner, Janet
Wilbur, William F.
Williams, Lucile and Ronald W.
Wilson, Robert and Valentine
Wolter, Judy
Wooten, Barbara Stearns and Rike
Wotkyns, Jeannette and Roger, III
Wulsin, Pamela Macdonald
Zemach, Peggy Millett

~ Index ~